ORAL
IMPLANTOLOGY

PERSONAL HISTORY

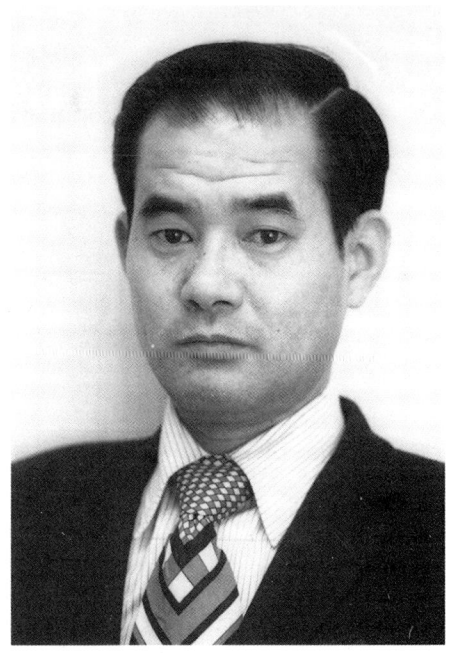

Shumon Otobe, D.D.S.   July 27th, 1928 in Tokyo

Professor of Hagi Womans College, 1977-1979.
D.D.S. from Nihon University School of Dentistry in 1954.
Tokyo University School of Medicine, Department of Oral Surgery, 1954-1956.
Practiced in Central Tokyo.
Associate Editor of Journal of Japan Dental Association, 1960-1973.
Founder and Past-President of Clinical Implant Society of Japan.
Over Sea Editor of Newsletter of American Academy of Implant Dentistry.
Active Member of the American Academy of Implant Dentistry, 1975.
Fellow Onorario: Gruppo Italiano Studi Implantari, 1974.
Honorary Member of the British Implant Association, 1977.
President of Asia Implant Academy, 1984.
Lectured on Implantology to the American Academy of Implant Dentistry
        in Washington 1974, Chicago 1975, Las Vegas 1976, Miami
        1977, Las Vegas 1978, Texas 1979, New Orleans 1980, Kansas
        City 1981, Las Vegas 1982, Washington 1983.
Lectured on Implantology to the International College of Oral Implantolo-
        gists in New York 1974, Kyoto 1975, Paris 1979.
Lectured on Implantology to the Gruppo Italiano Studi Implantari,
        International Meeting at Bologna 1981, 1982, 1983.
Lectured on Implantology to the British Implant Association 1977.
Lectured on Implantology to the Korea Academy of Oral Implantologists
        in Seoul 1983, 1984.
Lectured on Implantology to the Swiss Society of Oral Implantology, 1977.
Lectured on Implantology to the Japan Society of Implant Dentistry in
        Hakata 1974, Okayama 1976, Tokyo 1977, Gifu 1978, Ube
        1979, Kyoto 1980, Niigata 1981.
Lecturer, Instructor and Author.

Shumon Otobe D.D.S.

ORAL
IMPLANTOLOGY

PICCIN

ISBN 88-299-0263-2

Printed in Italy

CONTENTS

FOREWORD

Implantology from its very roots, was started by only a very few men - men with vision, courage, humility, and willingness to go against the wind, and thus against the so called conventional dentistry approach.

They were dreamers ready to work hard to see their dreams become realities. It is because of the perseverance and endurance by those very few that we have today a discipline in implantology that has passed the scrutiny of time and can show predictable results for hundreds of thousands of needy patients throughout the world for as long as thirty or more years with subperiosteal implants and as many as nineteen years with endosseous bladevent implants, thus placing dentistry among the most advanced disciplines of medical science.

During the past thirty-three years, I have lectured and shared my experiences and have taught thousands of open-minded dentists the theories and techniques of implantology - as a predictable method in oral rehabilitation.

In Japan, Shumon Otobe was one of my earliest students who showed excitement, tremendous interest, and human feelings to help those dental cripples for whom the conventional dental approach was hopeless.

Since those earlier years, Dr. Shumon Otobe has started practicing implantology successfully in his own country and also formed his own implant society sharing his knowledge with other peers, and therefore opening the way for modern dentistry. Unrested in his activities in this field, he has raised his stature high among the ranks of implantologists throughout the world.

As a true man of science, he never stopped being interested in improving himself and in the continuous development of Oral Implantology. He attended most of the implant congresses throughout the world. Dr. Shumon Otobe continues to lecture and teach throughout the far eastern countries. His engagements in that direction are too numerous to be mentioned.

Respected as a practitioner and teacher by his fellow dentists, the Clinical Implant Society of Implantology in Japan holds him with the highest respect and admiration.

All his activities demonstrated his dedication and devotion and helped implantology to make a step forward and thus help humanity.

It is hard for me to draw his complete image as a professional in the limited space of a foreword, but I can say that "There have not been too many outstanding implantologists that emerged from their countries, and that Shumon Otobe is one of those rare few."

DR. LEONARD I. LINKOW
Clinical Professor
Temple University
Philadelphia, Pa. USA

PREFACE

Great advances have occurred in dentistry in the past 200 years. Particularly, in the field of dental implantology, remarkable progresses have been achieved, through the persistent efforts of many pioneer implantologists, in the last 30 years. Their common objective has been, I am sure, the realization of successful implants clinically enabling patient to have dependable "Third Teeth".

By ordinary dental treatments, some kind of failure made by the dentist would be considered less serious since modification and redoing are possible in most cases, for example, readjusting the denture.

By implantological treatments, on the contrary, we have to perform not only dental but also the surgical operation for inserting the blade into bone, or under the periosteum. No failure is, therefore, permitted to implantologists. Osseous tissues around unskillfully inserted blades, for example, might cause destruction and great pain to the patient. And, even after removing the blade, the alveolar crest, once lost, will never rebuild, leaving only miserable cicatrix in the site; and, therefore, the ordinary type of denture can no more be applied either.

Ever since I have studied implantology with Dr. Leonard I. Linkow at his office in New York from April through October 1972, I have been striving hard to introduce this revolutionary art and science of Oral Implantology into Japan. How to minimize possible failures in the implant operation has still been my first concern.

It is my greatest honor and delight that this book could meet the requirements of dentists, dental surgeons, and odontologists, who should be taking interest in the field of Oral Implantology. To clinical implantologists, or implantologists-to-be, I hope, this is the book for them, giving practical suggestions and tips, for them to share my own experience with many clinical cases.

I would like to express my sincere appreciation to Dr. Linkow who led me most friendly and educated me rather sternly, so that I can be what I am and write this book today.

"I am proud of you, Dr. Linkow, of being a student of yours, of being your best friend in Japan as well."

March 1989   SHUMON OTOBE

Part 1

Theory
and
Concept

1. Essential Areas of Expertise for Implantologists

1.0 INTRODUCTION

What is oral implantology? In the field of dentistry, this is a comparatively new art and science developed over the last 40 years. It is capable of giving many patients their "third teeth", much more dependable than those supplied by earlier methods. But, as occurs with any new science, implantology has met with great opposition. And in fact, there have been several cases of failed implants, performed by insufficiently experienced dentists.

What are the prerequisites for being an implantologist? To begin with there are *four essential areas of expertise.* An implantologist must have:

(1) Sufficient knowledge of *oral anatomy*
(2) Practical experience in oral surgery
(3) Training in radiographic diagnosis
(4) Clinical skill in designing dental prostheses

1.1 ANATOMY

Anatomy in general, oral anatomy in particular, is an absolute prerequisite to clinical implant activities. Consider as an example the maxillary bones. The implantologist should be able to answer all the following questions:

(1) What shape do the bones have?
(2) How thick are these bones in the palatine, front teeth, and molar areas?
(3) Through what alveolar canals do the posterior-superior alveolar nerves pass?
(4) Where are the alveolar foramens located?
(5) How large an area is affected by the posterior-superior alveolar nerves?
(6) What would happen should these nerves accidentally be cut?

(7) Where is the junction line between the maxillary bones?

(8) What bones are the maxillary bones sutured to?

(9) How are these bones sutured?

(10) How long and how thick are the junction lines?

(11) How solid are the opposite suturing bones?

(12) What are the corresponding muscles?

(13) Where are origin and insertion of these muscles?

(14) Are they extensor or flexor muscles?

(15) How are nerves and blood vessels distributed in these muscles?

(16) What functions do these muscles have?

(17) What kinds of tissue are the maxillary bones made of?

(18) What is the composition, rigidity, viscosity and solidity of the maxillary bones?

(19) Where are the maxillary bones located relative to the maxillary sinuses?

(20) How does this location change over time?

(21) How are the maxillary bones located relative to the nasal fossa?

The above deal only with essential knowledge about the maxillary bones, the mandibular bones. The point is that knowledge of oral anatomy is indispensable for the implantologist.

1.2 SURGERY

Also indispensable to the implantologist is the theory and clinical art of oral surgery. When the mucosa is stripped profuse bleeding naturally occurs. Insufficiently trained operators have panicked on seeing such bleeding during implantation fearing that a vessel had been inadvertently cut. In contrast well-trained operators with sufficient knowledge and experience in surgery, could remain unperturbed in such cases. Normal bleeding represents no problems for them.

Several years ago a case was reported in a conference of dentists in Japan presenting a subperiosteal implant for lost front teeth in the maxillary bone. The operator stripped the mucosa from both sides of the front teeth area leaving mucosa around the incisive foramen. This made both the operation and impression-taking of the bone troublesome. It also made designing the substructure and the insertion procedures more difficult. Furthermore the prognosis of the case was unfavorable. Why then did the operator not strip the palatal mucosa without excluding the area of the incisive foramen? Apparently the operator selected the significantly more complicated procedure because he feared he should accidently sever or cut the nasal palate nerve; such a fear is unfounded as long as the operator has a knowledge of oral surgery and oral anatomy.

Generally speaking, by observing the dimension of stripped mucosa, we can estimate (or judge) the surgical skill and experience of the operator analogically; they are also important factors in evaluating the ability of implantologists.

In any clinical operation, experience is crucial. In performing implants the operator faces a range of cases. Unless he has sufficient experience, he will not be able to perform the operation confidently. In fact, stripping palatal mucosa from the maxillary bone is similiar to *palatorrhaphy*; stripping mandibular mucosa is analogous to the amputation of the mandible itself.

Suturing techniques are also essential in implant operations. Unfortunately this is another area where dentists tend to be insufficiently skilled.

Suture does not merely mean mechanically joining together the edges of a surgical or accidental wound. It is a fundamental technique as it is a means of healing mucosa injured by incision. Moreover wasted time in unskillful suturing prolongs the operation, necessarily exhausting the patient. In general, ability to correctly allocate time is another component of the knowledge of oral surgery that is a prerequisite to successful implant operations.

1.3 RADIODONTICS RADIOLOGY

1.3.0 General

The most important procedure preceding the implant operation is precise diagnosis. This is true, of course, not only of implants, but of any medical treatement.

In the case of implants, a basic aid to correct diagnosis is the interpretation and analysis of radiograms usually taken by pantoradioscope. Without sufficient knowledge of radiology and radiodontics, even well-taken radiograms are less useful. Mastering the operation of the pantoscope is one of the qualifications for an implantologist. It is far preferable for the implantologist to take the radiogram himself than having it done by somebody else. The implantologist knows best how the finished radiogram should look in order to enable a correct interpretation.

The developing process including the condition of the developing solution, also affects the quality of the radiogram. The best results are thus obtainable when the implantologist himself takes charge of the entire process of radiography. If the x-ray seems less than satisfactory, the process should be repeated until a radiogram is obtained that enables correct interpretation and precise diagnosis.

It is important to be familiar not only with the specifications, but also with the characteristics of the machine, particularly its magnifying power. Some models of pantoscope have a 1.1 ratio whereas others have a 1.5 ratio. Magnifying power also varies with the superior-inferior and mesial-distal direction of the jaw. Such factors should always be taken into account and compensated for.

There are several anatomic areas in which pantoradiogram are especially important for implant diagnosis.

1.3.1 Junction line of pterygoid process of sphenoid bone with maxillary bone

Interpreting radiograms of this area is not easy because the area is often hidden behind the malar bone and is usually overlapped by the coronoid process of mandibular bones in radiograms. When resorption of maxillary bones has progressed beyond a certain point, care must be exercised to obtain a clear image of this area in the radiogram. Interpreting radiograms of this area is indispensable to diagnose for a pterygoid implant.

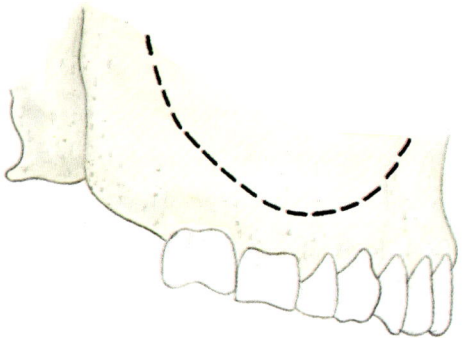

Fig. 1. Posterior wall of maxillary bone sutured with pterygoid

1.3.2 Posterior wall of maxillary bone

The area near the posterior wall of the maxillary bones, particularly between the palato-alveolar crest in the rear of the second molar and the posterior wall of the buccal flange, has a relatively large space. Moreover there is usually a considerable amount of remaining osseous tissue especially around the maxillary molar teeth. However, if the maxillary posterior wall has been injured or fractured by extraction of molars or lost through resorption, there may be less osseous tissue.

The question of whether the posterior wall of the maxillary bones is still intact or not is an important one. Interpretation of a pantoradiogram of this area may require extensive training and experience on the part of the implantologist.

1.3.3 Location of maxillary sinus

The appropriateness of inserting an implant blade into the maxillary bone in any given case will depend largely on the location of the maxillary sinus. If the blade penetrates the sinus, serious consequences may follow.

The question is how much clearance is there between the surface of the alveolar bone and the maxillary sinus base. In other words how much osseous tissue remains in the inferior area of maxillary sinus base to receive occlusal pressure. If the osseous tissue is too thin, it can easily be crushed or broken. This is of course very dangerous. Furthermore broken pieces of bone left in the maxillary sinus could cause undersirable effects or even serious diseases.

The thinnest and, therefore, most vulnerable area in the maxillary sinus base is usually on the palatine side of the molar teeth. The buccal side must be protected against external forces. There it is formed with thick and hard osseous tissue. On the contrary, stimuli given to palatine side are limited to occlusal pressure and to those associated with intake. Such stimuli are usually weaker. This is why in human anatomy the palatine side of bone is weaker on the buccal side.

When performing an implant operation in mandibular bone, care must be taken to avoid contact between the implant head and the thinner area of the maxillary sinus base. Before the implant operation, the patient most likely had a tendency to bite harder than necessary since his lost tooth side has no corresponding tooth on the opposite jaw. This way of biting will continue even after the implant operation has provided a new denture.

The stronger occlusal pressure naturally reacts with the corresponding tooth or the area around the tooth. The implantologist must confirm this by locating the maxillary sinus before he performs an implant operation in mandibular bones.

For any implant operation, a radiogram that does not show a clear image of the maxillary sinus is of very little use.

1.3.4 Location of nasal fossa

Before performing an implant in the front teeth area of the maxillary bone, it is important to know the exact location of the nasal fossa. The maxillary alveolar bone below the nasal fossa base is formed of very hard osseous tissue for several reasons:

(1) This bone is firmly sutured to both sides of the maxillary bone.
(2) It is protecting the nervous tissue of the nasal palatal nerve contained in the incisive canal located in mid-palatal area above the alveolar crest.
(3) It is also sutured with the vomer forming the septum nasi; further the vomer is sutured with the caner perpendicolaris and lamina cribrosa leading to the cranial base.

The high-power occlusal pressures exerted by the inserted blade can effectively be dispersed through this area of hard bone when the appropriate insertion point is selected. The implantologist should therefore know the exact thickness of the osseous tissue in this area before performing the operation.

Should the edge of the inserted blade penetrate the nasal cavity (Fig. 2), the patient might then suffer every time his nose is touched. Such a mis-

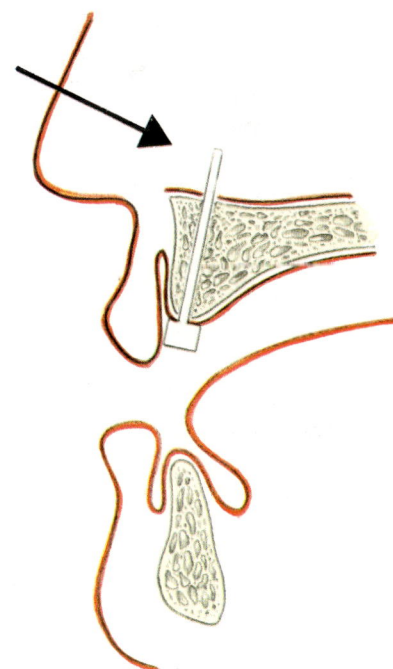

Fig. 2. Exposed blade edge in nasal fossa

take should never occur. In most cases it stems from the fact that the operator did not, or possibly could not, confirm the exact location of the nasal sinus base by interpreting radiograms during the process of diagnosis.

1.3.5 Location of mandibular foramen

The mandibular foramen is the opening for the mandibular canal. By confirming its location the operator can judge the direction of the mandibular nerve. Further, from its location, relative to the alveolar crest of the mandible, he can judge the depth of the mandibular canal.

The saying "what begun is half done" is quite valid with respect to locating the mandibular canal. Locating the mandibular foramen, that is, opening of the mandibular canal, makes to find the exact location of the canal itself much easier.

In subperiosteal implants, the substructure is inserted under the periosteum at the level of the mandibular foramen. Thus to ascertain the exact location of the mandibular foramen is of most importance. Should the substructure be inserted incorrectly, even slightly below the mandibular foramen, there is danger of injuring or cutting the alveolar nerve of the mandible.

In short, as with the areas discussed earlier, the mandibular foramen must be shown clearly in radiograms and implantologists must be able to precisely interpret the relevant radiograms.

1.3.6 Location of mandibular canal

The precise location of the mandibular canal in the mandible must also be ascertained with the aid of a pantoradiogram before performing an implant operation. The distance between the alveolar crest of the mandible and the mandibular canal is calculated by multiplying the distance measured in the radiogram by the magnifying ratio of the pantoradioscope used.

If the patient still has teeth, it is useful to compare the length of the teeth as shown in an ordinary dental radiogram, assuming a magnifying ratio of 1.00, with the length of the same teeth as shown on the pantoradiogram. Determining the practical magnifying ratio in this way makes it possible to limit error in measuring factor-distance to fractions of a millemeter; otherwise, the magnifying ratio obtained is less useful for correct diagnosis.

The magnifying ratio also varies depending on whether the length to be measured is superior-inferior or medial-distal. It is important to be completely familiar with the practical use of the pantoradioscope. Accurate magnifying ratios are indispensable to correct diagnosis and especially to correctly locate the mandibular canal.

I once was shown a radiogram of a clinical implant performed by a dentist and at first glance the lost teeth seemed to have been beautifully replaced with a denture. However, closer inspections revealed that a L-10D type of blade with a short body had been inserted in the alveolar bone of the mandible, leaving a considerably large space (approximately 10 mm) to the mandibular canal. The area of the implant, the condition of resorption in the alveolar bone, and the position of the prosthesis all argued for the use of a blade with a longer body tie L-8D, E-14D, or E-22D. The reason for my criticism here is very simple: effective dispersion of occlusal pressure would have been obtained by using a longer blade.

The possible causes of an unsatisfactory implant like this one are several:

(1) The operator did not or could not estimate the exact distance from alveolar crest to the mandibular canal.
(2) The operator lacked the clinical skills needed to perform an implant operation.
(3) He simply misselected the blade, either because of lack of basic knowledge in implantology or because of a mistaken fear that would cause excessive bleeding.

1.3.7 Location of mental foramen

The mental foramen is at the end of the mandibular canal. Determining its location is therefore helpful in determining the location of the mandibular canal.

When however, the mandibular bone has been resorbed, as usually happens in patients of advanced age, the radiographic image of the mental foramen may overlap with the alveolar crest of the mandible. In such cases the mental foramen cannot be accurately located by interpreting the pantoradiograph.

1.4 PROSTHETICS

An implant operation that is well done loses some of its value if followed by unsuitable prosthetics. In my opinion, most claims of short duration of implants can be explained by inadequate or defective prostheses.

Similarly when patients complain of pain following an implant, the cause generally lies in mis-designed prostheses.

However correct the occlusal surface of the prosthesis looks like, however correct it is made theoretically, pain may occur if occlusion exerts too much pressure on the implant blade supporting the prosthesis. Prosthetics should be designed to disperse occlusal pressure, that is, to achieve maximum occlusal function with minimum occlusal pressure.

There is currently a world-wide tendency to take occlusal theory more seriously. Surely, without full understanding of occlusal theory, no useful implant prosthesis could be prepared. Modern dentistry insists on the need to protect natural teeth on the basis of occlusal theory. This necessity is all the greater in the case of implant dentures, artificial substitutes for lost teeth. Care must be exercised, however, in applying occlusal theory. Application of the pure theory of occlusion can result in too much occlusal pressure on implant dentures.

One of the most unfavorable prosthesis for implant dentures is the so-called bucket crown, including that made of gold. Fixing this type of bucket crown to the denture base usually requires a generous amount of dental cement. When combined with a primitive prosthesis like this, an implant can have very little effect. Implantology is a coordinated, integrated art and science which draws on many arts and sciences in the broad field of dentistry. If one of these is lacking, a perfect implant becomes impossible.

Prosthetics is the final stage of the implant procedure and the application of modern prosthetics is indispensable.

2. Alveolar Bone and Implant: Hypotheses

2.1 NATURE OF ALVEOLAR BONE

The most essential precondition for a successful endosteal implant is accurate and complete records of the nature of the alveolar bone.

Clinically speaking, a blade can be inserted in the alveolar bone only if a sufficient amount of osseous tissue remains. A blade implant should not be applied in cases where the alveolar bone is already resorbed or resorption has progressed to a considerable extent. Even if mechanically inserted, the blade would not remain in the oral cavity to function as a reliable denture support.

The standard criterion for a successful operation is that the blade has functioned in the oral cavity for more than 5 years. In other words, minimum durability of 5 years is to be assured in any case of clinical implant treatment.

Because this is possible only when a sufficient amount of osseous tissue remains in the alveolar bone, implantologists must be fully familiar with the nature and characteristics of the alveolar bone.

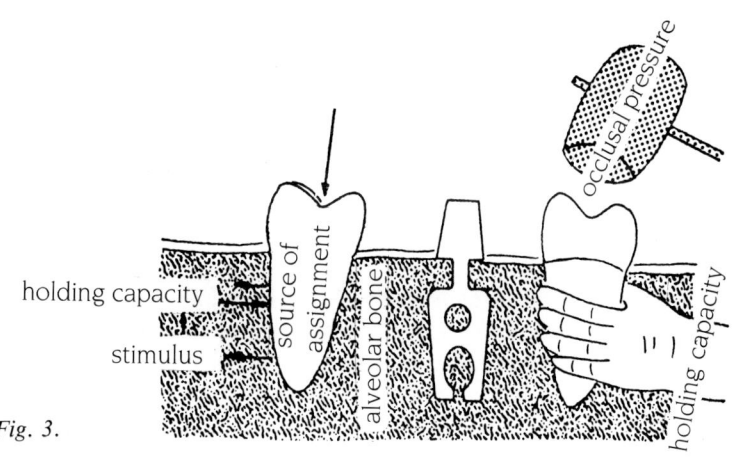

Fig. 3.

The basic function of the alveolar bone is to support teeth firmly in the maxillo-mandibular bones. The alveolar bone must therefore be sufficiently rigid and yet flexible to hold the teeth safely in place and bear the pressure exerted on the teeth. The outer force of the occlusal pressure exerted on the teeth and the inner capacity of the alveolar bone supporting these teeth must balance each other.

When this balance is lost, the roots of the teeth become loose and move frequently, destroying the alveolar bone in this area. Once begun, this process of destruction accelerates rapidly, until the bone loses its holding capacity and the teeth eventually fall out.

It is generally recognized that bones become involuted when pressure is continuously exerted on them. Dentists are very aware of this especially from their experience of fitting dentures to fully edentulous patients. The surface of the oral mucosa changes in shape as the alveolar bone is absorbed. This follows from the fact that the denture base is pressing continuously against both the mucosa and alveolar bone of the maxillary area. The matter is virtually self-explanatory as shown in figure 4.

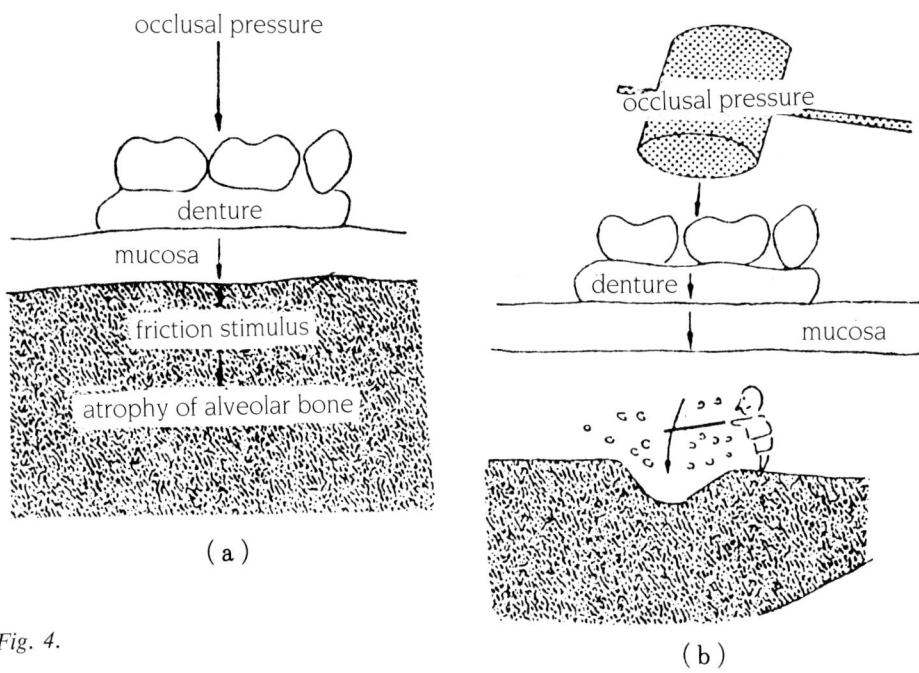

Fig. 4.

(a)

(b)

HYPOTHESIS (1): *The alveolar bone is always resorbed as a result of outer pressure.*

The function of the alveolar bone is to fix teeth firmly to the maxillo-mandibular bones as mentioned earlier. When the teeth come out this function obviously no longer exists. The alveolar bone has in effect become a useless structure in the oral cavity. In human anatomy, we know that our body tends to lose useless tissues.

The alveolar bone therefore has to take on a new function namely that of being resorbed and vanishing as quickly as possible.

HYPOTHESIS (2): *The alveolar bone has two functions: first, to support teeth firmly to jaw bones; second, after loss of these teeth, to disappear immediately.*

The latter process is specifically known as disuse atrophy. The effect of disuse atrophy and pressure exerted by outer forces accelerate the degeneration of the alveolar bone.

Let us now look at how the alveolar bone reacts to inner pressure, or, stated more precisely, to the pressure exerted outward from inside the bone. Here we have to consider the medium that transforms the pressure exerted inward from outside the bone by outer forces into outward pressure from within. This medium is, in the normal healthy oral cavity, nothing more than the natural teeth supported by the alveolar bone. Let us return to the hypothesis (1): Alveolar bone is always resorbed by outer pressure. Outer pressure, including occlusal pressure, is transmitted repeatedly to the alveolar bone at the root of each tooth. The following question therefore arises: "Does the alveolar bone degenerate in a short time particularly around the teeth root area?" Clearly, the answer is "No". If it were "Yes", human teeth would be lost much earlier than they actually are through resorption of alveolar bone.

There must be a reason for the durability of human teeth; remember that our second set of teeth are also called "permanent teeth".

One explantation is that pressure exerted outward from inside the bone is transformed into a kind of stimulus, distinguishable from pressure exerted inward from outside the bone. This stimulus militates against resorption. Furthermore stimuli transmitted to the inside of alveolar bone are changed to the message of supporting the source of this stimulus, namely, the roots of the teeth. The osseous tissue forming the alveolar bone thus begins to work in accordance with the objective of supporting the teeth firmly in the jaw bones.

This then is the relationship between the teeth and the alveolar bone. Permanent teeth would literally be retained permanently in the bone were it not for other factors such as accidents, disease and senility. As indicated here these factors include senile resorption of the bone as well as pyorrhea and decalcification of teeth caused by decay.

The force of the stimulus transmitted to the alveolar bone must also be considered. A stimulus of moderate force not greater than the supporting capacity of the bone has a positive or constructive function. In contrast, a high pressure stimulus exceeding this limit constitutes a negative and potentially destructive factor.

Insofar as occlusal pressure and supporting capacity are well balanced, outer forces including occlusal pressure are transformed into favorable stimuli (fig. 4b).

This theory of balance is highly significant in designing the implant superstructure, that is the prosthesis to be attached to the implant head. When occlusal pressure exceeds the holding capacity of the alveolar bone, balance then is lost and the pressure works as a destructive force.

The loosening of teeth by alveolar pyorrhea is a case of this lost balance. Necrosis of the alveoli is accelerated by the destructive effect of osteoclastic activity around the roots of the loosened teeth.

In conclusion, occlusal pressure has a positive function in the alveolar bone as long as it is well balanced within the holding capacity of the bones. Once this balance is lost, however, occlusal pressure causes destruction of the osseous tissue of the alveolar bone. This fact must always be taken into account in selecting the size and shape of the implant blade for the tooth replacement.

2.2 FUNCTION OF PERIODONTAL MEMBRANE

Traditionally pericementum has been considered nothing more than a buffering device or shock absorber preventing direct transmission of occlusal pressure to the alveolar bone. Is this view in fact accurate?

When an implant blade is inserted in the alveolar bone, does the new membrane that forms around the blade have the same nature and function as the pericementum? A leading scholar of dentistry in Japan once answered my question affirmatively. According to him, the new membrane had the same buffering and shock-absorbing function.

However, clinical observation revealed that an implant blade properly tapped into the alveolar bone stood firm; outside pressures did not move it a fraction of a millimeter even at the beginning of the implant procedure. If the new membrane had the same function as the pericementum, the blade would be moved by occlusal pressure. Thus it appears that the new membrane formed around the inserted blade is not a substitute of pericementum. Recall, by the way, that one of the important conditions for successful implants is stability of the inserted blade throughout the implant operation.

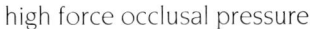

high force occlusal pressure

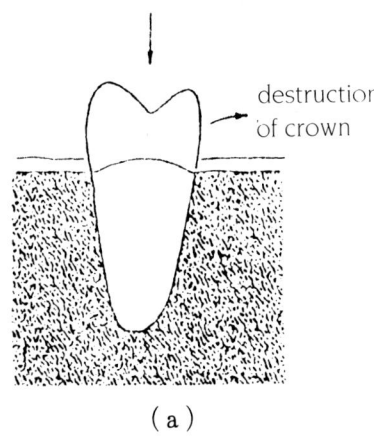

destruction of crown

(a)

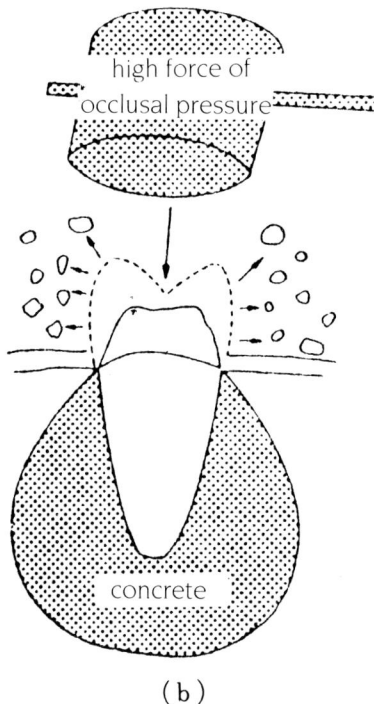

high force of occlusal pressure

concrete

(b)

Fig. 5.

At this point, we should return to our question of whether the pericementum itself is to be primarily limited to buffering function. The membrane formed around the implant blade does not serve as a buffer, yet the blade is retained for a long time acting as a dependable denture base.

What then is the real function of the periodental membrane? I have tried to solve this problem by looking at the new membrane's relation to the implant blade.

HYPOTHESIS (3): *Pericementum is a buffering device serving mainly to protect the crown fracture, which could be caused by excessive occlusal pressure.*

If extraordinarily strong occlusal pressure is exerted on a tooth, the crown of the tooth will be fractured into pieces unless an adequate buffering device absorbs the pressure properly (Fig. 5). The pericementum plays just this role. This is the conclusion I have arrived at on the basis of various clinical observation.

In addition I have recently recognized a second major function of pericementum.

HYPOTHESIS (4): *Pericementum is the basis of an organic reflex of nerve and muscle controlling occlusal pressure.*

When an extraordinarily strong occlusal pressure is exerted on the teeth exceeding the limit of rigidity of the crown, the nerve in the pericementum at once commands the relevant muscle to stop or lessen the occlusal pressure. This is a kind of "feedback system", or "servo-mechanism" or, more specifically, an organic nerve and muscle reflex.

How can this organic reflex control occlusal pressure when an implant blade is inserted in the alveolar bone rather than a natural tooth? There is of course, no organic reflux with the implanted blade. In other words, there is no reflux of stopping or lessening excessive occlusal pressure.

In short, implant blades in alveolar bone cannot be controlled by the organs. When we are comparing blades with natural teeth, the major difference between them is the lack of pericementum in the former.

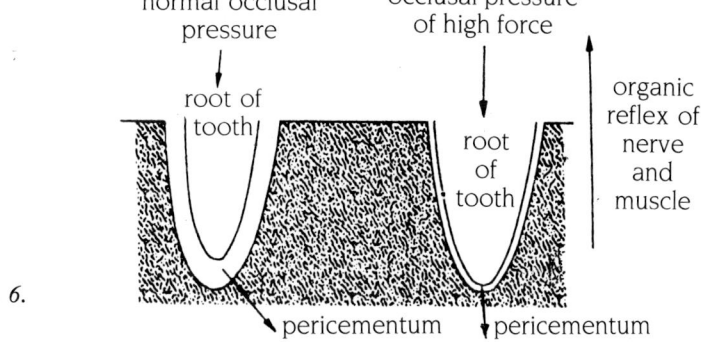

Fig. 6.

Clearly we must change our concept of the function of pericementum. It works as a buffering device; its major function however, is that of controlling occlusal pressure through an organic nerve and muscle reflex. Although both hypotheses (3) and (4) are valid, the latter is the more important.

This new concept has important practical repercussions and we must always take both functions of pericementum into account. First, since implant blades have no natural protection, the prosthesis must be made in such a way that occlusal pressure is dispersed as widely as possible with the implant head receiving minimal occlusal pressure. Second, use should be made of natural teeth whenever possible in designing implant bridges, to give the organic nerve and muscle reflex mechanism to the bridge.

The old method which attached each prosthesis to an implant blade has been rendered obsolute.

Further information on prostheses is given in the following chapter.

2.3 NEOPLASTIC MEMBRANE

Within a certain period following insertion of an implant blade, a new membrane, the so-called neoplastic membrane, forms around the blade. As already discussed, this new membrane cannot be considered a substitute for pericementum.

What then is the function of this neoplastic membrane?

When an implant blade is inserted into the alveolar bone, it always digs a ditch in the bone, that is, the alveolar bone is temporarily and artificially cracked or fissured. In any bone, including the alveolar bone, when a crack or fissure is made, osteoclasts are generated and these then change into osteoblastic cells. Finally the crack is filled with osseous tissue and the wound is completely healed. All human bones have a regenerative ability and it is of vital importance in maintaining a healthy life. Thus the crack in bone is filled with osseous tissue; however, no neoplastic membrane is generated here.

Yet when an implant blade is inserted into the crack, neoplastic membrane is regenerated around the blade. What for? Is its function to separate blade from bone? If the surface of the metallic blade was such that it dissolved in the bone, producing a chemical irritant, then the newly generated membrane would serve to protect against this irritant; yet none of the modern implant blades uses harmful metals. We can conclude that the objective of neoplastic membrane cannot be that of protecting against chemical irritants.

Making a crack in a bone has the same physiological effect as cutting the bone in two. Sections of dead bone naturally generate nothing; sections of living bone in a living body, however, are restored with osteoclasts and osteoblasts. The inner substance of bone, namely, bone matrix, is made of comparatively hard tissues. In other words, it normally has little fluidity. If the bone matrix were more fluid, the inner substance of the bone would easily flow out, like an uncorked bottle full of wine that is placed on its side (Fig. 7).

But although the bone matrix is made of hard tissues and has little mobility in the bone when an end of bone is cut or the bone is partially cracked, bone matrix will gradually flow out. This would of course, be quite determinant to the bone. To protect against the escape of bone matrix, a new membrane is regenerated at the section.

HYPOTHESIS (5): *Neoplastic membrane is regenerated not as a substitute for pericementum, but to protect against possible outflow of bone matrix.*

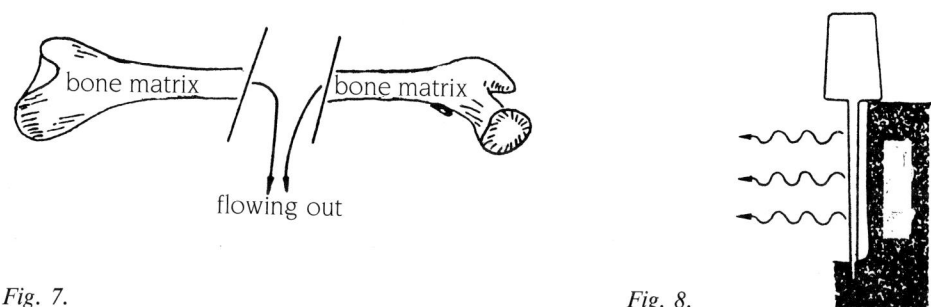

Fig. 7.   *Fig. 8.*

2.4 VITAL REJECTION

Vital rejection is frequently discussed in conjunction with implants, and the discussions are usually critical. Nonetheless I believe that, according to the strict definition or narrow sense of the word, no vital rejection is observed with implants.

There are certain scholars who insist that implanted blades can cause a reaction of rejection. Although readily observable in most soft tissues, when alien material is introduced in hard tissues like bone tissue, vital rejection is seldom seen. One apparent exception in the field of dentistry or dental surgery is the falling out of the remaining root from the alveolar bone. This situation is interpreted as being due to vital rejection.

Let us consider then the problem of vital rejection with clinical implants. If the inserted blade always causes vital rejection, rejection must occur in the maxillary or mandibular bone as soon as the blade is implanted, and the rejection would last for a long time. Clinical observations, however, fail to reveal any such rejection of implant blades or any rejective symptoms.

The upper part of Figure 9 illustrates the process by which the remaining root is discharged. The bottom of the root withdraws progressively from the mandibular border. The distance between the mandibular border and the bottom of the blade foot remains unchanged, as shown in the lower part of Figure 9. Resorption of the alveolar bone progresses from the surface to the inner portion. The falling out of the implant blade is caused by the atrophy of the alveolar bone. Can this be called rejection, or the result of vital rejective reaction?

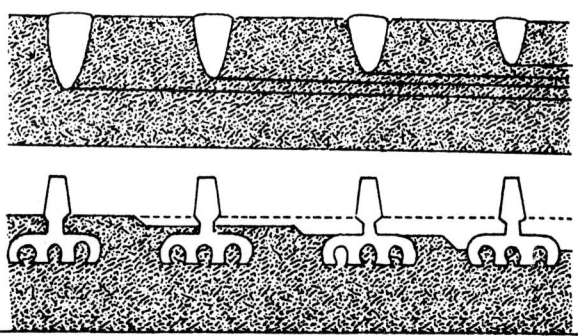

Fig. 9.   mandibular border

There have been reports that alveolar bone around the body of the implant blade changes into granulation tissue several months after the insertion. This is, however, not the result of a rejective reaction but of a failed implant operation, that is, of an inexpert insertion.

Let us recall the nature of the alveolar bone.

The bone is not resorbed by stimuli exerted outward from inside the bone. Therefore, the implant blade tapped in alveolar bone is supported firmly with ossified tissue. Osteoblast cells help this ossification.

Neoplastic osseous tissue of the cortical bone, generated above the blade shoulder, holds the blade firmly should vital rejection try to drive it out. The fact that neoplastic osseous tissues were generated above the blade shoulder clearly shows that there was no rejection of the implant blade inserted in the alveolar bone.

We cannot declare definitely that no rejective reaction occurs in osseous tissue but we can at least state that no rejection takes place when the implant blade has been properly tapped in by an expert implantologist. Should a rejective reaction be observed, it would be explainable in terms of a specific factor operation, extraordinarily great occlusal pressure which exceeds the holding capacity of the alveolar bone, etc.

Most objections to implants stem from a lack of knowledge. They can easily be answered in terms of the four topics of this chapter:

(1) The nature of the alveolar bone
(2) The function of the pericementum
(3) Neoplastic membrane
(4) Implants "vital rejection"

In closing I stress that my four point refutation of criticisms of implants is based on many years of experience with a wide range of problems.

2.5 FIXING CAPACITY

It is commonly thought that mechanically an implant is done by hammering a metal post into the jawbone and fixing the denture to it. The implant blade is supported physiologically rather than mechanically. Otherwise, its durability would be impossible.

The fixing capacity of the implant mainly depends on, and is enforced by, the vital reactions and curative properties of the human body. In an endosteal implant, the inserted blade partly fractures the jawbone. It is because we make use of the healing process of fractured bone that the blade is supported firmly in the bone.

The human body experiences vital rejection: any extraneous substance that is brought in is rejected and driven out. Contact lens can be placed on the surface of eyeball; it is impossible, for the time being, to install the lens in the eyeball. Indeed, it is difficult to put artificial mechanically prepared substitutes into any part or organ of the human body.

When implants were first introduced in the dental field, small metal pins, 1 mm in diameter, were inserted into the jawbone through the pulp canal for the purpose of fixing the loosened tooth. This is the idea behind the pin implant. Neither Linkow nor myself are in favor of this old type of pin implant.

Initially the tooth is fixed mechanically. However, as result of occlusal pressure, it soon comes loose. The alveolar bone and jawbone around the roots of the teeth are destroyed until the pin stands alone in the gingiva, isolated and with no holding capacity.

When a construction worker wants to remove a pile from the ground, he pushes and pulls it back and forth several times. The pile comes loose and is easily withdrawn (Figure 10). It is just the same when a pin implant comes loose and drops out.

Today the pin implant has become obsolete among leading implantologists world wide. Unfortunately, however, it has not fallen into complete disuse. It is therefore worth looking at the reasons why the pin implant should be avoided.

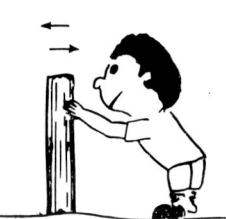

Fig. 10.

(1) A pin of small diameter has no mechanical capacity to bear occlusal pressure. Moreover, the shape of the pin makes it unable to provide any physiological support.

(2) The pin is inserted through the pulp canal and the root of the tooth into the jawbone for the purpose of fixing the tooth mechanically (Fig. 11).

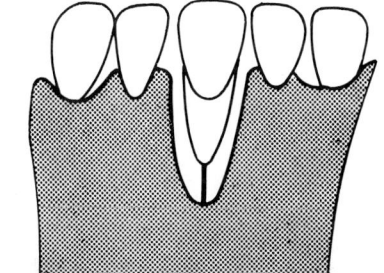

Fig. 11.

(3) The operative procedure of boring a small hole through the pulp canal into the jawbone leaves behind irregularities and fragments, which are rather difficult to remove. Organic chips and splinters that are left over might degenerate, causing destruction of osseous tissue in the area (Fig. 12).

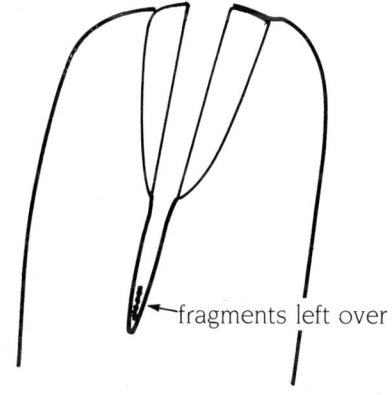

fragments left over

Fig. 12.

(4) The border of the pulp canal containing the pin and jaw bone is closed up by filling in dental cement. It is very difficult to perfectly

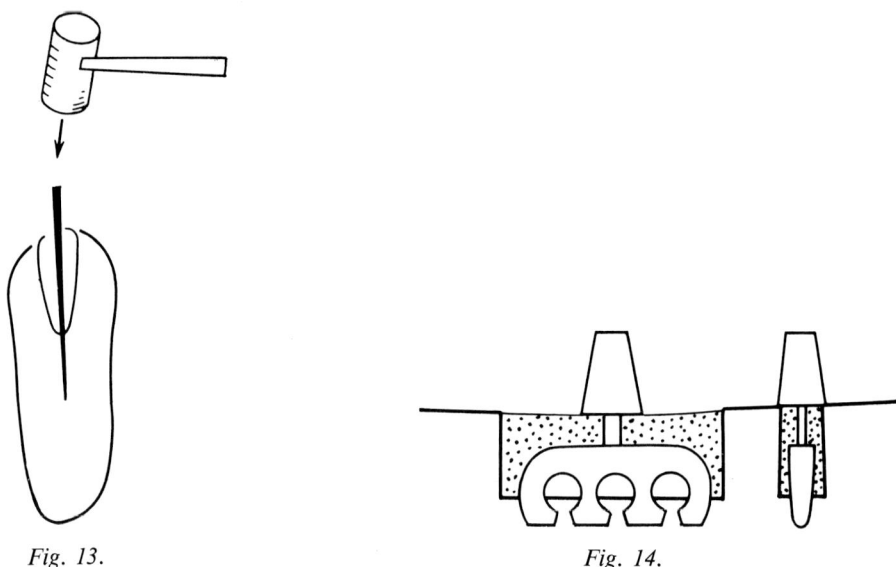

Fig. 13.   *Fig. 14.*

execute both the pin insertion and closing-up procedures. Incomplete closing up, however, may later cause disease in this border area.

(5) Finally, as the pin implant depends on mechanical capacity alone, durability cannot be expected, as explained above.

The blade implant is inserted by being tapped into the jawbone; this fixes the blade temporarily until ossification around the blade is completed in a month or more. The blade is then supported firmly, especially by cortical bone formed above the blade shoulder. The blade is thus physiologically fixed making full use of the body's vital healing capacity. This is the great difference between blade and pin implants.

A case report published in a Japanese dental journal included a radiogram showing an exposed blade shoulder. Such an outcome is no doubt an example of an unsuccessful operation caused by a misunderstanding of blade function.

Part 2

Clinical
Button
Techniques

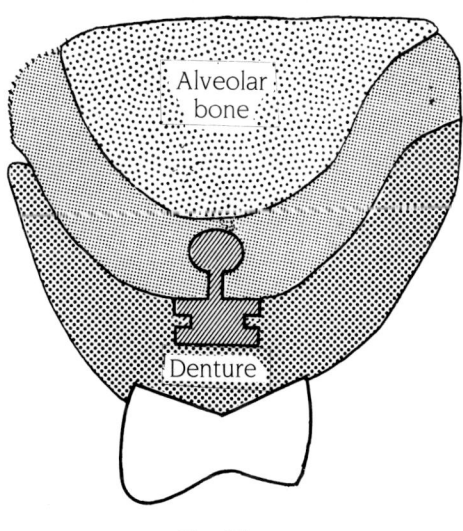

Fig. 15.

3. Intramucosal Insert Button Implant

3.0 GENERAL

Intramucosal inserts are gradually becoming popular in Japan under the name of "button implant" or "snap implant" as an effective means of dental treatment.

The method was introduced in Europe in the 1940s under the name of intramucosal implant a name which refers to mucosal insertion, reflecting improvements in the technique for clinical application. The first article on the subject written by Dr. Gutav, S.A. Dahl of Sweden, was published in 1943. Ten years later, Isaih Lew of the United States published a book entitled *Implant Button Technique for Denture Prosthesis*. Subsequently Leonard I. Linkow and Kenneth Yudy published important articles in the United States. Leading implantologists elsewhere including Ronald Cullen of England, Giordano Muratori of Italy and Richard Guaccio of USA have also reported their theory and art.

In Japan, Setsuzo Okino, a professor at Nihon University, was a pioneer in the field. He had brought several pieces of dental button from Europe but unfortunately World War II interrupted his studies. In 1960, Toshitaka Kaketa clinically applied the intramucosal insert and reported the case.

Recently, since the establishment of the Japan Society of Implant Dentistry, Akira Mori of Nagoya and Hidemaro Ohzeki of Tochigi have reported on the subject every year. Wataru Nemoto of Tokyo published an important booklet: "Intra-Mucosal Inserts Manual" in 1975.

There are therefore three chronological phases in Japan with the mucosal insert: (1) the 1950s during which this new art was introduced into Japan; (2) the 1960s of experimental applications; (3) the 1970s of clinical applications. In my beliefs lack of availability of implant materials posed a problem. In recent years, however, the circumstances are much improved. Several companies provide materials: Tokyo Dental Supply Co. import implant from Howmedicam Inc.; Morita Co., from Implants International; and Yoshida Co., from Implant Research Corp. Implant materials are now also made in Japan. Their quality is comparable to that of imported materials and they cost only one-third or one-fourth as much.

In Japan as elsewhere there are compelling motives for trying to produce as good a denture as possible. The average life span has greatly increased now we have many more elderly people in our society. The natural teeth have not become more durable. Thus the number of denture-wearers is also increased. And most of these people experience some degree of discomfort, primarily because of the looseness of their denture. Their desire to overcome this discomfort is reflected in the numerous materials and fixing pastes for dentures advertised daily on TV. As a dependable aid for fixing dentures over the long term, button inserts are welcome and have come into wide use in Japan.

3.1 INDICATIONS

The application of button inserts is limited to the maxillary dentures. Corresponding attempts for the mandibular dentures are still in the experimental stage. Button inserts are of little use for lost front teeth (3.-3). They are of most use for lost molar teeth of the maxillary bone. There are no restrictions on the physical condition of the patient, nor are there any contraindications. Button inserts can also be used in the patient with a cleft or flat palate, a flat alveolar crest, etc., where ordinary dentures could not be applied.

The intramucosal insert gives far greater stability in fixing the denture than does any other method; hence, it also helps in recovery of the dental function. A patient need never again worry about losing his denture upon sneezing or coughing.

Nonetheless any dental arch with a dental plate, no matter how carefully designed and produced, will loosen after a certain period of time mainly due to resorption of the alveolar bone, and eventually lose its balance and fall out. This is particularly true when the stability of the denture was limited from the beginning because of the oral condition of the patient.

3.2 CONDITIONS

Prior to the intramucosal insert, the denture plate is carefully designed and prepared using ordinary dental techniques. If the plate is made of metal, the metal must be removed where buttons are to be attached.

When the button is being applied to a denture already in use, rebasing will be necessary to compensate for the change in the facing mucosa caused by the resorption of the underlying alveolar bone.

Cracked or defective structures should, of course, be completely repaired.

3.3 ADVANTAGES

3.3.1 Easy operation
A key advantage lies in the simplicity of the procedure. The operation is far simpler than injection and marrow extraction. No particular surgical training is required. The injection involved is very small. In fact, although the procedure is termed operation, the word is hardly warranted.

With patients it is best to avoid the word operation in view of the fear it can arouse. It is preferable to simply speak in terms of a treatment for applying a denture. The wound caused by the operation is very small; the operation site comprises what is required for holding a small button in, and no more.

3.3.2 Reinforced fixing capacity

With buttons now the patient need no longer worry about losing his denture when biting and chewing, sneezing and coughing, and so forth. Inserts greatly increase the fixing capacity of the denture. As already mentioned loose dentures are the greatest source of unpleasantness and anxiety for denture-wearers.

3.3.3 No looseness

With the button inserts the dental plate will never loosen or move. Since the obstacle to articulation caused by loosening dentures is eliminated, the patient derives the benefit of a clearer articulate pronunciation. As we have seen, the natural resorption of the alveolar bone occurs after losing natural teeth from the bone even if no denture is attached. But looseness of dentures accelerates the process. They become loose within relatively short periods of time, usually 1-3 years, until the denture is liable to fall out easily.

Dental plates with buttons, however, never come loose; hence resorption of alveolar bone is limited and the progress of disuse atrophy is very slow, keeping the alveolar bone in good condition for much longer, nor will troublesome rebasing be required.

3.3.4 Smaller dental plate

Because buttons greatly reinforce the holding capacity of dental plate, the dimensions of the dental plate can be kept as small as possible within the supporting limit for occlusal pressure. It is now possible to design non-palate dentures for fully endetulous maxillas. Such dentures have several merits:

(1) No physical discomfort caused by artificial plate in oral cavity
(2) Recovered sense of taste caused by open palate
(3) Better pronunciation
(4) Increased appetite

3.3.5 Better appearance of dental plate

Because of the greater holding capacity of the dental plate, the buccal side of the front teeth area can be designed so as to eliminate artificial gingiva and resemble natural teeth. Non grasp dentures are also possible; eliminating the grasp improves the appearance of the dentures.

3.3.6 No need to rebase

However precisely made, dentures may loosen and fall out in 1-3 years' time. This follows from the fact that the surface of the dental plate, which is made of resin or metal, is solid and undeformable, whereas the gingiva deforms and degenerates with the resorption of the underlying alveolar bone. The gingiva itself also changes its shape slightly in a short period of time. Thus the original fit between the dental plate and the palatine gingiva is lost, causing the denture to be loose while in use, that is, during chewing, swallowing and speech. A loose dental plate rubs against the alveolar bone accelerating its degeneration. The dental plate facing the gingiva must therefore soon be rebased. Dentures with buttons rarely require rebasing as already explained.

3.3.7 Simple implanting procedure

When the proper method is followed, implanting buttons in the dental plates is very simple. Neither complicated tools, nor technical training are necessary.

3.3.8 Protecting natural teeth

A further advantage stems from the fact that there are no clasps on the remaining natural teeth. Ordinary dentures are usually held by the neighboring natural teeth with a clasp, and the occlusal pressure exerted on the dentures is supported by the remaining natural teeth; this can cause the loss of these teeth. Buttons on the denture make it possible to eliminate clasps so that the natural teeth are not involved. In this way, button inserts are helpful in protecting the natural teeth.

3.4 NATURE OF METAL

In World War I, many soldiers suffered injury to the bone. As surgeons sought effective surgical and medical remedies, rapid progress was made in the field of oral surgery. World War II gave rise to similar problems and progress. And in general surgery faced the problem of suturing fractured limb bones. The search for substitute material for damaged bone led to the development of surgical metal.

Surgical metal must meet two requirements for safe use in the human organism: chemical stability and minimun liquefiability. Most surgical metal is made of a cobalt-chrome alloy or pure titanium, which meet these requirements.

Generally speaking, no allergic reaction is found when surgical metal is implanted in osseous tissue. There is a slight possibility of a rejective reaction. This possibility can be eliminated however. The implanted surgical metal is not liquefiable. Although some have casually speculated that any metallic material implanted in the human body may cause cancer, numerous clinical observations have proved that no change occurs in organic tissues around implanted surgical metals of minimum liquefiability. Except for the liquefactive tendency of the metal, there is no possibility of generating cancerous cells. No medical or dental report has ever made a linkage between surgical metal and cancer. The button used for the intramucosal insert is a kind of implant; it is therefore made of surgical metal. There is no doubt about its safety from the biochemical point of view.

3.5 FUNCTION: BUTTON AND SOCKET

How is the inserted button supported in the gingiva? The button is convex in shape, whereas the corresponding socket of the gingiva is concave. They thus fit together just like a snap used for fastening. The next question is: how to puncture the gingiva?

A hole is made in the gingiva that is just the same size as the button, which is then inserted. The hole made in the gingiva is, of course, an incised wound, enveloping the inserted button.

The button socket is thus formed as a result of the properties of the human body.

Any implant including an inserted button cannot remain permanent if fixed only mechanically without the back-up of the body's vital reaction. It will eventually drop out, giving pain similar to that characterizing the last stage of alveolar pyorrhea.

If a 2 mm hole is bored in the gingiva, a vital reaction occurs to fill up the hole. When a metallic button is inserted in the hole, the button is enveloped completely through the process of cicatrization, as long as the metal is of minimum liquefiability so that rejection does not take place (Fig. 16).

When the button is incorrectly shaped, that is, when its corners form acute angles as shown in Figure 17, cicatrization is incomplete, leaving hollow areas adjacent to the corners. The shape of the button is, therefore, of critical importance for effective functioning of the intramucosal insert.

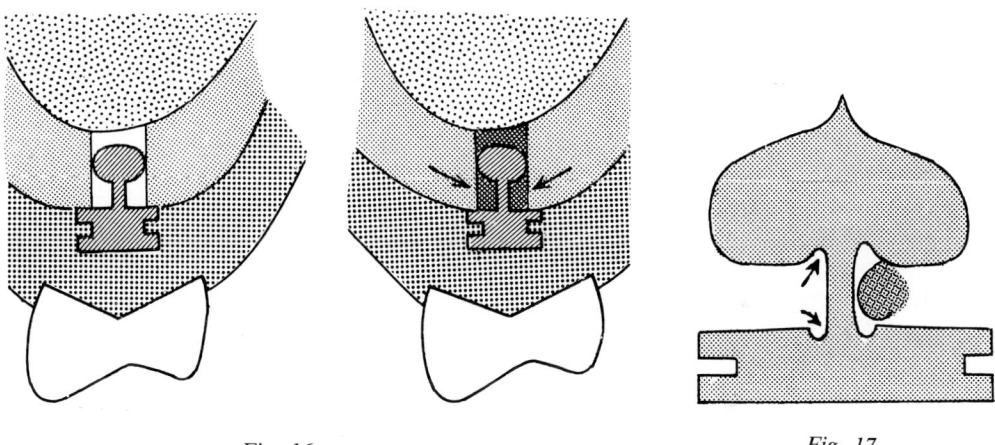

Fig. 16.   Fig. 17.

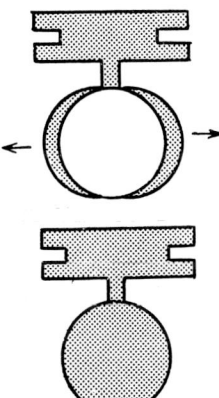

3.6 SHAPE

The button must be shaped in such a way that it will remain firmly in the socket formed by the healing process. In terms of both easier healing and more effective holding capacity, a ball type button, with the smallest surface, would seem the most appropriate. Clinical experience, however, has shown the ellipsoid-type button to be most effective for pratical use (Fig. 18).

Buttons that are too flat and ellipsoid, however, are not desirable, given the pain and difficulty associated with them in attaching and removing them. The neck connecting the ball and the base for the prosthesis should not be too thick in terms of the holding capacity of the gingiva. The overall size of the ball and neck should be, of course, less than the thickness of the gingiva, preferably two thirds of its diameter (Fig. 19).

Fig. 18.

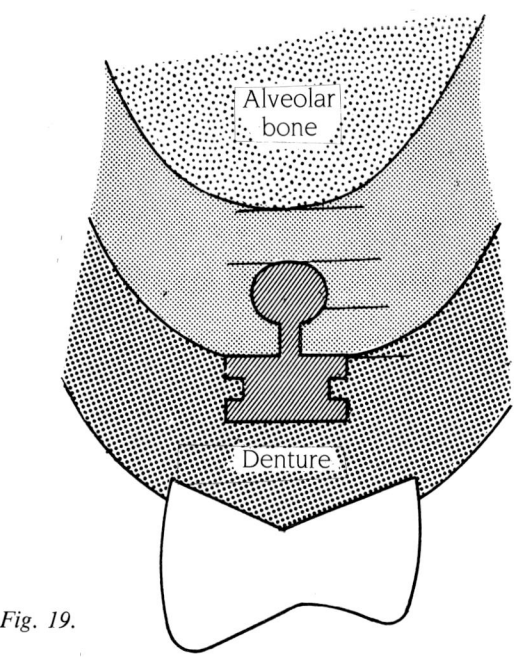

Fig. 19.

3.7 INSTRUMENTS

3.7.1 Bur for scraping hollows in the dental plate.

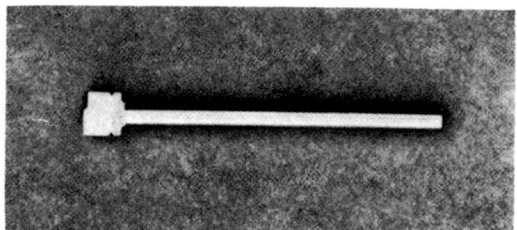

Fig. 20.

3.7.2 Bur for incising gingiva. This bur has a hollow edge of the same diameter as the ball. The incised portion of the gingiva fills the empty edge for purposes of easy removal.

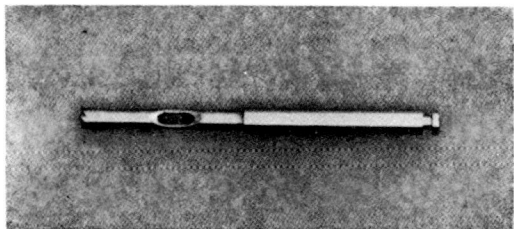

Fig. 21.

3.7.3 Bur for incising portion of the alveolar bone when the ball is touching the bone.

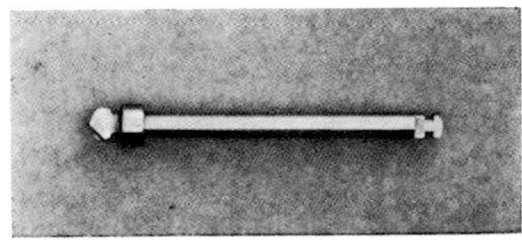

Fig. 22.

3.7.4 Round bur for general dental use. This type of bur is also used for the purpose of incising a portion of the alveolar bone.

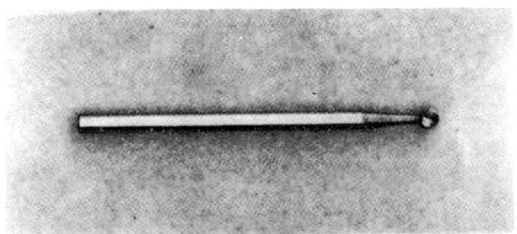

Fig. 23.

3.8 CONDITIONS AND RESTRICTIONS

3.8.1 Flabby gums

Button inserts should not be applied in patients who have flabby gums. After the mucosa has been improved the button may be inserted. When mucositis fires, (inflammation of the mucous membrane is found), tissue conditioner should be applied before inserting the balls.

3.8.2 Restricted areas

Button inserts should not be used in the 3/3 front teeth area. They should not be used anywhere except in the area on either side of the oral pharynx.

In particular, buttons should never be inserted in the median palatal side of 1/1, where the opening of the incisive canal containing the nasal palatine nerve is located. Nor can they be inserted in the palatal side of the second molar 7/7 (Fig. 25). This is the area with the openings of the major and minor palatal nerves. Insertions here could cause functional disorder of the nervous tissues.

In Figure 24, no button should be inserted within the area bordered by Line X and Line X'. This restriction includes buttons to be used for partial dentures.

3.8.3 Location of buttons

In Figures 25 and 26, Line A is the vertical line passing through the alveolar crest. Buttons inserted on Line A are generally able to hold the dentures against vertical external pressures.

Line B passes through the palatal side of the alveolar crest. Buttons inserted on Line B are generally able to hold the dentures against horizon-

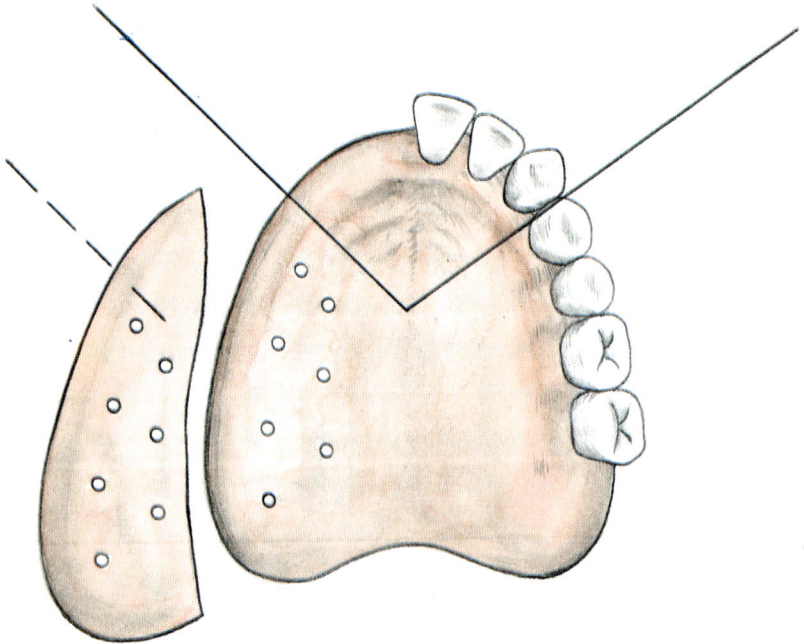

Fig. 24.

tal external pressures, preventing the loosening of the denture in the buc-
cal-palatal direction. If the purpose is solely that of preventing lowering of
the denture, buttons inserted on Line A are sufficient. On Line A, Point a
indicates the location of the first premolar; Point b, the location of the second premolar; Point c, the first molar; Point d, the second molar. Buttons can be inserted at these four points.

Point e is located at the apex of the equilateral triangle whose base is

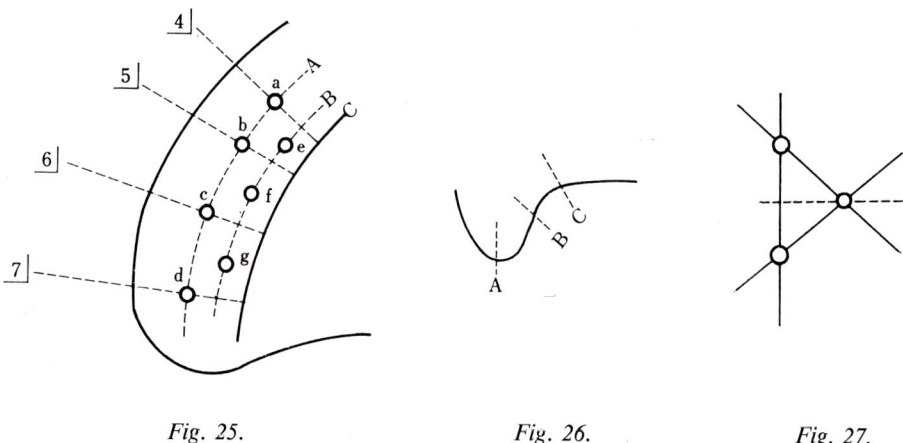

Fig. 25.   *Fig. 26.*   *Fig. 27.*

ab (Figure 27); Points f and g are determined in the same way, in relation
to *bc* and *cd* respectively. Buttons can be inserted at Points e, f, and g.

Points A-G illustrate the general rule for determining insert positions.
They can be modified according to the patient's condition. Points c, d, and

g are the most important, because they are the points where the greatest occlusal pressure is exerted. If sufficient holding is to be provided, capacity points must be carefully calculated.

Figure 25 shows one side only; in full denture cases, of course, it is just necessary to reverse the figure to set the other side.

3.8.4 Position of button

Buttons should be implanted in the denture so as to form a right angle with the gingival surface. This 90° applies to all buttons on Line A and Line B. Buttons inserted in the wrong direction would have less holding capacity.

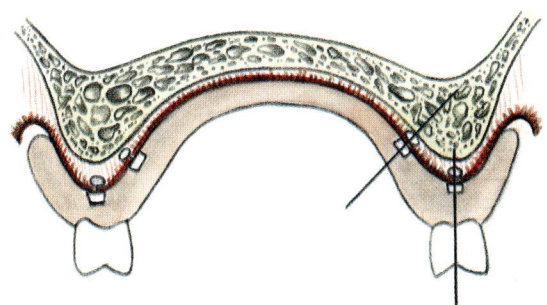

Fig. 28.

3.9 INSERTING PROCEDURES

3.9.1 Examine the condition of the denture carefully by fitting it in the oral cavity of the patient. In particular, inspect the fit between the dental plate and the oral mucosal membrane.

3.9.2 Draw Line A on the oral mucosal membrane beginning from the alveolar crest, with a soft copying pencil such as the "Kopierstift" or "Dermatograph". Then attach the denture, transferring Line A on to the dental plate surface. Line B is to be transferred in the same way.

3.9.3 Set Points a, b, c, d, e, f and g on the dental plate surface using the above method. The number of points may be increased, or reduced depending on the condition.

3.9.4 Set these points on the palatal mucosa. Carefully confirm that they have been correctly placed.

3.9.5 Make the hollows for fixing the buttons in the dental plate, using the special bur designed for this purpose (Fig. 29). The hollows should be made just a little deeper than the height of the button base. Test the hollows through a trial application of the buttons. This trial test is always crucial in obtaining the best result.

3.9.6 Fix the buttons in the hollows by filling in with a quick hardening resin (Fig. 30). Care must be exercised to keep the correct direction of the button. After hardening the resin, dip the denture in hot water, to eliminate harmful residual monomers.

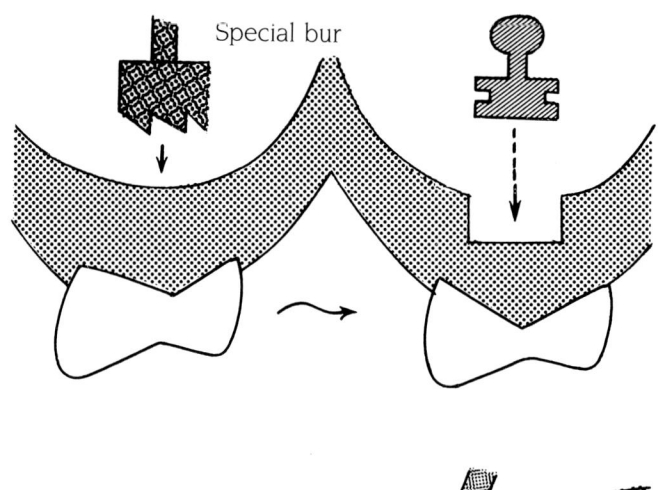

Special bur

Fig. 29.

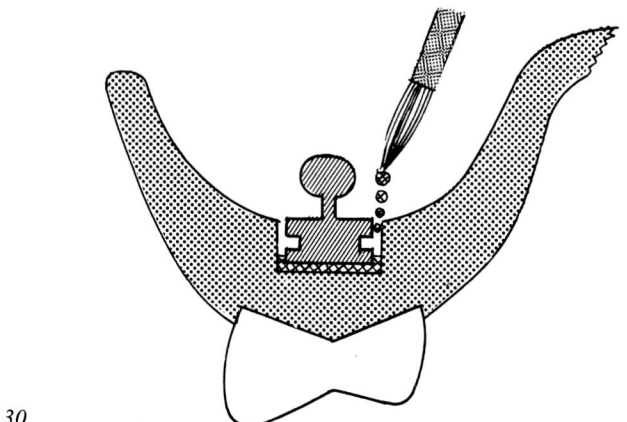

Fig. 30.

3.9.7 Excess resin should be planed with the round bur (Fig. 31).

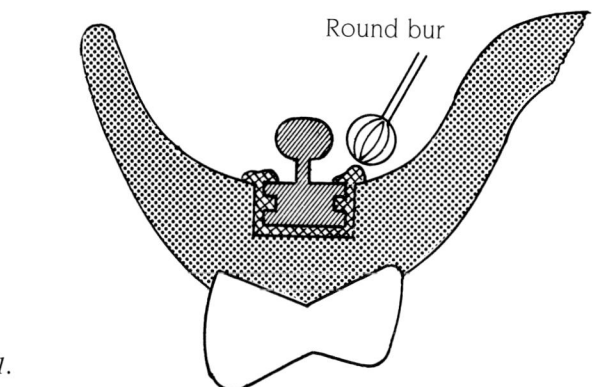

Round bur

Fig. 31.

3.9.8 Polish the inserted portion of dental plate with a Robinson brush (Fig. 32). Be careful not to bend the buttons accidentally at the neck.

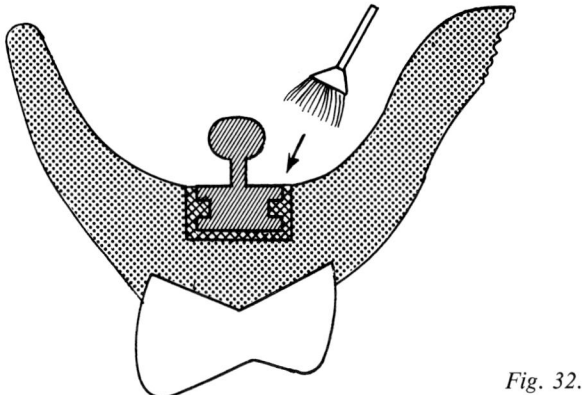

Fig. 32.

3.9.9 Mark the tops of the buttons with ink or with a copying pencil. After cleaning the oral mucosa, attach the dental plate in the oral cavity. Do not exert high pressure on the dental plate in attaching it.

This would push buttons into the mucosal membrane, causing considerable pain. It is a good idea to use iodine tincture to mark the point, instead of ink or pencil; points transferred on to the membrane with iodine tincture last much longer (Fig. 33).

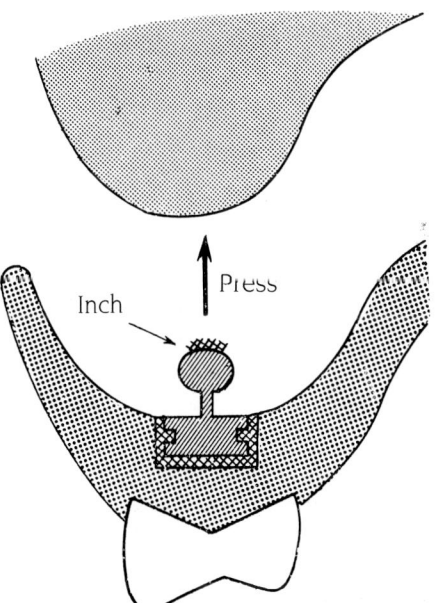

Inch

Press

Fig. 33.

3.9.10 Apply a very small quantity of anesthesia to the marked portion of the mucosal membrane. If a mizzy syrijet system is available, the anesthetic to be administered will usually be sufficient and an injection will probably not be required (Fig.34).

3.9.11 Incise the oral mucosa through to the alveolar bone, using the special bur for this purpose (Fig. 35).

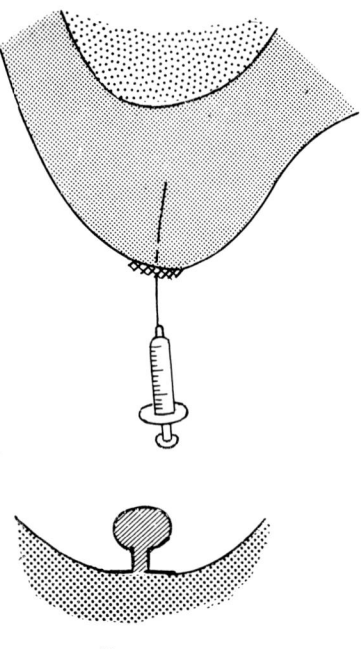

Denture   *Fig. 34.*

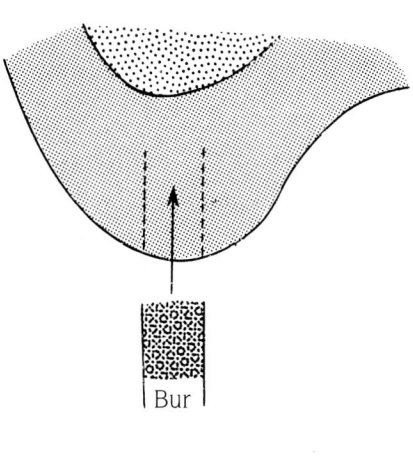

Bur

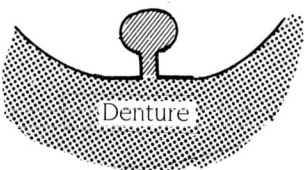

Denture

Fig. 35.

3.9.12 After the incision, apply the dental plate in a trial test. If any button is in direct contact with the alveolar bone, the denture base will become loose and cause pain.

A similar result will follow, if soft tissue is left between the dental plate and the membrane (Fig. 36). In that case, the thickness of the mucosal
membrane is less than the height of the button head. As explained above,
the gingiva should be 50 percent thicker than the height of ball; to thicken
the gingiva, incise the contacting portion of the alveolar bone (Fig. 37).
This will eliminate the problem of touching the bone. There is no reason
to be conservative in determining how much bone to incise; this procedure
can greatly improve the prognosis.

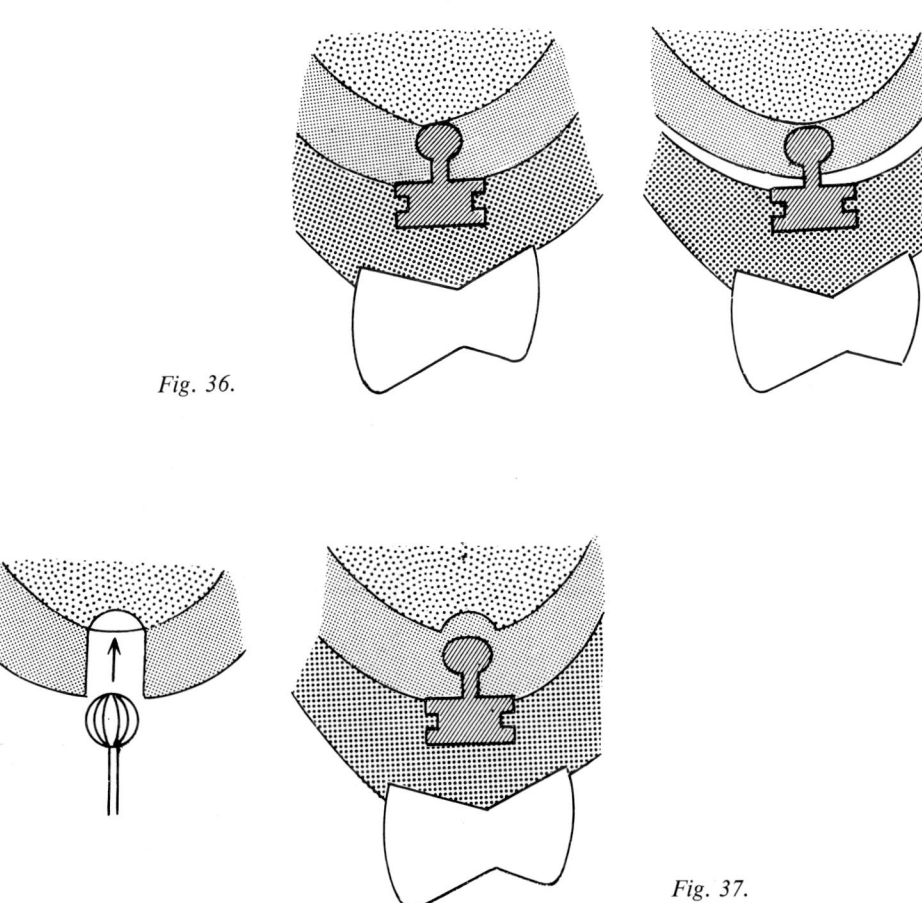

Fig. 36.

Fig. 37.

3.9.13 On completion of the operative procedures, attach the dentures
with fixing paste to the oral cavity.

3.9.14 Instruct the patient not to remove the dentures for two days after
the operation. It usually takes at least 5 to 7 days before the mucosal membrane around the operation site is completely healed. Until that time, the
buttons have no holding capacity; the fixing paste is a temporary aid for
this period.

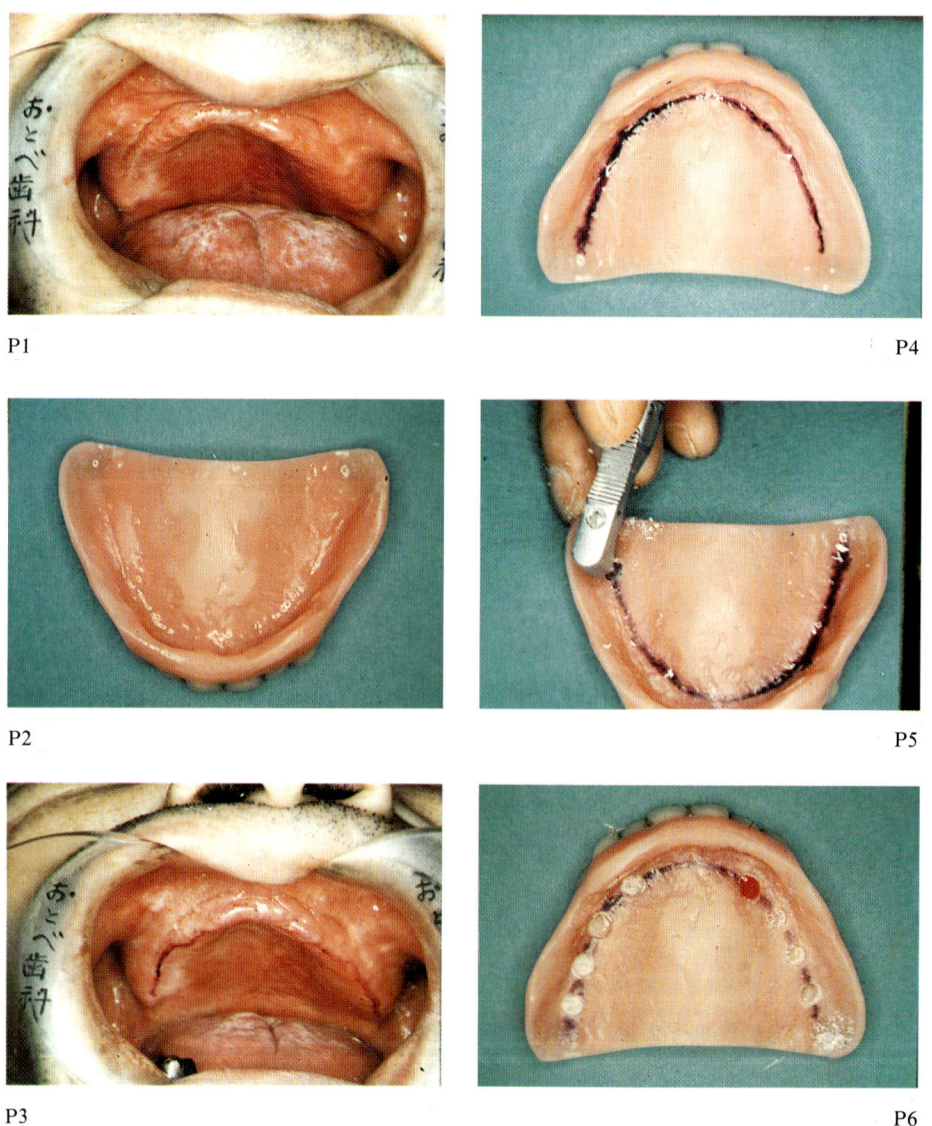

P1

P2

P3

P4

P5

P6

Case 1a

P-3 - The alveolar ridge is most suitable for insertion of buttons. Hence the location of the alveolar ridge is indicated in ink on the mucosa. The points are printed on the inside of the denture when it is pressed to the mucosa.

P-4 - Holes to insert the buttons are made according to the marks.

P-5 - Holes for the buttons are made on the mucosa.

P-6 - Holes for the buttons are made on the denture.

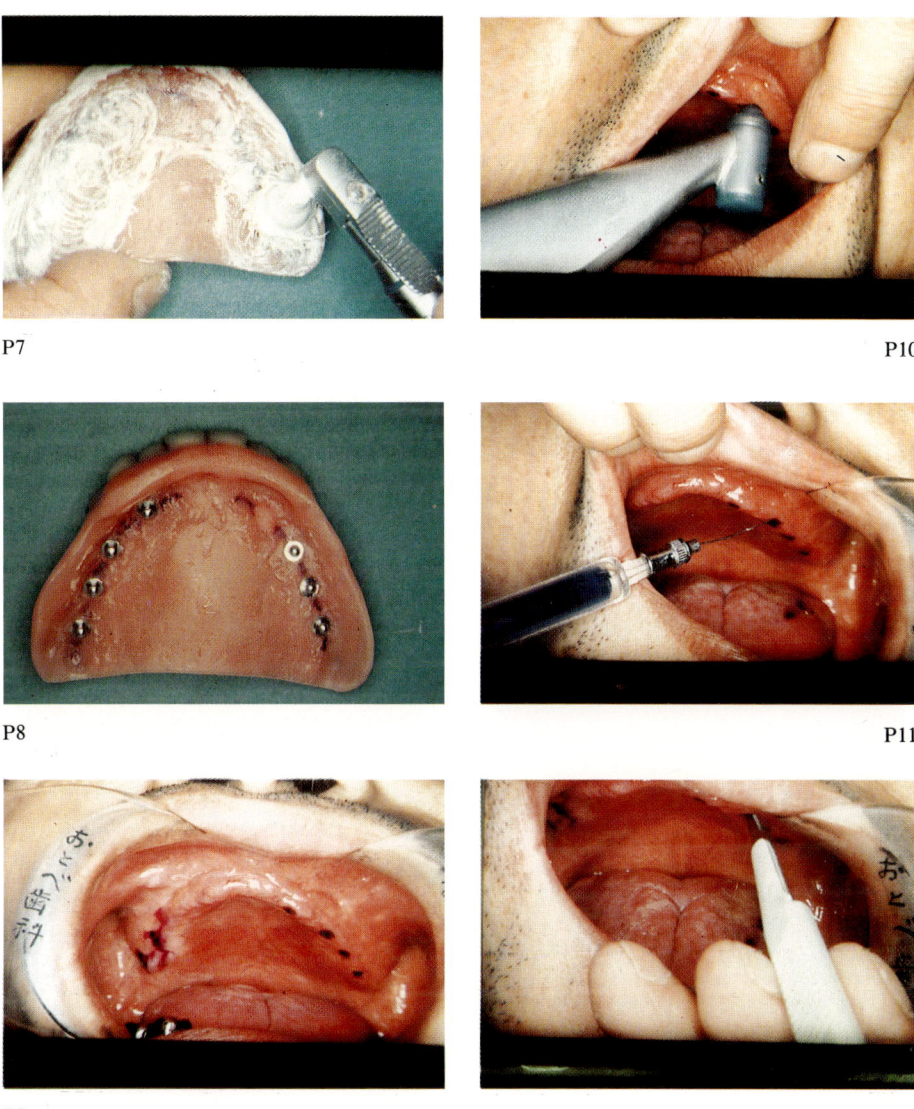

P7

P10

P8

P11

P9

P12

Case 1b

P-7 - The buttons are cemented to the denture with acrylic resin. Excessive resin is removed and polished.

P-8 - Ink is put at the top of the buttons.

P-9 - Marks are made on the mucosa.

P-10 - Local anesthesia is administered by mizzy.

P-11 - Local anesthesia can be administered by injection.

P-12 - Holes are made on the mucosa using special instruments. If not available made cross-cuts with a surgical knife.

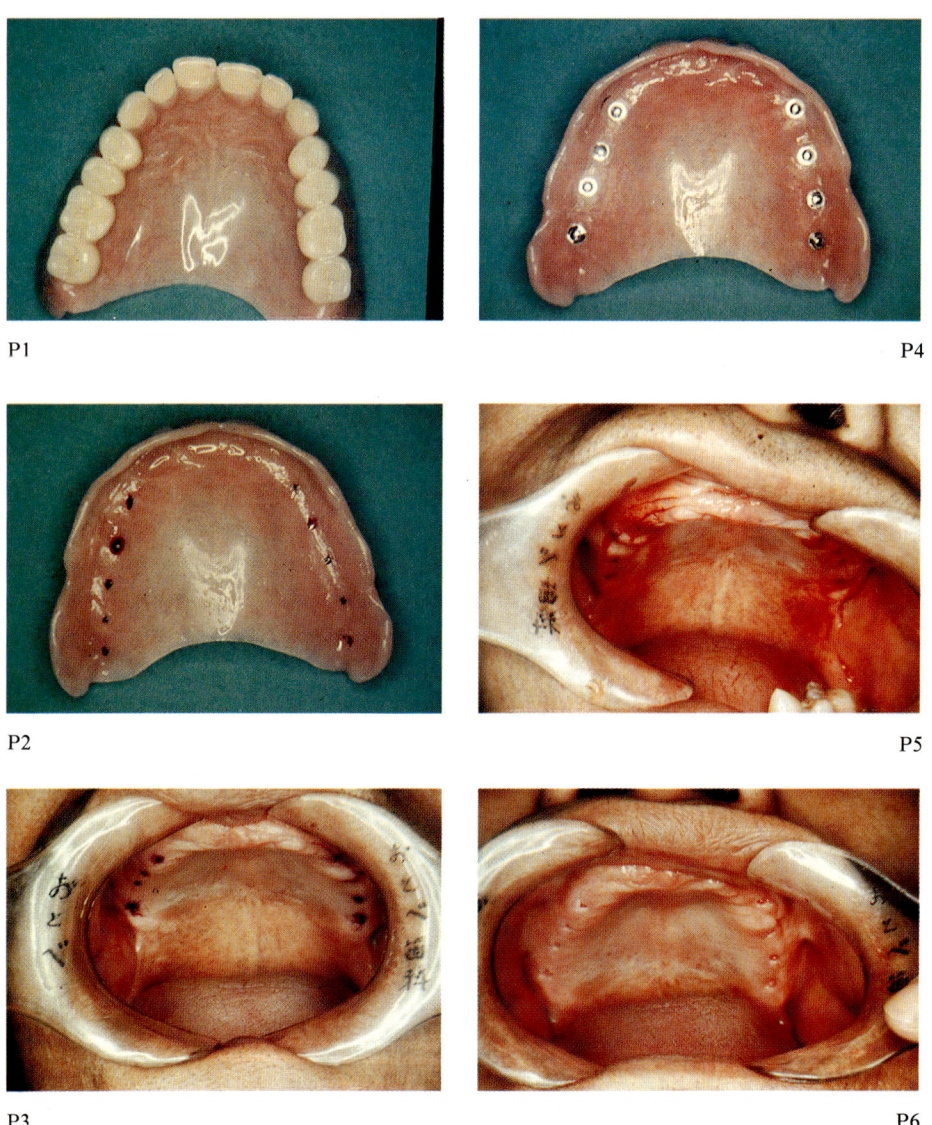

P1

P4

P2

P5

P3

P6

Case 2
P-6 - Holes are formcd properly on the mucosa.

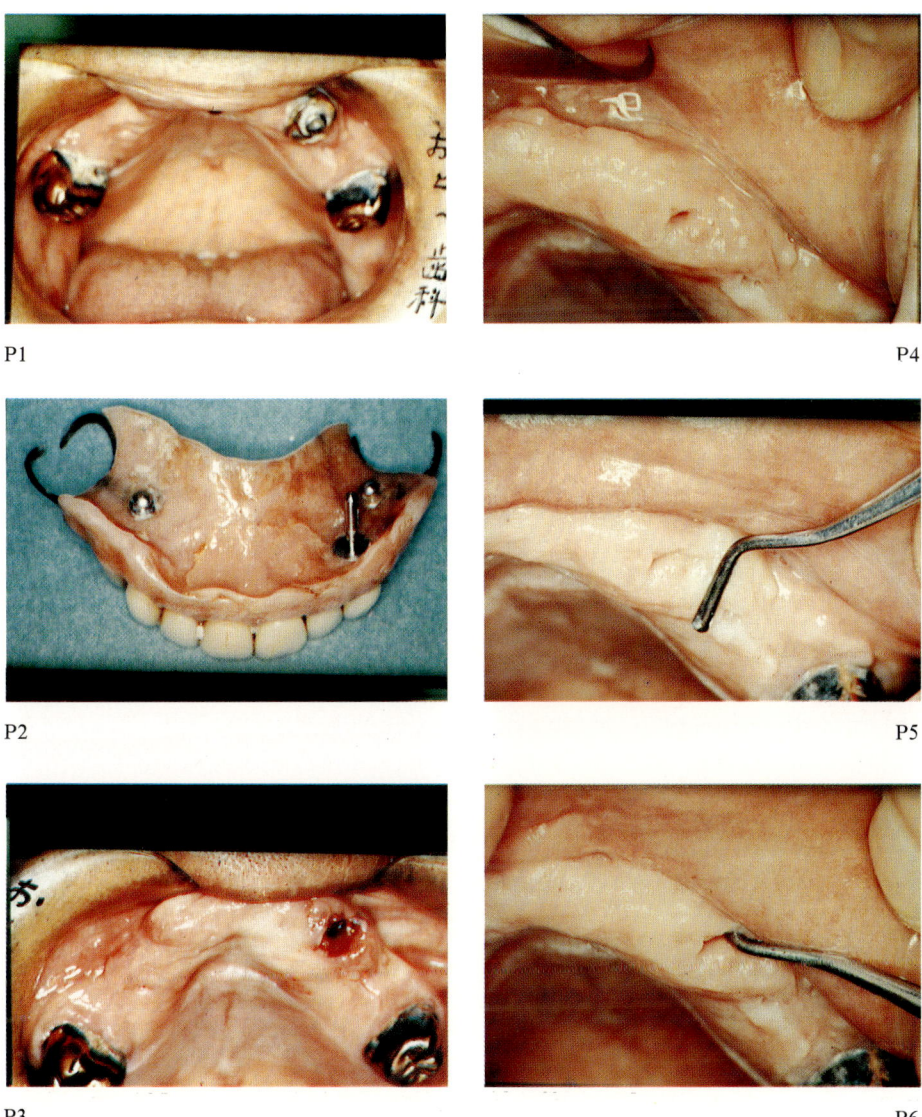

P1

P2

P3

P4

P5

P6

Case 3
P-1 - Left cuspid is unstable and planned to be extracted.
P-2 - The denture is corrected at the position corresponding to cuspid. Big button (8 mm) is attached.
P-3 - Left cuspid is extracted. Denture is placed right after extraction.
P 4 - Holes on the mucosa one month after the operation.
P-5 - The depth of the holes are examined by the depth gauge.
P-6 - The depth is found about 10 mm.

3.10 BIG BUTTON TECHNIQUE

In case of full edentulous maxillary bone, when resorption of the bone progressed to certain state, blade implant can not be applied in consideration of the necessary thickness of bone.

Some patient would hate operation for subperiosteal implant and, at the same time, he might want to have reliable denture.

Up to now we have had to rely on Intra Mucosal Insert using ordinary small-sized button.

This method has, however, proved causing several problems, including less durability of denture and possible pain to the patient.

It is well known that the Button Implant was invented by Gustav Dahl in 1943 and introduced to dental field.

The size and shape of Button have been modified and improved by many implantologists to the present model. Method of clinical application of Button Implant has also established now, although there are several problems to be studied and solved.

The author invented and developed the new method, the Big Button System; clinically we have got very favorable results. This is the first report of Big Button for improved Intra Mucosal Implant Dentistry.

3.10.1 Explanation of the Shape of Big Button

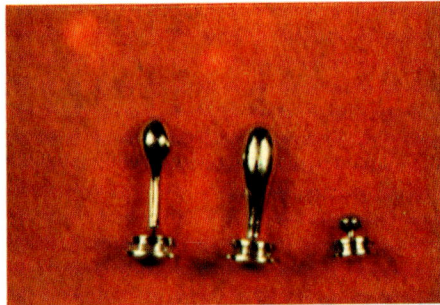

Fig.- B1 Photo of Big Button

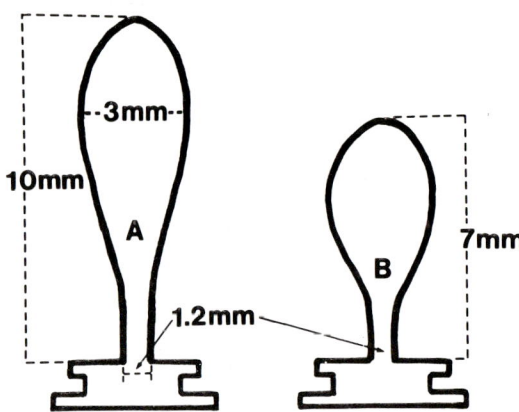

Fig.- B2 Dimension and specifications of Big Button

A type   B type

3.10.2 Merits of Big Button compared with small button
(1) Fewer buttons, usually less than four, will do.
(2) Much more durability and reliability of the denture can be expected.
(3) Less possibility of causing pain to the patient.
(4) Easier search for pain-causing button treatment.
(5) Shorter period of time for examination.

Those who had tried Intra Mucosal Inserts had also faced and experienced the above points, 2-3, 2-4, 2-5, in particular.

3.10.3 Location of Inserting Button
(1) Left and right maxillary tuber region
(2) Left and right cuspid region

Full Edentulous Case

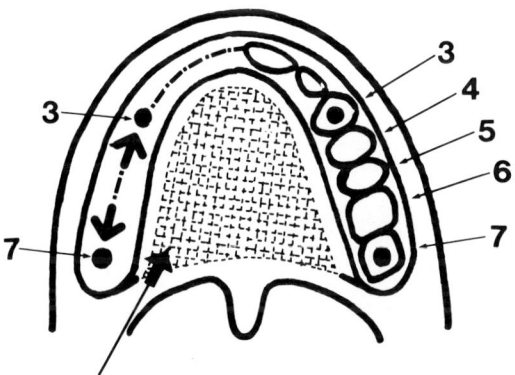

Remove palatal parts of denture

Fig. - B3

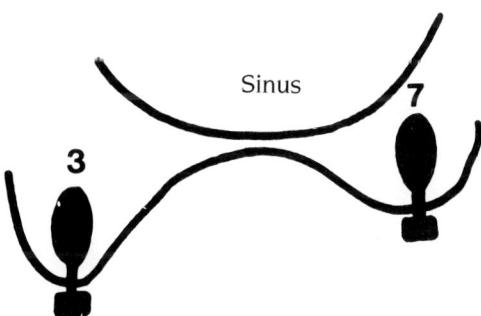

Fig. - B4

Avoid inserting buttons in maxillary sinus and its surroundings.

Case of Mandibular Application

Generally speaking, application of Standard button to the mandible would be very difficult; application of Big Button, however, is comparatively easy even to the mandible.

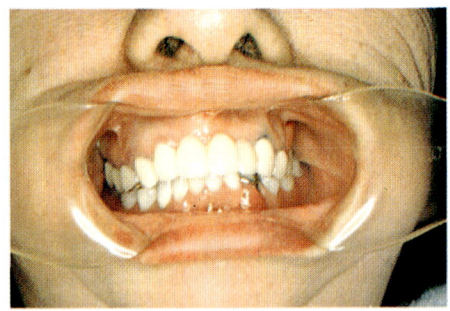

Before operation

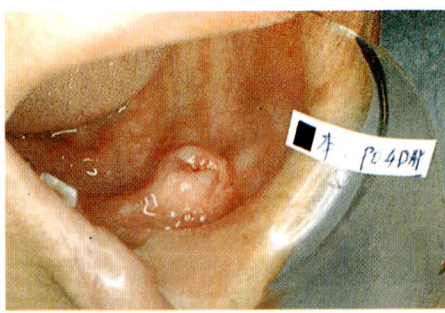

4 days post operation

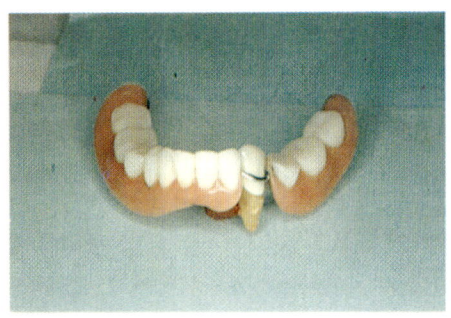

Extraction

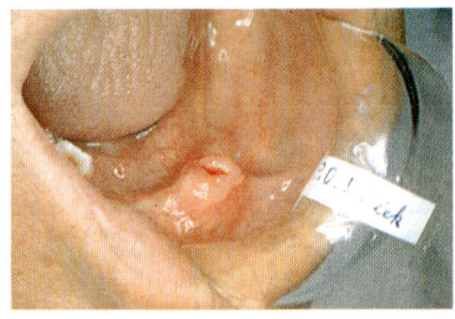

5 weeks post operation

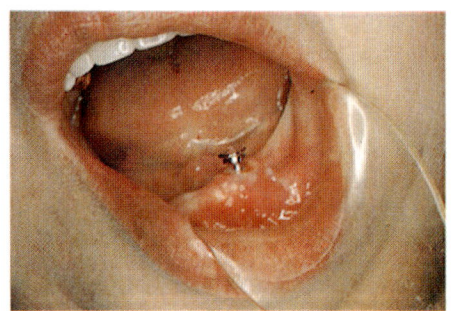

Put for extraction hall

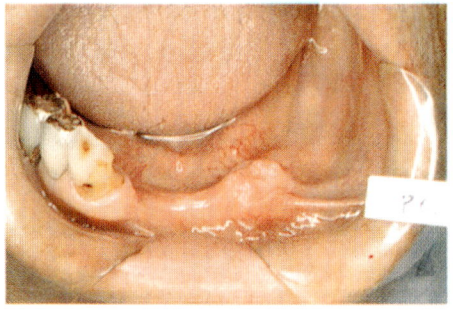

3 years post operation

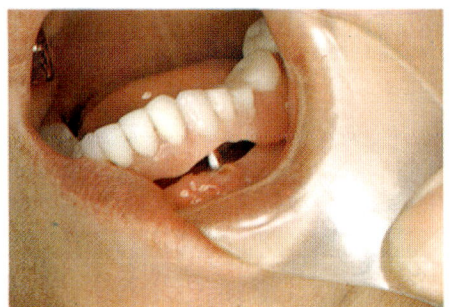

Long Button set for denture

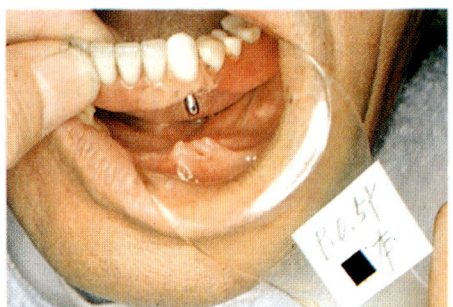

5 years post operation

Only One Cuspid Case

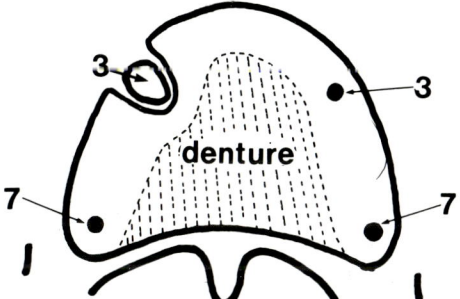

Fig.- B5

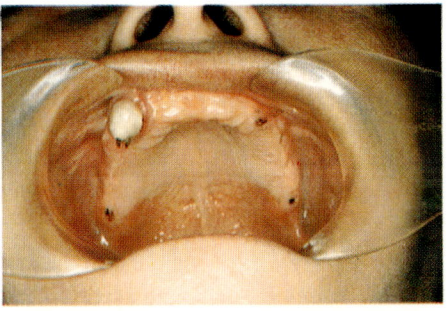

Steps to make a hole in mucosa to put in button. First, mark the spot with color pencil.

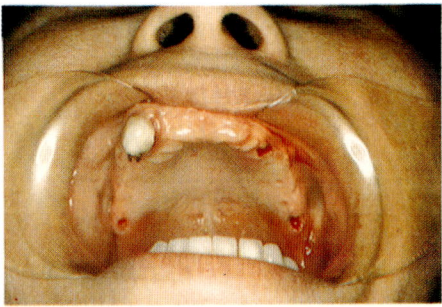

Make a hole with bur.

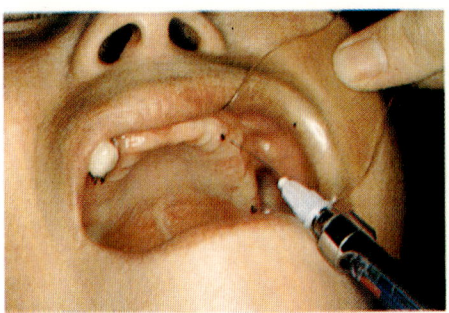

Apply infiltration anesthesia.

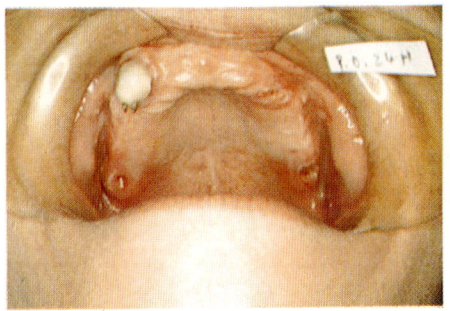

Hole after the operation. Favorable recovery mucosa around the hole.

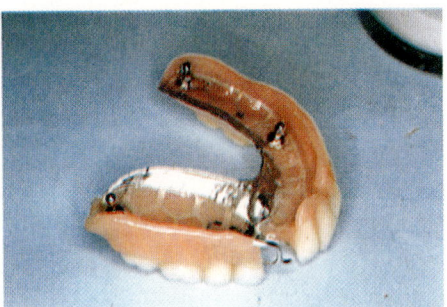

Denture with button.

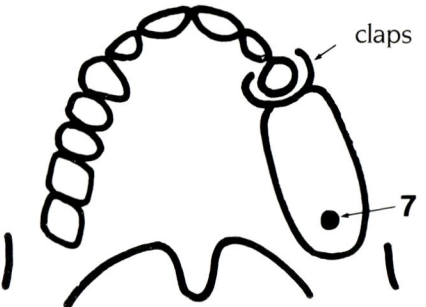

Fig. - B6

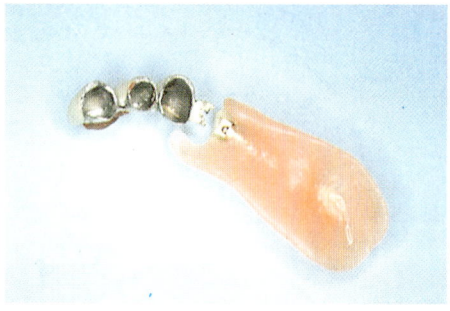

Denture for lost molar and bridge with attachment.

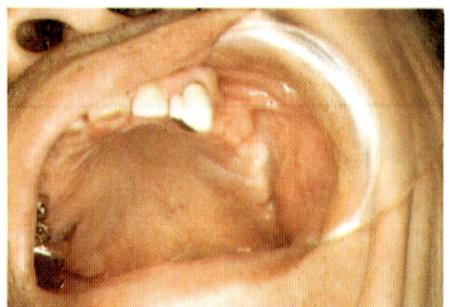

Lost part on right side.

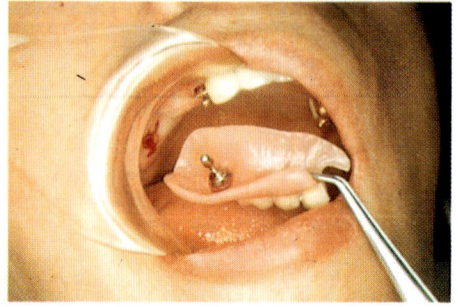

Fix the bridge by cementing, then make button hole.

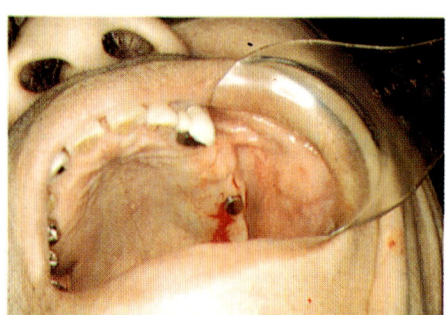

Make a button hole at 21/.

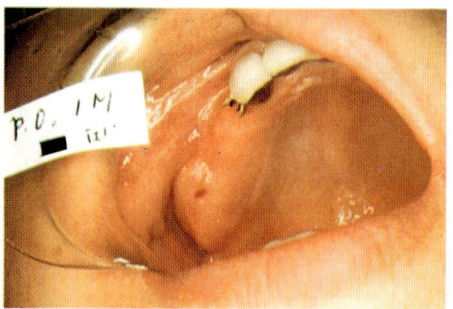

Button hole a month after the operation.

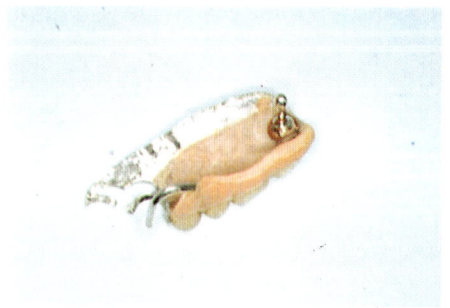

Denture with Button.

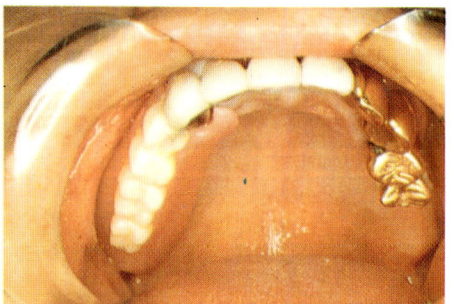

Only One Molar Case

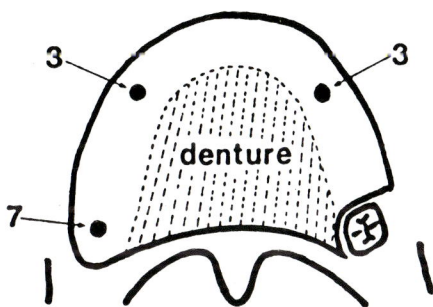

Fig. - B7

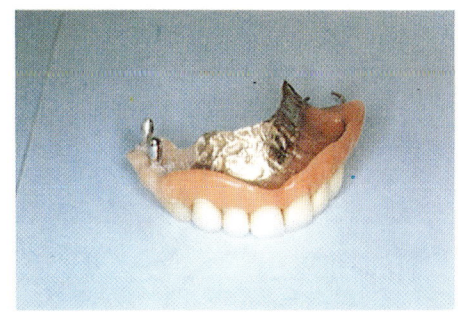

Fix button to denture.

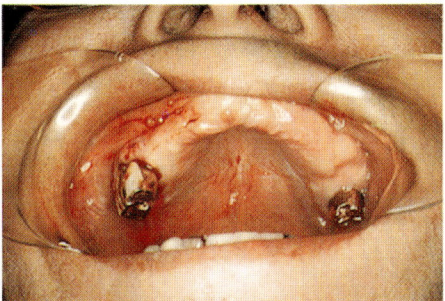

Right-side gold crown being shaky.
Needs extraction.

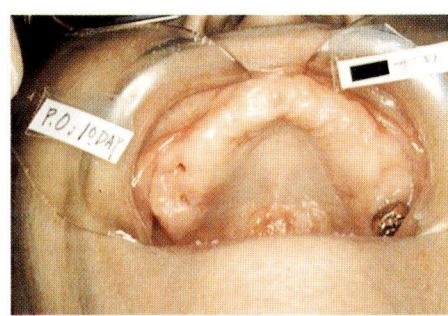

Ten days later.

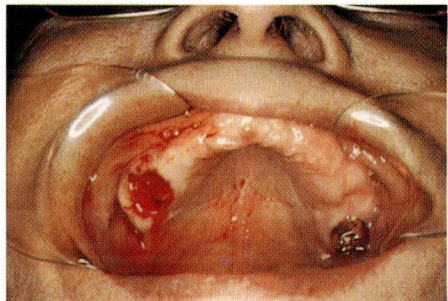

After extraction.

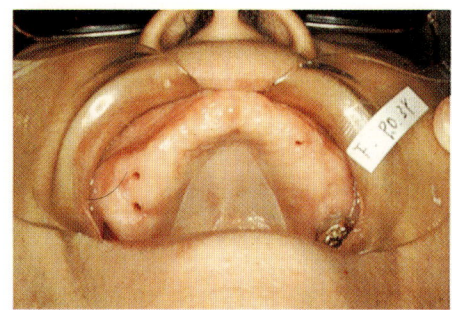

Make a new hole in left cuspidate mucosa
for button.

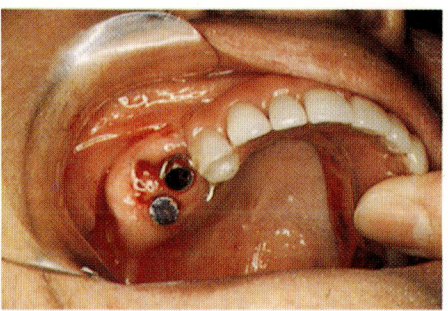

Apply button in the hole immediately after the extraction.

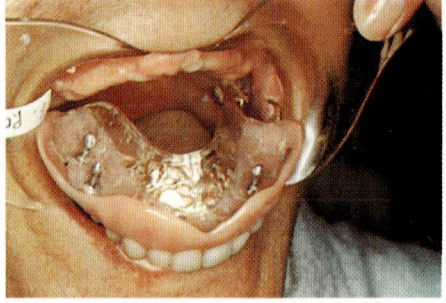

Denture prepared.

3.10.4 Inserting Operation (Bone Perforation Method)

(1) Perforate the denture for putting-in buttons by a 700 bur.

Step 1

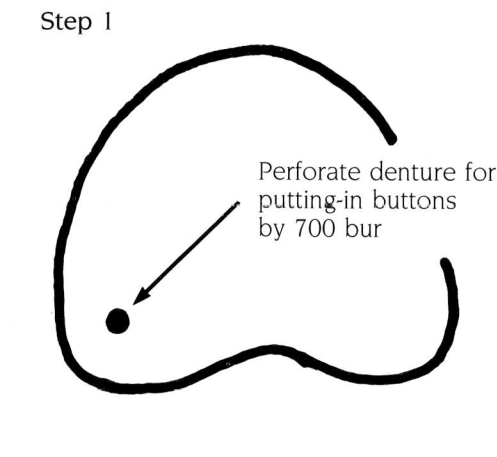

Perforate denture for
putting-in buttons
by 700 bur

Fig. - B8

Step 2   Denture into mouth

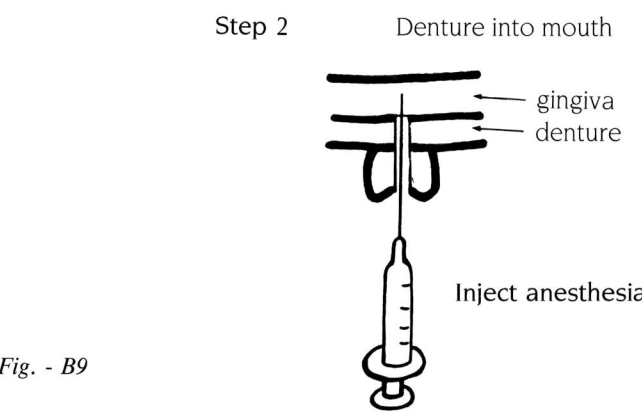

— gingiva
— denture

Inject anesthesia

Fig. - B9

(2) Insert the denture into the mouth. After fitting the denture, inject anesthesia (permeating) through the perforations prepared in the preceding step.

(3) Take out the denture.

Step 3   take out denture

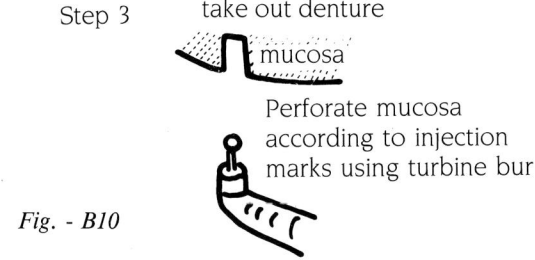

mucosa

Perforate mucosa
according to injection
marks using turbine bur

Fig. - B10

(4) Perforate the mucosa according to the injection marks using a turbine bur. Holes should be just a bit larger in dimension, deeper in depth, for inserting the expected buttons.

(5) Try fitting the buttons. If necessary, adjust perforations by re-boring them wide and deep enough to hold buttons; or, by making the buttons shorter.

It is recommended to place sanitary cotton around the buttons as illustrated, for the following purposes:

to prevent excess bleeding.

to locate the buttons at the center of perforation,

to prevent direct contact of the buttons with bone, consequently,

to lessen the patient's pain after the operation.

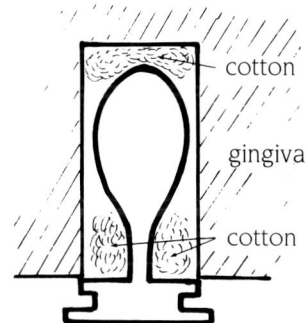

Fig. - B11

(6) Fit buttons to the denture.

CAUTION TO THE PATIENT:

Never take off the denture two days after the operation.

Let him come to the clinic on the third day; then, remove the denture and sterilize the wounds; examine and adjust the buttons if the patient undergoes pain.

3.10.5 Remove Palatal Parts of Denture

There are several advantages for the patient when the palatal part of the denture is removed.

Remove method of palatal parts

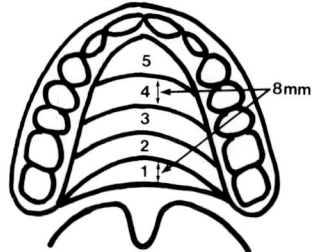

Fig. - B12

The ordinary denture completely covers palatal mucosa and, as a result, the sense of taste would largely be handicapped.

In English, they say "he has a delicate palate," praising somebody who is considered being a gourmet. In the Japanese vocabulary, there is a word "Fuhmi" which literally means "wind (or, air) and taste". This word originates in Chinese; both in Japan and China, people enjoy not only tasting by tongue, but also feeling warmth/coolness and aroma/fragrance by palate. Removing the palatal part of the denture therefore enables the patient to recover the organ of human taste, once lost by wearing a normal type of palatal full denture.

Instinctively the patient would recognize the fact that the most important factors of this tasting ability thus come back a certain time after the operation. The Big Button system is helpful to hold denture tighter and longer; at the same time it recovers the gourmet's taste.

The removal of palatal parts of the denture is to be done when the denture fits well and is stabilized, usually after two weeks from the operation.

The diameter of the area of possible removal is ca. 40 mm. It is better to remove this area step by step, in five times, 8 mm each at a week's interval.

Thus, the patient would realize that he is recovering his sense of taste and that pronunciation difficulties are decreasing. His appreciation would be larged than it he had the area removed in one time.

3.10.6 Applying the Hole of Extracted Tooth
When a hooking tooth comes to the condition of being extracted, (Figs. F, G) the button can be inserted directly, after the extraction, in the extracted hole.

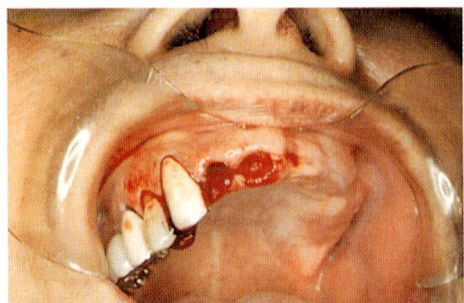

Extract 32/.

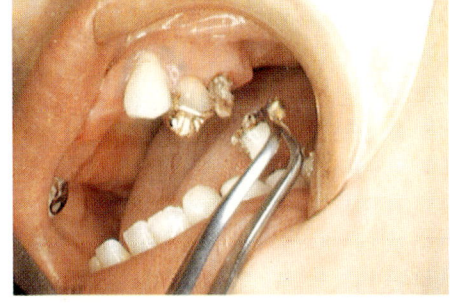

Broken hook; needs extraction.

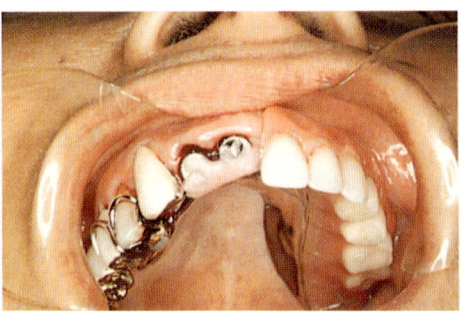

Put button in the hole immediately after extraction and connect button to denture.

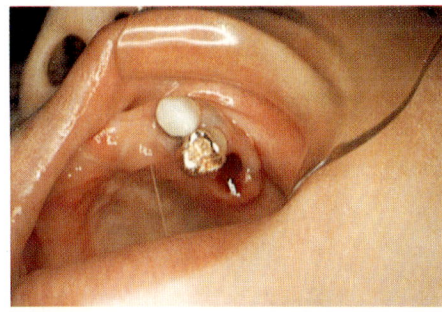

Immediately after extraction.

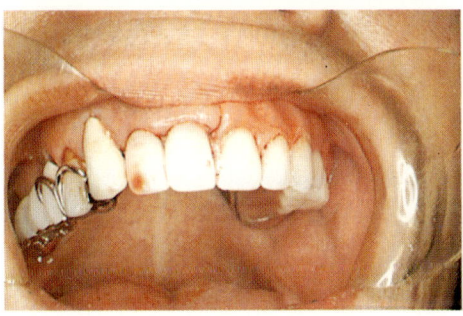

Fix resin tooth to denture.

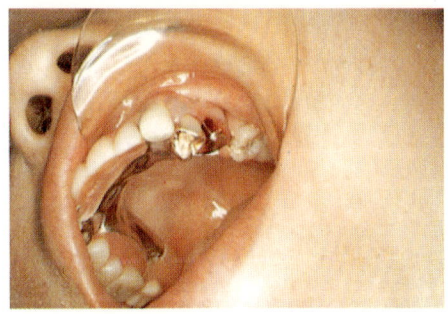

Button applied in the hole.

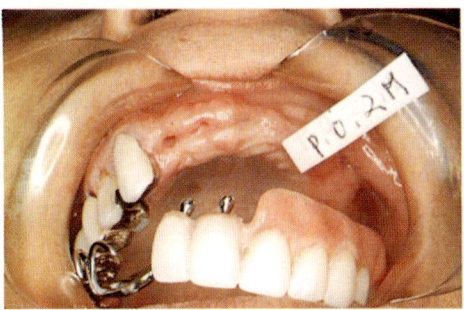

Favorable condition of the button hole two months later.

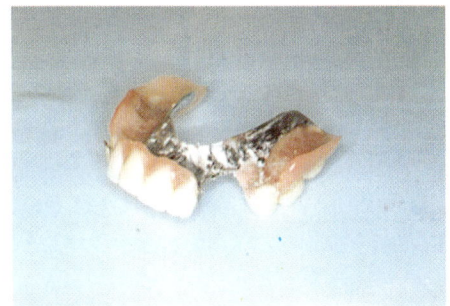

Denture.

Smaller "Standard" button replaced by Big Button.

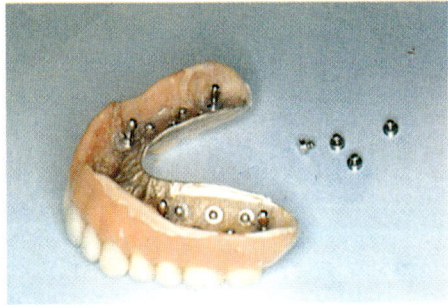

"Standard" button took off from denture.

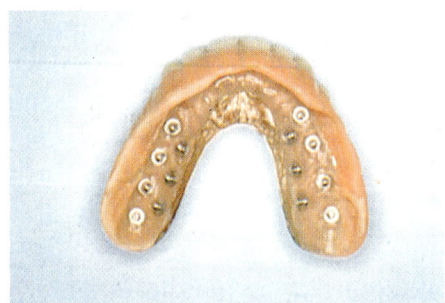

Button denture with smaller "Standard" button.

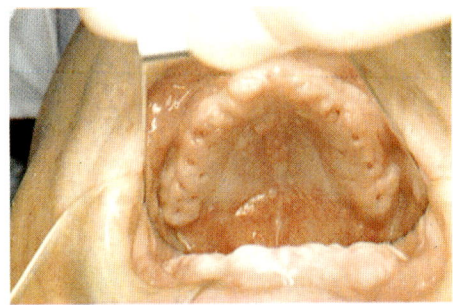

Three days later, all "Standard" buttons took off.

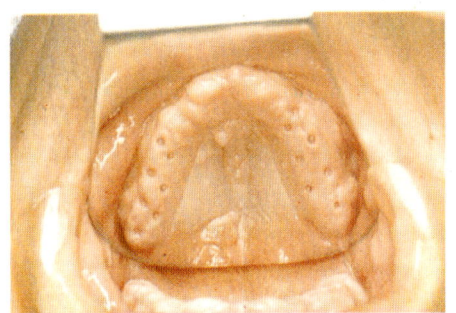

Loose button hole; cranky denture.

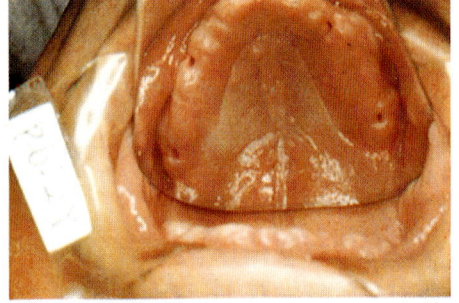

Very favorable condition of the Big Button hole one year later.

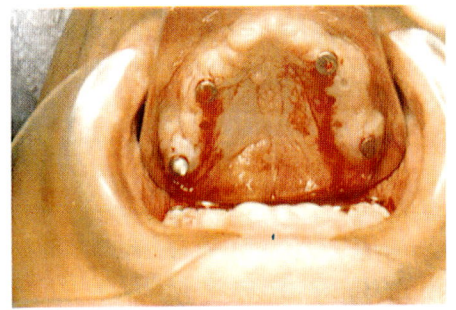

Make a new hole for Big Button at 73/37; apply button in the hole to check the depth.

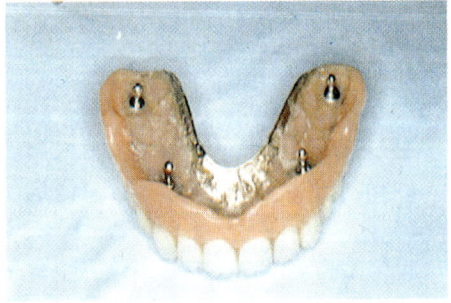

Denture.

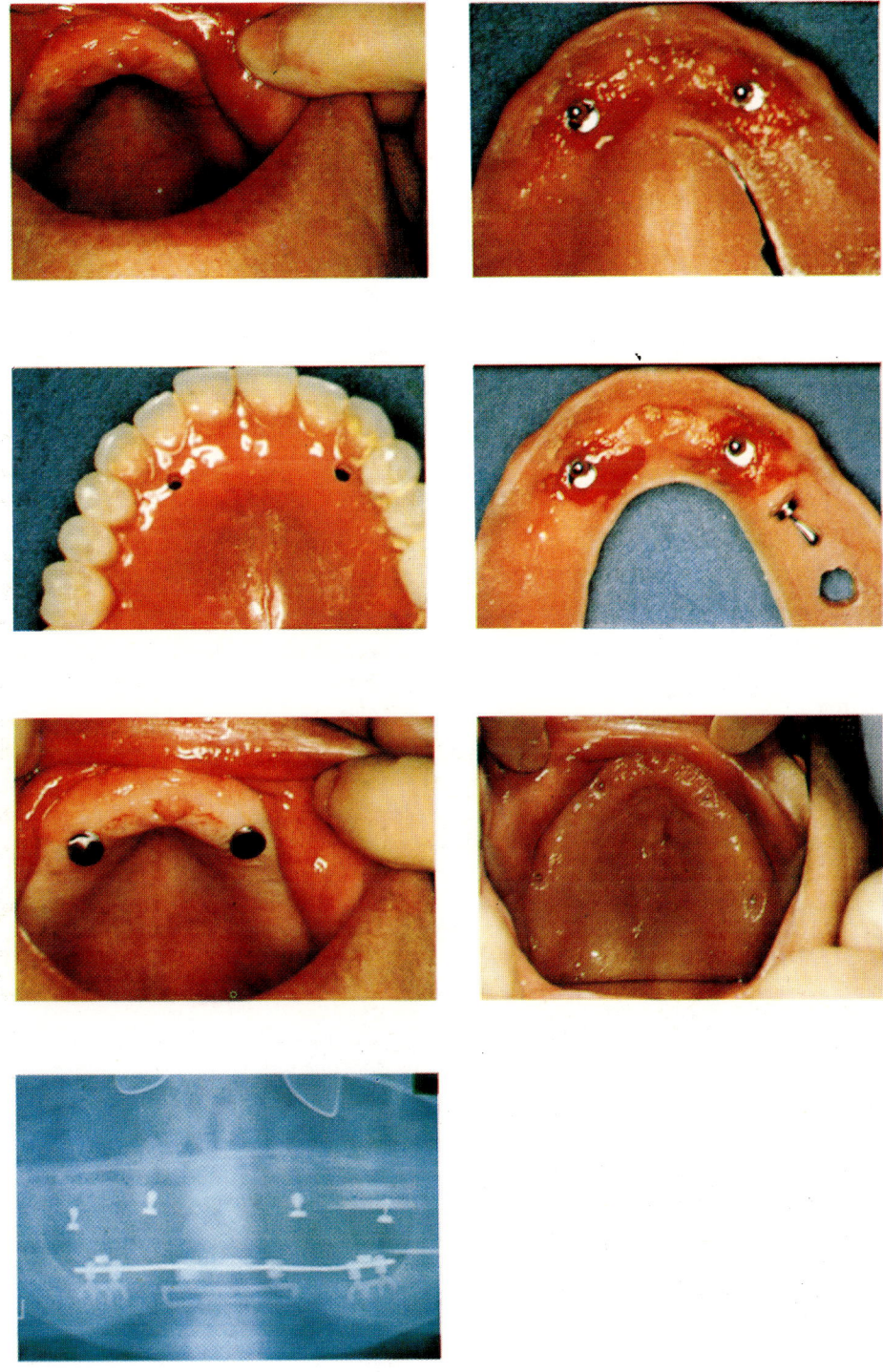

3.10.7 Application to the Mandible

In case of edentulous mandible, the applications of ordinary mucosal insert have been rather limited, because of the smaller thickness of mandibular mucosa and of the surface location of mandibular tract. By the use of long buttons, it is now possible to insert two long buttons at 3 3 position, boring the mandible cuspidate region.

The long button method can also be helpful for stabilizing the denture to all edentulous mandible as well.

Long buttons can be inserted avoiding the danger of hurting mandibular tracts and mandibular nerves.

3.10.8 Conclusion

To sum up the advantages of Big Button compared with ordinary "Standard" button, the following six points are to be recognized:

First, with less pieces of button, much greater holding power is to be expected. Only four pieces of Big Button are quite sufficient for a full denture.

Second, less pain for the patient. The location of the pain in also easily found, because of lower number of buttons.

Third, it is appliable to flabby gum. The "Standard" button, when applied to flabby gum, usually causes pain and has little holding power. Big Button, on the contrary, can hold denture much better, and, is painless.

Fourth, it is appliable successfully immediately after extraction.

Fifth, it is appliable to the maxilla. There are very few successful cases of "Standard" button applied to the maxilla; Big Button can be applied to the maxilla, even to the cuspid part.

Sixth, the operation is simpler, easier and shorter.

I have reported the basic method of my Big Button implant system; on the basis of your personal creative research and careful experience, you shall be able to find better uses of Big Button.

3.11 SUMMARY

3.11.1 The ball should be inserted so as to form a right angle with the gingival surface.

3.11.2 When the gingiva is incised, a portion of the underlying alveolar bone should also be incised, for better results.

3.11.3 Use of a loosened denture plate of an unrebased denture always leads to a failure.

3.11.4 The buttons should not be applied to flabby gum. Proper pretreatment is required in this case.

3.11.5 Successful intramucosal insertion of buttons does not cause pain.

3.11.6 Particular care should be taken in locating the buttons on Line B as well as in incising these points.

3.11.7 The denture must be attached very shortly after the incision. Should a couple of days elapse, the incision sites would close, and it would no longer be possible to attach the denture.

Part 3

Endosteal
Blade
Implant

4. Endosteal Implant: Material for Implant Blades

4.1 VARIETY OF BLADES: MANUFACTURERS AND PRODUCTS

4.1.0 Introduction

Various kinds of implant blades are currently manufactured and marketed. This section reviews their characteristics and provides a critical evaluation.

4.1.1 Chercheve blades

Chercheve blades are made of titanium (Fig. 38). In shape they are similar to the later Linkow-type blade. They are slightly smaller, however, having been designed with the average French man in mind. Thus, for nations like Japan where people are comparatively small, Chercheve blades are usually appropriate from the standpoint of size.

However, the narrow blade head of only 1 mm square would cause the difficulty in designing prostheses later.

It can be noted in passing that, before he designed this blade-type implant, Chercheve had also produced screw-type or spiral-shaft implants, including those with interchangeable gold copings.

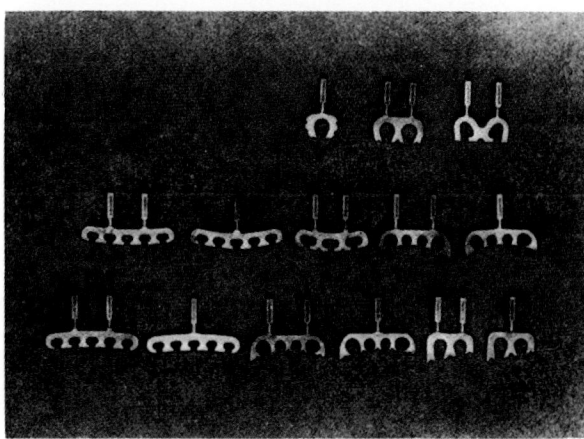

Fig. 38.

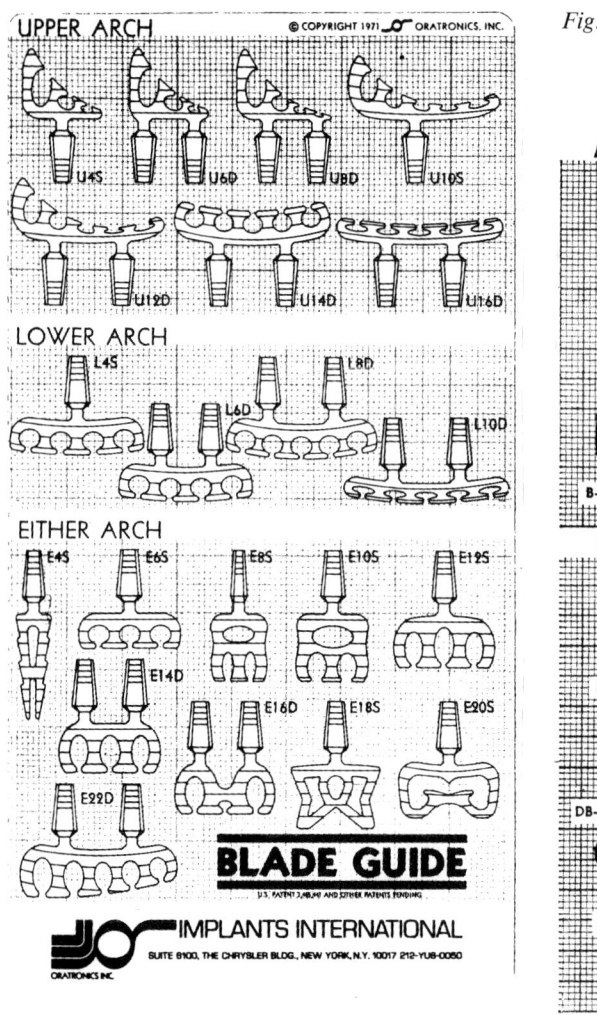

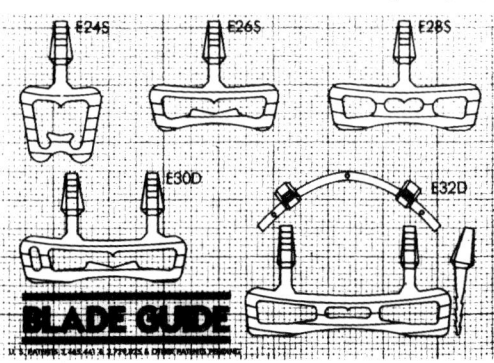

Fig. 40

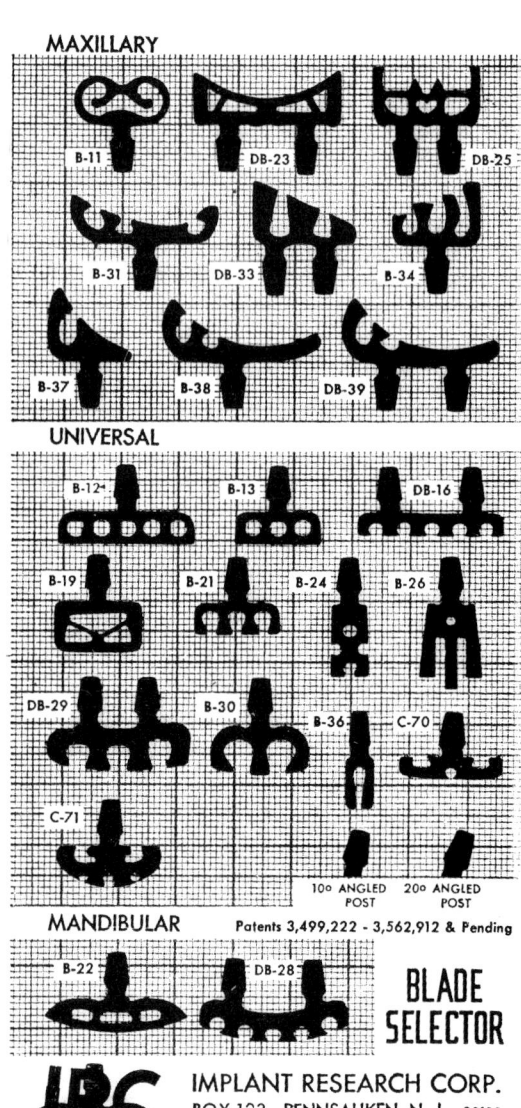

Fig. 39

Fig. 41

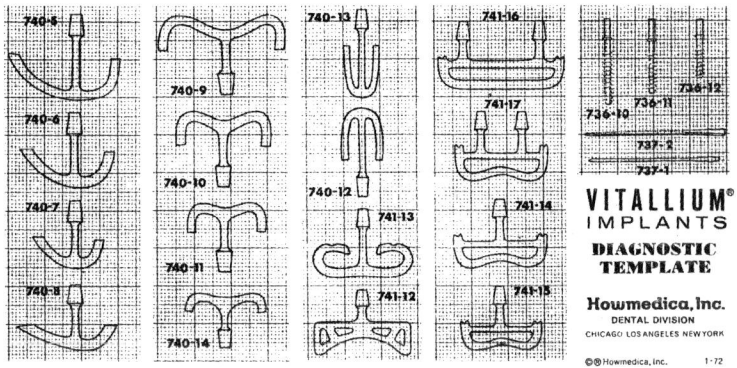

The visual aid has been designed to enable you to select an appropriate implant. The implants are divided into five categories and indicating their most common uses.

Pass the visual aid over radiographs of a potential implant site until the most suitable implant design is found. You will be able to clearly relate the shape and depth of each blade with that of the bone between the crest of the ridge and any crucial and/or critical point. Soft tissues must be retracted to reveal the true width of the crest. However, this dimension is rarely a problem with the blade vent.

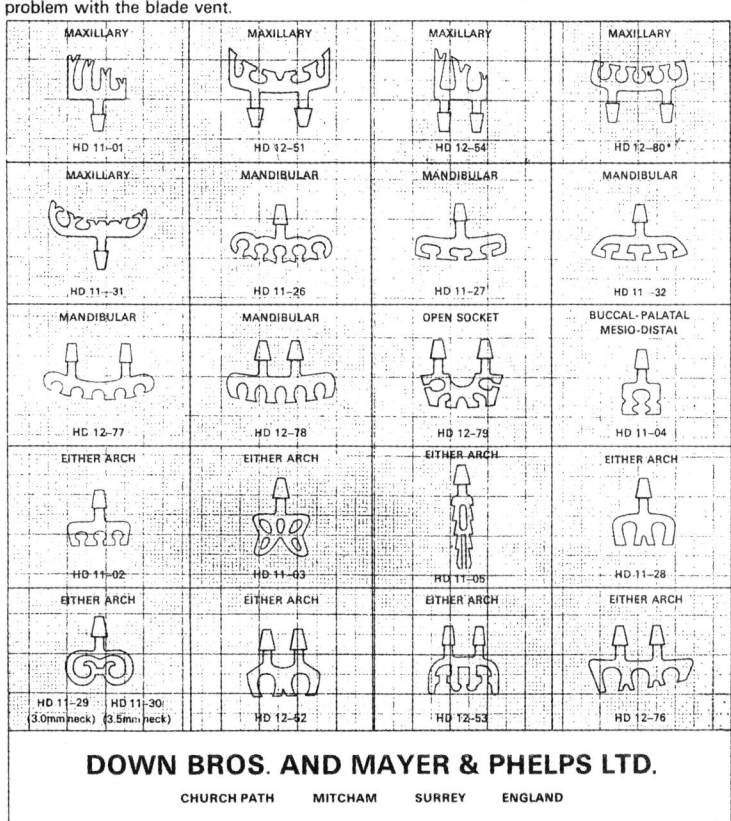

Fig. 42

4.1.2 Implants International Blades

Linkow developed a new type of blade, modifying the general shape and the size of the blade head, in particular (Figure 39). Implants International of New York later marketed Linkow's blade. I prefer these blades, both in terms of design and quality, as do many implantologists throughout the world. Recently, Implants International has begun the distribution of Lew-type blades.

In addition, Implants International distributes buttons for mucosal inserts, also developed by Lew and improved by Judy, as well as several kinds of pins for endodontic, endosteal implants. Given its various product lines, this corporation may well succeed in dominating the world market in the field of implant materials and equipment.

4.1.3 Howmedica, Inc.

Howmedica Inc. is the original American distributor of Vitallium alloy. Howmedica contributed a great deal to the rapid growth and development of implantology. At present, it supplies Lew-type blades only. Through Tokyo Dental Supply, its sole agent in Japan, Howmedica implant metal products have gained a reputation among Japanese implantologists as trustworthy clinical materials.

4.1.4 Implant Research Corp.

Implant Research Corp., of Pennsauken, New Jersey, supplies mainly Linkow-type blades, cast in Vitallium. Some blades have interchangeable heads which screw into the blade body. Implant Research also produces blades on request according to any design specified by the implant operator.

4.1.5 Down Brothers and Mayer & Phelps, Ltd.

In England, Down Brothers and Mayer & Phelps are suppliers of Linkow-type blades. However, as I am not familiar with these blades, I cannot evaluate their quality.

4.1.6 Muratori blades (Fig. 43)

Professor Giordano Muratori of Italy produces free-design blades primarily for his own use. I have had the opportunity of inspecting and using Muratori's blades. The body is made of titanium. Both the size and the shape of the blade are effectively designed for practical application, reflecting Muratori's extensive clinical experience. In short, these are quite recommendable as a free-design type of blade.

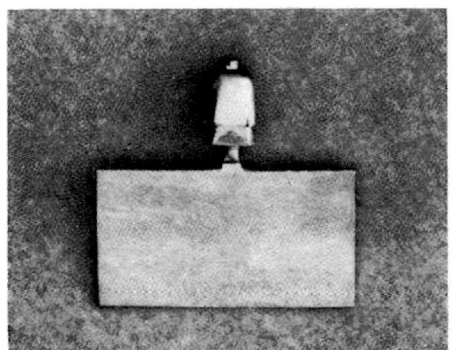

Fig. 43 Free design. Blade by Prof. Muratori

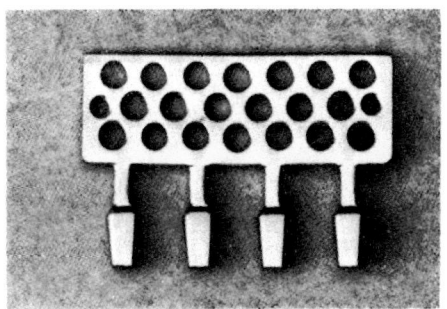

Fig. 44 Prof. Ugo Pasqualini
Free-design Blade

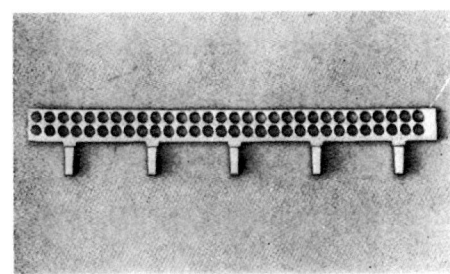

Fig. 45 Park Dental (New York)

4.2 PARTS OF THE BLADE AND THEIR FUNCTIONS

4.2.0 Major parts of the blade

The major parts of the implant blade are the head, safety stop, neck, shoulder, body, and foot (Figure 46).

4.2.1 Head

When an implant blade is inserted into the alveolar bone, most of the blade is embedded in the bone, leaving only the head exposed in the oral cavity. The head supports the prosthesis firmly after the implant site is healed.

The bottom end of the head should always be in close contact with the surface of the alveolar bone; the lower area, including the bottom end of the head, is specifically called the "safety stop" (Y in Figure 46).

Implants International blades have a cubic head. Cylindrical heads resemble natural teeth in shape and, therefore, might seem more suitable for supporting the prosthesis. In fact, however, the cubic head has proved much more practical and effective. There is a reason for this, of course.

The direction of the implanted head is naturally determined by the direction of the inserted blade. Frequently, the direction of the head is not parallel to that of the remaining teeth (Fig. 47). In designing prostheses, of course, it is desiderable that both directions be parallel. Therefore, before

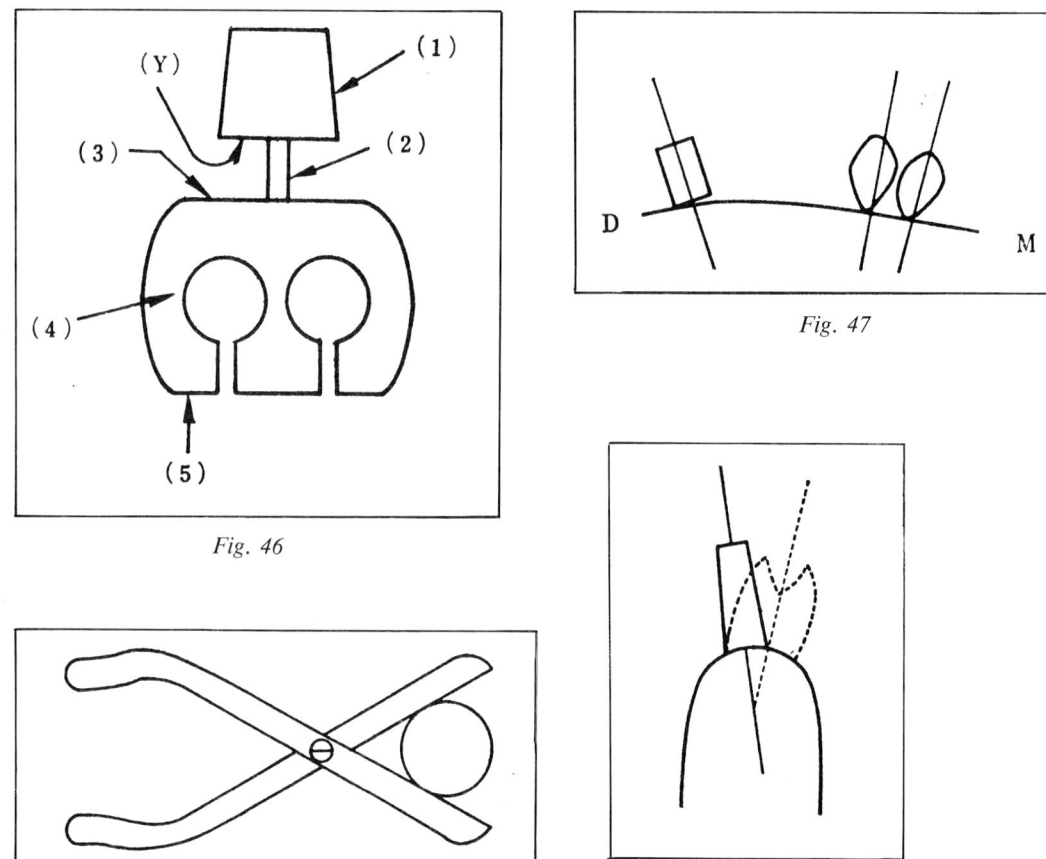

Fig. 46

Fig. 47

Fig. 48

Fig. 49

the operation, the head should usually be bent at the neck in a mesial to distal, or buccal to lingual, direction so that it lies parallel to the remaining teeth when the blade is inserted into the alveolar bone. For purposes of this bending procedure, a cylindrical-shaped blade head is rather inconvenient. It is too slipperly to be grasped or held with pliers. A cubic shaped blade head, in contrast, can easily be grasped firmly and lightly. It should be noted in this connection that the blades supplied by Howmedica and Implant Research still have cylindrical heads. Implants International blades are the most recommendable; not only have they been improved in size and shape, but, most importantly, they have cubic heads. Traditional Chercheve blades are less recommendable, because, as mentioned above, their heads are too small.

The standard head length of Implants International blades is 8 mm from the top surface to the bottom end, that is, to the safety stop. This length was apparently designed on the basis of the average physique of Europeans and Americans. For people of comparatively smaller physique, 8 mm usually proves a little too long. My clinical experience, with most Japanese patients, points to 6.5 mm as the appropriate head length.

The teeth in the jaw opposite the implant site descend over time, leaving a smaller space, of approximately 8 mm, between the surface of the alveolar bone and the top of the opposing tooth. Consequently, after the blade is implanted, the top of the head may touch the opposing tooth when the jaws are closed. The operator is thus required to adjust the head level by scraping it to provide enough space for the intended prosthesis. Scraping the head of an already inserted blade may be difficult for the operator and painful for the patient.

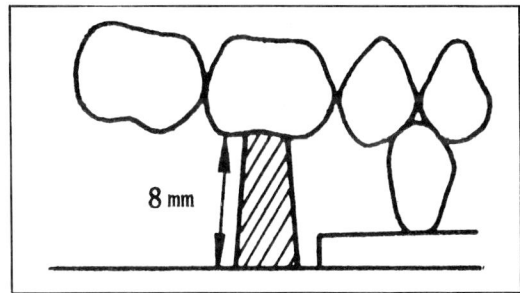

Fig. 50

A head that is too long can be adjusted to the proper size by cutting or scraping before the operation. Plastic copings attached to the head cannot be used, of course, when the head has been adjusted, yet the following procedures for prosthetics depend largely on the usefulness of the copings. Further, if combined with an adjusted head poorly finished, no valid prosthesis is possible. The only solution, therefore, is to carefully select the blade with the appropriate head length for the individual patient through precise diagnosis.

I know, for instance, of a failed operation an inexpert implantologist had done who, before the operation, shortened the head too much. After the blade had been inserted into the alveolar bone and the oral mucous membrane sutured, he found the head completely covered by the mucosa. His implant operation was all in vain.

Several years ago Dr. Linkow held a seminar in Nagoya, Japan. Linkow energetically demonstrated his marvellous technique of blade implantation on a long line of patients. A Japanese doctor, who had volunteered himself the previous day, took his turn. After inserting the blade, he scraped the head of the blade unsparingly, since he thought the top of the head might touch the opposing tooth upon occlusion. Tapping would have brought the blade deeper into the alveolar bone to just the desired position, he thought, with the safety stop touching the surface of the bone. Unfortunately, however, after the suturing the head disappeared from sight under the mucosa. There would have been no need to scrape the head, had the blade been inserted to the correct depth. This was, I thought, at the time a failure typical of an operator with insufficient knowledge of blade implantation. And I, therefore, wrote an illustrated manual, "Clinical Techniques of Oral Implant Operation", (text in Japanese) hoping to prevent failures of this kind.

4.2.2. Safety stop

The bottom end of the blade head is called the safety stop. There are certain *must* and *must nots* that are crucial to the functioning of the safety stop:

(1) When the blade is inserted, the safety stop *must* be in close contact with the surface of the alveolar bone. This contact means that the blade shoulder will be 2 mm from the surface of the alveolar bone. This is the most

important point. If the blade is not inserted deeply enough, so that there is a space between the safety stop and the surface of the alveolar bone, then the ossified tissue that forms around the upper area of the normal blade shoulder will be too thin and too weak to bear normal occlusal pressure.

A few years ago, I had the opportunity of inspecting several radiograms showing blade implants performed in Japan. To my great surprise and disappointment, most of the radiograms showed blades that were incompletely inserted, with certain amount of space between the safety stop and the alveolar bone surface. It appears that most of the operators had not understood the function of the safety stop of the head.

(2) The safety stop *must not* be tapped into the alveolar bone. Should the safety stop portion of the blade penetrate into the alveolar bone, then it is possible that occlusal pressure will force the blade deeper and deeper into the bone, which could have dangerous consequences. In mandibular molar implants, a blade that is inserted too deeply could reach the mandibular canal area, and eventually even touch and cut the canal. In such implants, then, several serious effects are possible:

(a) The blade could enter the mandibular canal, amputating the mandibular nerve (mandibular division of trigeminal nerve). This leads to paralysis of the whole mandible, on that side.

(b) Contact between the blade and the mandibular canal can cause persistent nerve paralysis of the mandible.

(c) The blade's approaching the mandibular canal leads to instantaneous nerve paralysis of the mandible upon occlusion.

To summarize shortly, keeping close contact with the surface of the alveolar bone, the safety stop will prevent the blade from entering the bone. If, however, the blade is inserted too deeply, embedding the safety stop portion, the outer pressures will bore the alveolar bone and the blade will enter further the bone. After the tissue around the blade has ossified to some extent, of course, the blade will be held firmly and no longer be pushed into the bone by occlusal pressure exerted on the blade head during the early period of ossification. However, occlusal pressure on the head is carried directly to the foot of blade and stimulates and irritates the osseous tissue around the blade, and even causes injury to these tissues.

The safety stop must not be inserted into the implant channel. If this occurs and the safety stop portion becomes embedded in the channel, then the blade head enlarges the channel mechanically by acting as a wedge.

An enlarged channel means an enlarged ossified area around the blade, a development that is not at all favorable. In the worst cases, a blade head inserted deep into the implant channel could, under repeated occlusal pressure, gradually penetrate the alveolar bone, causing injury and even fracture of the bone.

Thus the safety stop *must* always be placed correctly in close contact with the surface of the alveolar bone, since this portion of the blade head is designed to function literally as a "safety stop", stopping the intrusion of the blade head into the bone for safety purposes.

4.2.3 Neck

The neck connects the head of the blade with the body. Occlusal pressure exerted on the head is transmitted to the body through the neck. The neck must therefore have at least enough rigidity to withstand this occlusal pressure. Necks that can readily be bent should be avoided, since they might be bent and deformed externally by force, such as occlusion.

Adjusting the angle of the head to keep it parallel to the remaining teeth requires bending the head at the neck. Thus, in addition to being sufficiently rigid, the neck must be flexible and unbreakable enough to bend. From this standpoint, Implants International blades are excellent, meeting the requirements of both rigidity and flexibility; the necks of these blades withstand any external force including occlusal pressure. In my experience practically no breakage has occurred, even when the neck has been bent as much as 90 degrees in angle. Howmedica blades and Implant Research blades are made by casting. They are sufficiently rigid and are of uniform quality, having undergone individual inspection with an industrial radiological testing device. Their neck will sometimes break in two when trying to bend it with a pliers. Their metal appears too hard and consequently, insufficiently flexible for the preadjustment procedure of bending.

When an operator designs and makes his own implant blade, in casting the surgical metal he must be careful not to make the undesirable porosity overall, particularly in the neck portion of the blade.

The length of the neck is invariably 2 mm; it can be neither longer nor shorter. The reason why this is so will be discussed in relation to the function of the blade shoulder.

4.2.4 Shoulder

The upper portion of the blade body is called the shoulder.

Suppose an external pressure is exerted directly onto the head of blade, shortly after its insertion into the alveolar bone (Fig. 51). Point A is pushed downward and Point B is pushed upward, pivoting the central axis toward Point C'. Conversely, due to external pressure exerted in direction Y, Point A is pushed upward and Point B downward. This is the phenomenon that occurs when external forces are exerted on the blade head, in a mesial to distal direction.

After ossification of the tissue around the inserted blade has progressed so that the blade is firmly held in the bone, the osseous tissue formed through ossification in the upper area of the blade shoulder, from A to B, prevents A or B from being driven upward. The blade body as a whole is held by ordinary softer osseous tissues. The stability of the blade against outer forces from the direction of X or Y, depends mainly on the osseous tissue at the upper area of the shoulder, where ossification has occurred.

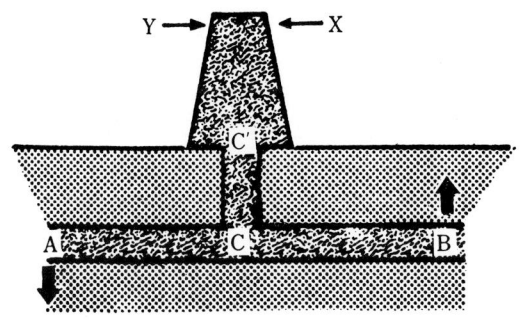

Fig. 51

If, where a blade was inserted into, the bone formed only ordinary soft osseous tissue, it could not bear strong occlusal pressures for a long period of time. This is why blades inserted into maxillary bone usually do not last as long.

In any event most of the occlusal pressures exerted on the blade are supported by the cortical bone around the shoulder.

In order for the shoulder of the blade to be embedded into the cortical bone effectively, the neck should be 2 mm in length. If the neck were shorter than 2 mm, the osseous tissue formed against the shoulder would not be sufficiently hard to support the blade against the forces from directions X and Y. If, however, the neck were longer, the shoulder would be embedded below the cortical bone tissue and, consequently, would be unable to bear occlusal pressure for a long time. Far from being arbitrary, the length of the blade neck is carefully determined both theoretically and clinically.

In the period following blade insertion, the blade shoulder may sometimes move up or down, particularly if the insertion procedures were incomplete. This situation is, of course, an undesirable one. It would have negative repercussions on the smooth healing of the implant site and the progress of ossification that is necessary for fixing the blade. For this reason the blade should always be inserted firmly in the alveolar bone by tapping. There is no alternative. This is a *must*.

Some Japanese implantologists have misunderstood the method for inserting the blade. According to them, the blade must be carefully placed in the channel formed in the alveolar bone, then nothing more is needed. They have evidently understood Linkow as claiming that no tapping is needed for blade insertion. In fact, the reverse is the case. I have witnessed lines of blade implants performed by Linkow himself in his New York office; he always, without exception, used a mallet to insert the blade by tapping. During an operation, he once told me "Try to move the blade just inserted here, Otobe, with your fingers", after he had finished tapping.

If the inserted blade could easily be moved with a finger or fingers, the implant could not be expected to be successful. Tapping is an indispensable procedure for implanting a blade. The fact that any kit of implant instruments includes a tapping mallet clearly demonstrates the necessity of tapping.

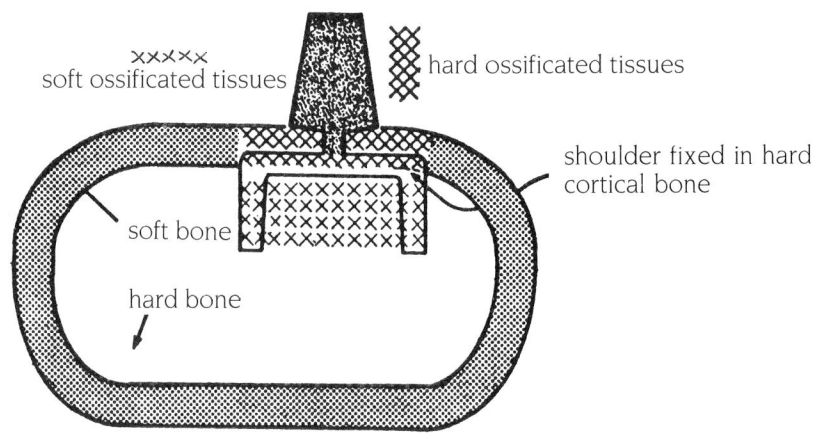

×ₓ×ₓ× soft ossificated tissues   ⊠ hard ossificated tissues

shoulder fixed in hard cortical bone

soft bone

hard bone

Fig. 52

Care must be taken when inserting blades to insure that Points A and B are embedded at the same distance from the surface of the alveolar bone. Neither point should be deeper than the other. Above all, the shoulder should never be bent in, up or down, but usually in a buccal or lingual direction depending upon the prepared implant channel.

The area above a blade shoulder that has been properly inserted will then be formed of hard osseous tissue that is, cortical bone tissue, and, therefore, can serve as a dependable buccal anchorage after the blade ossification has been completed.

On inspecting the radiograms accompanying the case reports of blade implants published in a Japanese dental journal (*Sgikai Tembo* Dentical Overview), I was disappointed to see that in most of these radiograms the blade shoulders were exposed above the surface of the alveolar bone. Such cases cannot be termed successful.

It should be noted in passing that the so-called anchor-type blade of Lew* had no shoulder but the bottom was shaped like an anchor (Fig. 50). As can easily be seen from the figure, no hard osseous tissue is involved in holding this type of blade. Because it is held only by the soft tissue of the *inner portion of the bone, the blade* cannot bear occlusal pressure for a long time.

Whether an inserted blade can remain in the alveolar bone over time depends mainly on whether it can stand the high pressures repeatedly exerted in occlusion. Since in this case the anchor-shaped portion of the inserted blade is not supported by hard cortical bone tissue, the anchor would be moved upward or downward every time any external pressure is exerted on the blade head. Patients would experience pain in the oral mucosa around the implant head for the same reason that a tooth loosened as a result of pyorrhea, would cause pain. In my opinion the anchor-type blade is a thing of the past. It is significant that among implant international lines of Lew blades, the anchor type is no longer included.

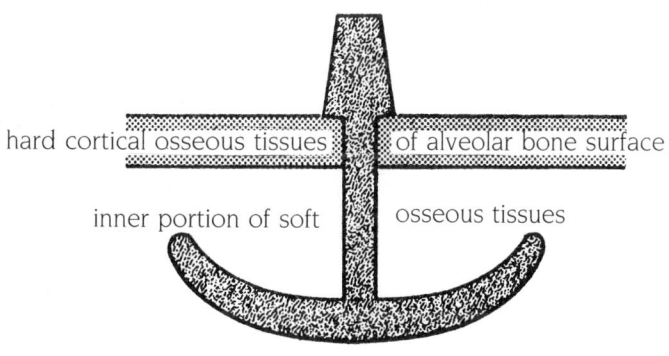

hard cortical osseous tissues of alveolar bone surface

inner portion of soft osseous tissues

Fig. 53

* Supplied by Howmedica. I feel that the original designer of this blade intended the anchor as an anti-dropping device in the early stages of ossification before the blade has become firmly fixed in the bone.

4.2.5 Body

The body of the blade is the portion that is inserted and fixed in the osseous tissue of the alveolar bone. Its size will naturally greatly influence the blade's capacity to withstand repeated occlusal pressure. It is true that by adjusting the surface of the prosthesis, occlusal pressure on the blade can be somewhat lightened. But the main factor determining the durability of the blade is the size of the blade body. The larger the blade, the greater the durability. The operator should therefore select as large a blade as possible given the amount of room of the patient's alveolar bone that had been determined through precise diagnosis with the aid of a pantoradiograph.

Carbon screws are not recommended for endosteal implant. They require a slot that is much greater in buccal-lingual diameter on the surface of the cortical tissue, instead of the inside tissue, of the alveolar bone for the blade channel. Healing and ossification will therefore take longer and the ossification might be incomplete. Consequently the durability of a carbon screw implant is less than that of a blade implant.

Windows bored into the blade body are very helpful enabling ossified tissue to envelope the blade buccal-lingually in the process of ossification. The implanted blade is to be sandwiched buccal-lingually in between bones with windows. The blade is wrapped up firmly, enabling the unification of blade and bone. Windows should be at least 2 mm in diameter. Smaller-size windows are not effective, since osseous tissue would not enter them in the ossification process. In addition windows should be round rather than square. Around the corners of square-shaped windows spaces or cavities are left in the ossified tissue when the ossification of other areas has been completed. Cavities within the alveolar bone are of course, not conducive to ossification.

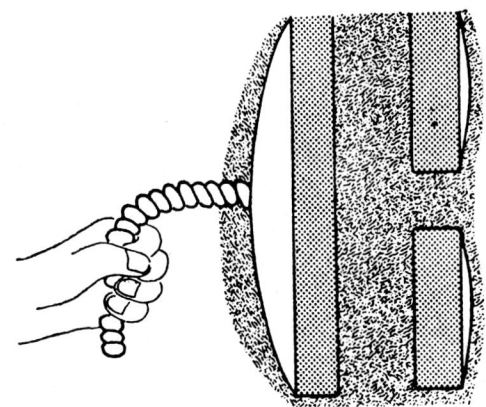

Fig. 54

4.2.6 Foot

The portion of the blade beginning 2 mm from the bottom is called the foot, which is appropriate, as it ends in acute angles.

The implant blade is inserted into the alveolar bone by malleting. If the foot of the blade had an obtuse angle or flat end, when malleted it would crush the osseous tissue. The tissue would then turn into decomposed bone, which would, of course, have unfavorable consequences.

Therefore, when the operator designs his own blade, the foot should always have an acute angle.

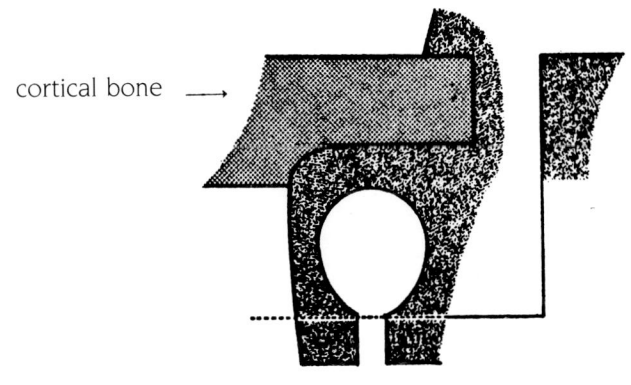

cortical bone $\longrightarrow$

Fig. 55

When the blade is inserted in the alveolar bone, it should always be tapped in so that all the 2 mm length of the foot lies within the bone. Simply placing the blade in the prepared channel is quite insufficient.

It usually takes 3-6 months for healing to be completed, that is, for the inserted blade to be supported and held firmly by ossified tissue formed in the implant site. Before that time, the blade can be loosened and moved by slight external forces, especially if it has been merely placed in the channel, instead of being tapped in.

To summarize the blade should always be tapped into the alveolar bone until the entire blade foot has entered the bone, that is, 2 mm deep. This is to implant the blade temporarily until the implant process is completed in 3-6 months.

4.3 DESIGNING OF THE BLADE

Tips for blades made by the operator.

4.3.1 Material
After mastering the basic knowledge and clinical techniques, the implantologist may want to design and cast an "original" blade for his personal use. There are, however, several basic rules to be considered. First of all, in selecting the cast metal, it is essential to use *surgical metal* and not *dental alloy*. Although both are commonly called cobalt-chrome alloy, they are quite different and have different uses. Dental cobalt-chrome alloy supplied for making the denture should never be used for casting implant blades. Only surgical alloy should be used.

4.3.2 Head
The head should, of course, be made larger than the neck; otherwise, the safety stop will not function properly. As discussed above, the safety stop is indispensable for any implant blade (Fig. 56). The head can be cylindric, ellipsoidal, or cubic. However, a cubic head is to be preferred, given the greater ease of adjustment for keeping the direction of the head parallel with that of the remaining teeth. Implants International blades have cubic heads; they can serve as a useful model.

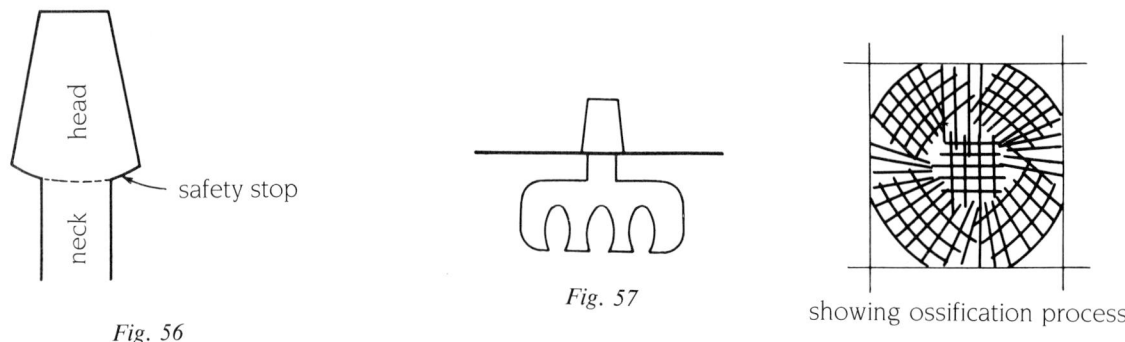

Fig. 56

Fig. 57

showing ossification process

Fig. 58

4.3.3 Neck

The neck must be 2 mm in length. In casting the alloy, care must be taken to avoid the presence of any porosity in the neck portion, which is the area where porosity is most likely. After the casting process, repeated tapping around the blade neck with a hard-metal should "tighten" the material.

4.3.4 Shoulder

The shoulder should be designed so that it will remain parallel to the surface of the alveolar bone after insertion. Should either the mesial or the distal portion of the blade be nearer than the other to the surface, the stability of the blade would be considerably lessened. The shoulder edges should be trimmed round, forming the so-called shoulder loop.

4.3.5 Body

The size of the body is determined by the space in the alveolar bone of the individual patient.

4.3.6 Windows

Round windows are recommended. Figure 58 shows the general process of formation of ossified tissue. Ossification begins in the central area of the window and then radiates in all directions. However the corner areas will remain unossified if square windows are used.

No portion of the blade body should form a right angle. Therefore, the corners of the shoulder should be trimmed as illustrated in figure 59.

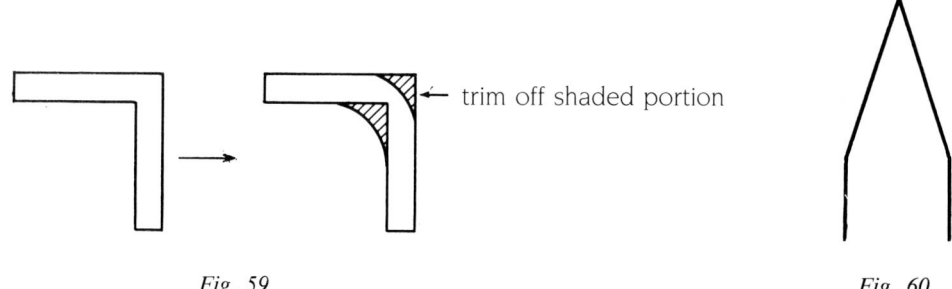

trim off shaded portion

Fig. 59

Fig. 60

4.3.7 Foot

The foot is the bottom end of the body and should have edges with acute angles so that it can easily be inserted into the bone by malleting (Fig. 60).

4.3.8 Finish

With the exception of the head the blade should not be burnished.

4.4 CONCLUSION

4.4.1 Evaluation

In my opinion the Linkow-type blades supplied by Implants International are the most highly recommendable blades in terms of both shape and quality. In clinical practice, they appear ideal. Howmedica blades and Implant Research blades are quite satisfactory; however they have a slight defect with respect to adjustability of head direction. Chercheve blades are not recommended because their head is too narrow and, above all, because have they no safety stop.

4.4.2 Summary

The main requirements of implant blades can be summarized as follows:

(1) The blade must have a safety stop.
(2) The blade must not be easily bendable.
(3) The blade must have a shoulder and this should be inserted 2 mm into the alveolar bone.
(4) Windows must be round and more than 2 mm in diameter.
(5) The neck must be 2 mm in length, neither longer nor shorter.
(6) The foot must have a wedge-like edge when a prefabricated blade. The edge should be sharpened then.

5. Diagnosis and Preliminaries

5.1. COMMUNICATION WITH PATIENT

Most patients have no idea what an implant is even if they have heard the term before. This is not surprising as there are too many dentists who are quite ignorant of this new art and science. But before performing any implant operation, it will be necessary to thoroughly explain to the patient what an implant is.

Communication has two aspects: understanding and being understood.

As occurs in medical or dental operations, prospective implant patients may experience anxiety and fear due to the uncertainty of this unknown experience. Besides, some patients hate injections and any operation that involves an injection. It is important to immediately emphasize to the patient that the implant procedure is simple and virtually painless.

Knowledge of oral hygiene is not sufficiently diffused. It is not unusual to have a patient insisting for example that the bone will be damaged by the inserted metal. Should the smallest shadow of a doubt remain in the patient's mind, the operation should not be undertaken. However try to get the patient understand the implant operation. Mutual understanding and the patient's full confidence are essential factors in successful implantology, which depends on the collaboration of the operator and the patient.

5.2. FINANCIAL NEGOTIATION

The implant operation changes and the prosthesis preparation expenses are usually not covered by the present National Health Service. Thus negotiation from the financial point of view between the patient and the operator is necessary before performing an implant operation. The patient must be given conditions he can accept and comply with. A patient should never be forced into undergoing an implant operation, even though he has the typical indications. Should the patient experience economic difficulties as a consequence of the operation he might complain he was coerced into it.

This would not only be unpleasant for the operator, but also could adversely affect his reputation.

In short, whereas an explanation of the procedure and financial negotiation are crucial, an aggressive sales pitch with suspicious patients should always be avoided.

5.3 OVERALL MEDICAL EXAMINATION

Like any dental treatment, the overall medical examination is essential. Naturally, the patients are elderly and have lost some or all of their teeth. Most fully edentulous patients are elderly.

Generally speaking, patients who have blood disease, tumors, chronic diabetes, renal diseases, or hyperplasia should be excluded. With such patients the implant operation could have unfavorable side effects. Patients who have stomatitis, that is, inflammation of the oral mucosa, should be examined carefully; in some cases this might indicate Bechet's syndrome.

Among diseases and changes in the jawbone, inflammation in the nasal fossae should be checked carefully. Patients who have these diseases should be excluded. Patients who have local facial paralysis caused by trigeminal disease should also be excluded.

The major factors in the general examination are blood pressure, blood precipitation, and coagulation time of blood, as well as urine analysis for sugar and protein. Although some of these examinations should be performed elsewhere, the operator should measure the blood pressure and analyze the urine for sugar.

5.4. PANTORADIOGRAPH

One of the indispensable devices for an implant operation is the pantoradioscope. Any of the makes available will function satisfactorily. It is important to note that the radiograms taken have different magnifying ratios. The operator should always be aware of this ratio; guesswork here is unacceptable. The operator should thoroughly know the specifications and characteristics of his machine, and how to teach the patient in order to take good radiograms: the best place to sit, the most suitable posture, etc. I simply do not believe in pantoradiograms taken by others. They can to some extent serve as a reference but that is all. The most important reason for this is that the magnifying ratio is unknown. At the very least pantoradiograms should indicate both the magnification ratio and model of the machine used. Taking a radiogram again with one's own pantoradioscope is never a waste of time.

One pantoradioscope can take the radiogram from inside the oral cavity. This system has a certain advantage in terms of the magnifying ratio, which is approximately 1.0. On the other hand, it has the disadvantage that it is difficult to interpret the overall relation of bones from the radiogram. This system is therefore not recommended for implantological use.

After natural teeth are lost the disuse atrophy of the alveolar bone would begin. Resorption goes on until the alveolar bone has completely disappeared. When observing the radiogram of fully edentulous patient carefully, projected mental tuber, as well as protrusive mandible, would be noticed. This results from the fact that the edge of the mandibular bone has an obtuse angle. In medical jurisprudence, by the way, the angle of the mandibular bone is used as a factor in estimating age.

The main reason for atrophy, and the disappearance of the alveolar bone, is one of human disuse reactions. After the teeth have been lost, the alveolar bone no longer has a function, as explained in Chapter 2.

Resorption begins with the decreased vitality of osteoblasts and then causes symptoms of osteoporosis, before further progressing. This however is a subject for the pathologist, not for the implantologist.

The osseous tissue forming maxillary bones and mandibular bones are different. The maxillary bone is sutured with other bones forming the base of the cranium; therefore, it can bear strong external pressure. The mandibular bone is stronger than the maxillary bone. It cannot be fractured by a temporary strong external pressure. The difference of osseous tissue is particularly evident in the Havers'canal, Volkman's canal, and cancellous crest.

In interpreting radiograms of the maxillary area, first confirm the image of the maxillary bone. Points of particular interest include the posterior wall of the maxillary bone in the molar teeth area, the exact location of the maxillary sinus and nasal fossa, and the location and thickness of the palate.

The thickness of the bone at the base of the maxillary sinus is of great importance when the implant blade is to be inserted in the molar area. The thickness of the bone of the nasal sinus base is also important. If a pin or blade that is too long is inserted, its edge might penetrate the nasal fossa; the operation then would fail as the result of incomplete radiographic diagnosis.

In general, the maxillary bones are less dense than the mandibular bones; one should use the radiogram to judge the density of the bone.

Check points in mandibular bones are the mandibular nerve and the mental foramen. Locating the mental foramen makes it possible to estimate the location of the mandibular canal. It also prevents the mistake of inserting the blade into the mental foramen area. Were a blade to be carelessly inserted into the mandibular canal, disorder such as mandibular paralysis would occur after the operation. The operator should therefore know the exact location of the mandibular canal, as well as the thickness of the bone between the alveolar bone surface and the mandibular canal, before performing the operation.

In a fully edentulous patient, the mental foramen becomes progressively closer to the body of the mandibular bone. Thus the mandibular canal shifts to the upper area of the mandibular bone near the surface of the alveolar bone. In the area around the mandibular ramus, the mandibular canal may be exposed since the surface bone has partly disappeared. Particular care must be taken in interpreting radiograms in such cases.

Interpreting pantoradiograms requires skill and the experience. These are the result of the study of many radiograms. A pantoradiogram should always be taken immediately after an implantology operation to check the location of the endosteal implant or the condition of the inserted subperiosteal substructure. This is, of course, to insure that the operation has been done correctly and to prevent possible adverse side effects.

It is very dangerous to perform an implant operation without having a pantoradioscope. At the same time, it is important not to trust the radiogram 100 per cent. For technical reasons, the images are always 1.20-1.50 times larger than the actual size, with considerable deformation. Both the magnification and the deformation must always be compensated for in radiographic diagnosis.

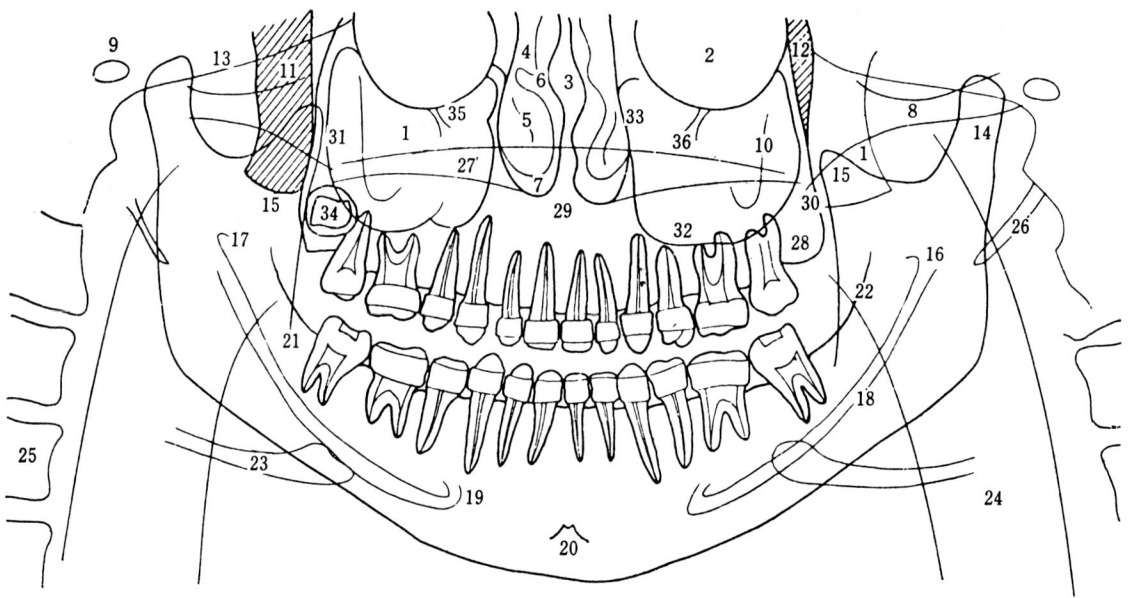

1. *maxillary sinus*
2. *orbit (orbita)*
3. *nasal septum*
4. *middle nasal concha (ethoidal bone)*
5. *inferior nasal concha*
6. *middle nasal meatus*
7. *inferior nasal meatus*
8. *zygomatic arch*
9. *external auditory foramen*
10. *tomographic view of zygomatic process*
11. *pterygoid process (sphenoid bone)*
12. *pterygopalatine fossa*
13. *basis cranii*
14. *articular process*
15. *muscular process*
16. *mandibular foramen*
17. *mandibular tongue*
18. *mandibular canal*

19. *mental foramen*
20. *mental spine*
21. *external oblique ridge*
22. *internal oblique ridge*
23. *hyoid bone*
24. *air-way (respiratory tract)*
25. *cervical vertebrae (IV)*
26. *styloid process*
27. *osseous palate*
28. *maxillary tuberosity*
29. *anterior nasal spine*
30. *posterior wall of maxillary*
31. *bone posterior wall maxillary sinus*
32. *interior border of maxillary sinus*
33. *medial wall of maxillary sinus*
34. *upper third molar tooth*
35. *infraorbital canal*
36. *infraorbital foramen*

Fig. 61

5.5 STUDY MODEL

It is now a common practice in the field of clinical dentistry to make a study model for any case. An implant operation is no exception.

What kind of blade and which blade should be inserted must be decided carefully, based on the characteristics of the corresponding tooth. How much occlusal space would be left to the corresponding tooth determines the height of the blade head.

Immediately after the insertion of the implant blade, a temporary prosthesis or bridge is attached. This temporary prosthesis or bridge can be made from the study model. Thus it can be easily prepared for immediate attachment.

5.6 RADIOGRAPHIC RECORDS

A radiographic record should be made and kept for each implant operation. Such a record is not only needed for future reference to the particular patient, but also provides the implantologist with useful study material.

In addition, use radiographic records as visual aids in explaining implants to new patients.

The relevant technical data should be attached to each radiogram. Engraving the operator's name ensures correct presentation of the radiogram.

5.7 TREATMENT OF REMAINING TEETH

In addition to the pantoradiogram, an ordinary dental radiogram should be taken to precisely determine the condition of the remaining teeth. Any caries found should of course be properly treated and cured. The pantoradiogram does not accurately indicate the size of the remaining teeth because of magnification.

If the remaining teeth are to be used together with the implant to support the prosthesis, they must be carefully inspected and, if necessary, treated.

The pantoradiogram taken after the operation shows not only the implant site but also the other teeth in the oral cavity; thus it does record the condition of the remaining teeth.

5.8 TABOO WORDS AND PHRASES

As already made clear, an implant operation should be performed only after the patient has understood what is involved and has agreed on his intention to the operation. Whenever even the smallest doubt remains, the operation should not be performed. Trouble can result if there is a significant discrepancy between the patient's prior concept of an implant and what he himself undergoes. A patient might subconsiously think that had he only been able to endure not having teeth or been contented with his loosened denture, he could have avoided a painful implant operation.

The operator must therefore explain what an implant is and why it will help the patient, making full use of visual aids such as slides. Under no circumstances, however, should the patient be shown pictures of the bleeding that occurs during the operation, particularly if these are in vivid color. Such pictures only serve to create fear. In general, fear and anxiety with regard to the operation, injection and incision are far greater for the patient than the operator imagines. Furthermore, the patient may worry about postoperative pain.

Actually, with anesthesia no pain is felt during the operation, as patients generally know. However, as the anesthetic wears away, the patient feels pain similar to that following the extraction of a tooth. Such pain is not at all serious and is easily relieved by taking an anodyne. Before the operation, the patient might be given an hypnotic suggestion such as the anesthetic will produce a good effect. "Take it easy. The implant will not cause you any pain". All that is possible should be done to remove the patient's fear of pain.

After the operation, the attachment of the temporary dentures will also lessen the pain.

The implant operation involves stripping of the oral mucosa. This process causes edema after the operation. Tell the patient, *not before, but after the operation*, that some swelling is to be expected and there is nothing to worry about.

With an implant in the mandibular molar area, swelling occurs around the root of the tongue causing some pain and difficulty in swallowing; a little bit of swelling is also found in the lymphatic glands. Tell the patient, again *not before, but after* the operation, that a little bit of swelling will begin in about six hours and will last for a week. "It's a natural consequence of the operation and is not serious".

5.9 DESIGNING PROSTHESIS

After the implant blade has been inserted, the prosthesis is attached to the blade head, in the shape of a bridge denture.

First, make a plaster of Paris study model. Inspect the last part carefully to decide whether a single-head blade or double-head blade is to be used. The bridge prosthesis is also designed at this stage. The remaining teeth are, of course, treated in advance, if any of them has the slightest defect. The remaining teeth should be used for attaching the prosthesis wherever and whenever possible. The prosthesis should not be supported by the implant blade alone. This is a general rule; attach the prosthesis to the combination of the implant blade and the remaining teeth.

The following is an example of an unsuccessful design. For lost tooth 76, a double-head blade is inserted in the alveolar bone at 76. Crown 76 is attached to the blade head.

With this design the inserted blade will come loose a week or so after the operation. Finally the blade will have to be removed.

Here is the correct design for this case: the blade is inserted at 76, and the abutment made using tooth 54 or 5. In other words the bridge denture is to be supported by the combined abutment of the implant and tooth 54 or 5.

The implant blade alone is usually insufficient for supporting denture.

Do not make vain efforts in implant operation followed by misdesigned prosthesis.

For the case covering wide area of the jaw bone, abutment is to be made combining all implant blades together with metallic material. The prosthesis should be made as a whole, in the shape of a full bridge denture, and not divided into two or three bridge dentures.

For a completely edentulous jaw, a full bridge denture should always be used. Some operators are still trying to use the blade head in the same way as the inner crown of a double crown. This is quite wrong. The blade would soon come loose.

The following is another example of failure. A blade is inserted at 3:3, attached to crown 3:3, making use of a crasp. Occlusal pressure exerted by the denture cannot be supported by the blade here.

5.10 TEMPORARY DENTURES

5.10.0 General
Temporary dentures, usually in the form of temporary bridge denture, are attached immediately after insertion of the implant blade. This procedure is now quite well established among implantologists. The form and shape of this temporary denture will depend on the ability and preferences of the operator. In any event the temporary denture should be easily made by the operator himself. It is held in place by temporary cement. There are several advantages to the temporary denture as described in the following subsections.

5.10.1 Recovering occlusion
Temporary dentures allow patients to recover occlusion to some extent immediately after the operation. This advantage is greatly appreciated by patients who now experience little inconvenience in ingesting food.

5.10.2 Covering operation site
The operation site of the implant is covered by the temporary denture; hence the incised wound is kept safe from external stimuli, such as the tongue or food. This means less pain for the patient. In addition, the pain that comes from an implant operation is usually much less than that caused by extraction of a tooth.

5.10.3 Preventing looseness of the blade
Initially the implant blade is held in only mechanically. When extraordinarly strong occlusal pressure is exerted on the blade, the blade will move. The use of temporary dentures, however, reduces this pressure. There is little possibility that the blade will loosen if it is held firmly in the ossified tissue.

5.10.4 Increased stability of the blade
Attaching temporary dentures increases the mechanical stability, while ossification is occurring in the blade channel formed in the alveolar bone.

5.10.5 Accelerating ossification
Occlusion is partly recovered by attaching the temporary denture. Through the temporary denture, occlusal pressure is exerted on the blade,

transmitting stimuli to the alveolar bone from within. These positive stimuli accelerate ossification in the implant operation site.

5.11. IMPORTANCE OF TEMPORARY DENTURES

5.11.1 Consequences of not inserting temporary dentures

Assume that an implant blade was inserted but the temporary denture was not attached. There must have been a reason for this situation: the operator was exhausted; the patient was exhausted; the temporary dentures did not fit properly; etc. In any event, if temporary dentures are not inserted, the implant blade is exposed in the oral cavity. Consequently, the blade may frequently be struck, which would cause it to loosen.

As already discussed, the inserted blade must be stable until the ossificated tissue can support it firmly. This usually requires at least a month, during which temporary dentures should be used with the remaining natural teeth. In any case, temporary dentures *must* be inserted whenever an implant blade is inserted; if not, the blade will loosen and the result may be a failure.

The insertion of a temporary denture is particularly crucial for implants in the maxillary bone because of the nature of the bone.

5.11.2 Incomplete insertion of temporary dentures

If incompletely inserted, temporary dentures may soon fall out. This can result in the sudden exertion of extraordinary pressure on the blade. The direction of the implanted blade will not always be parallel to that of the remaining teeth or of the other blades. If the temporary denture falls out, the pressure exerted on the newly inserted blade is quite unexpected in direction as well as in force. Even a blade that has been properly inserted in the alveolar bone by malleting might loosen, due to the pressure of this exceptional force. That is, under pressure, the blade could partly fracture the alveolar bone or enlarge the channel and eventually come loose. In the maxillary alveolar bone, the buccal side is particularly easy to fracture, due to its anatomical structure.

The operator must be extremely careful in fabricating temporary dentures and bridges. After the permanent denture or bridge is prepared, care must also be taken in removing the temporary denture or bridge. Removal must never be rough.

In short, the newly inserted blade is in a critical condition for at least one month. Thus the blade and the temporary denture attached to it must be handled carefully.

5.11.3 Occlusal imbalance of temporary denture

Occlusal harmony between the temporary denture and the remaining teeth is of great importance. This is true regardless of whether the denture is temporary or permanent. Extraordinary large occlusal pressures are usually due to occlusal imbalance. An implant blade cannot have a better holding capacity than the natural teeth. A newly inserted blade or a blade undergoing ossification cannot have a better holding capacity than a fully ossified blade. Holding capacity is particularly limited with respect to buccolingual pressure. This fact is unavoidable as it results from the shape of the implant blade.

When various blades are inserted simultaneously the temporary denture must be designed so as to disperse occlusal pressure evenly to each blade.

5.12 SELECTION OF BLADE

Which blade is to be used for the case? The operator must carefully select the blade most appropriate for the individual patient. The first step is usually to overlap the pantoradiogram on the blade guide, keeping in mind the magnifying ratio of the radiogram. The mesiodistal dimension is best measured on the study model.

The edge of the blade should never penetrate the maxillary sinus or the nasal fossa when inserted.

With blades to be inserted in the mandibular bone, there should be at least 2 mm between the end of the blade foot and the mandibular canal.

Blades can be modified prior to insertion; a modified blade must be finished perfectly and washed thoroughly.

Given the quality of blades marketed today, most failed implant operations are traceable to the operator's errors in diagnosing or in operating.

Figures 62 through 73 illustrate different cases and the different types of blades selected.

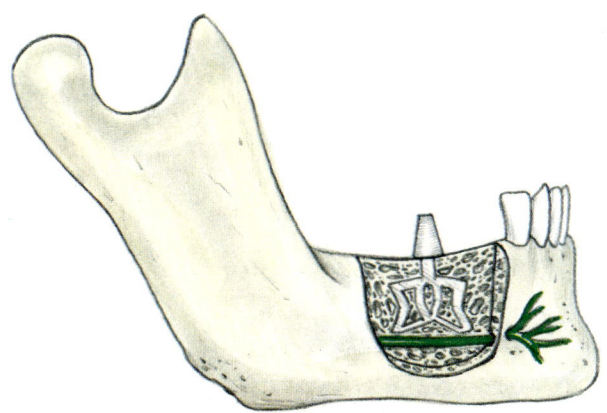

Fig. 62

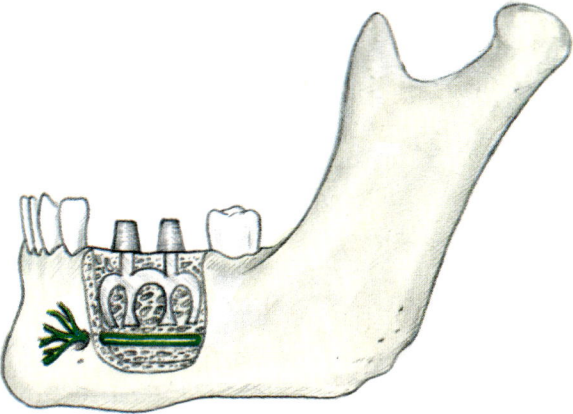

Fig. 63

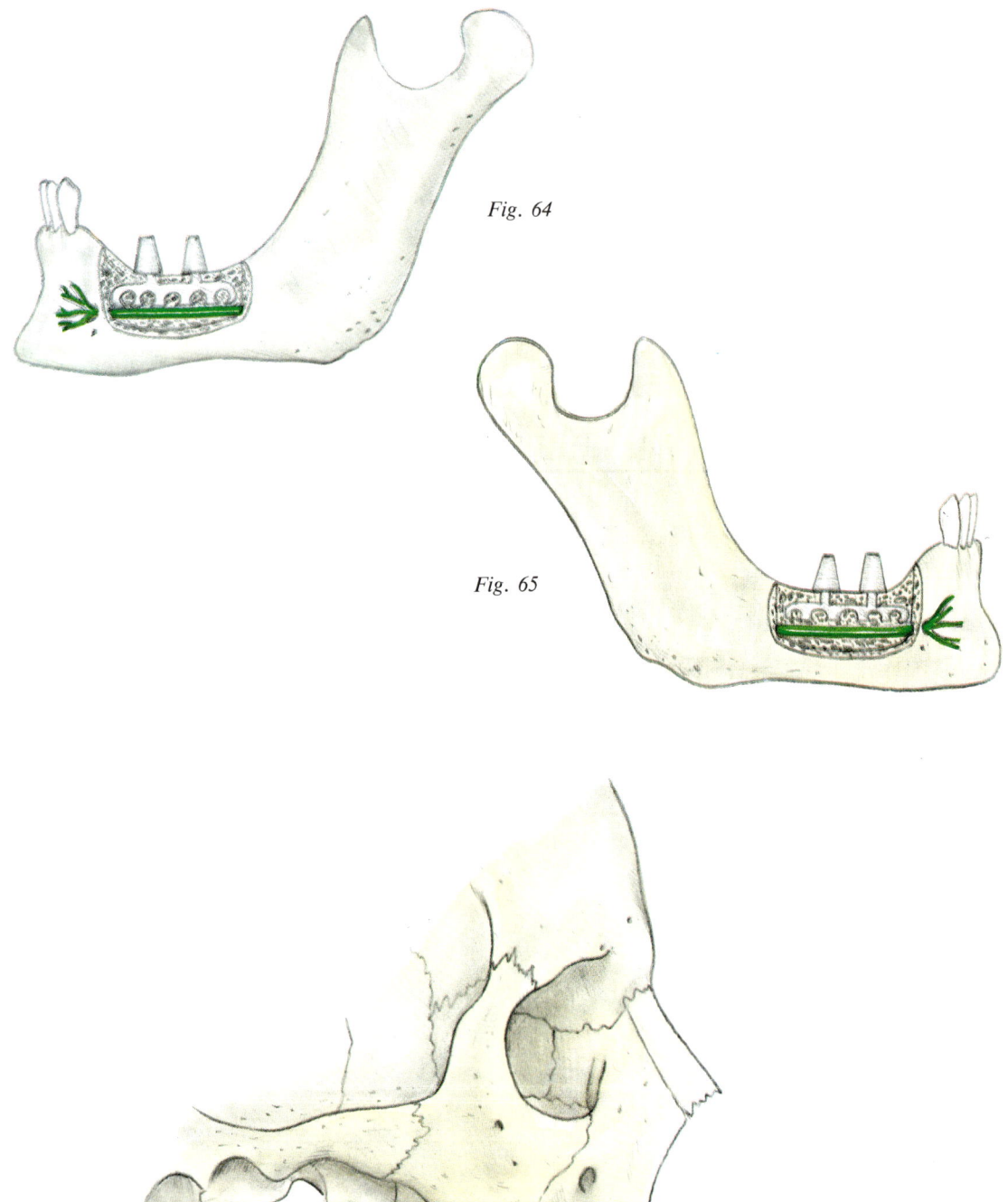

Fig. 64

Fig. 65

Fig. 66

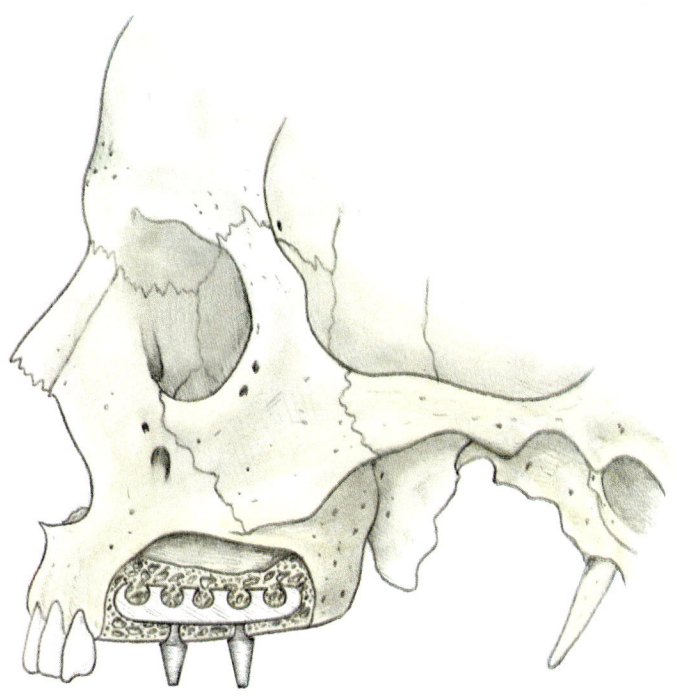

Fig. 67

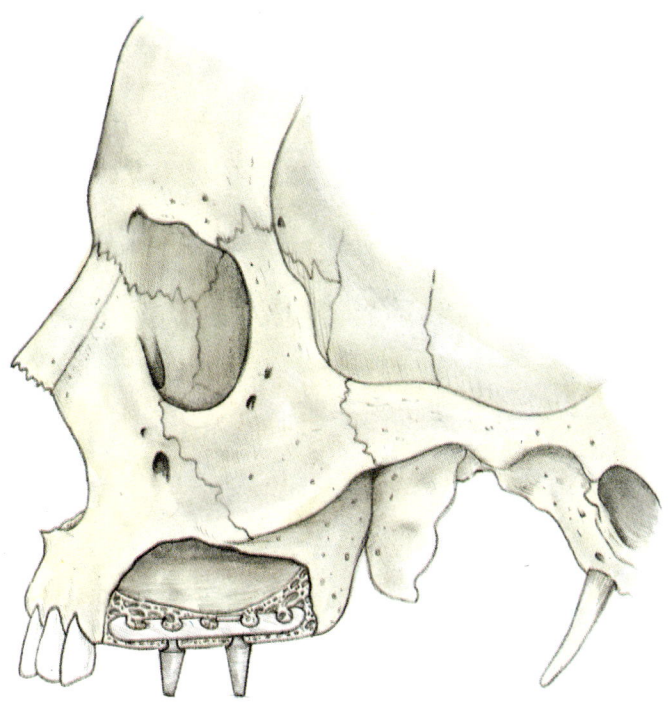

Fig. 68

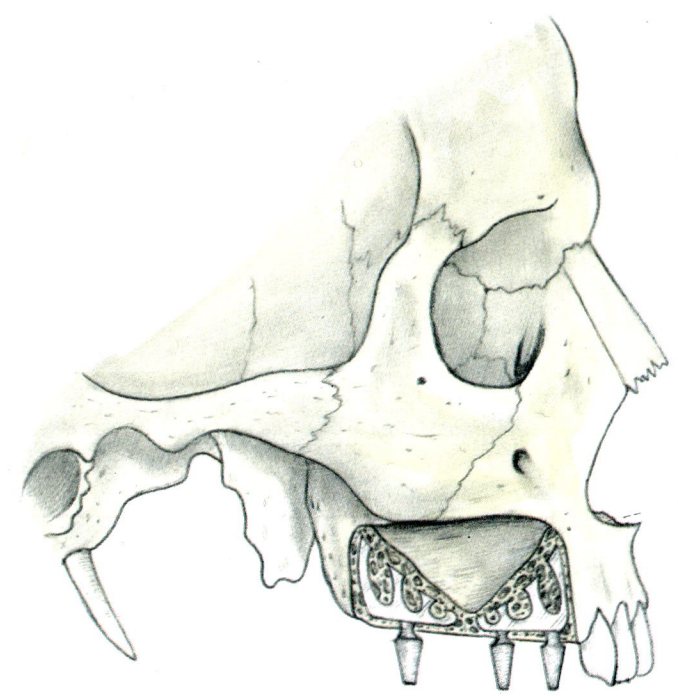

Fig. 69

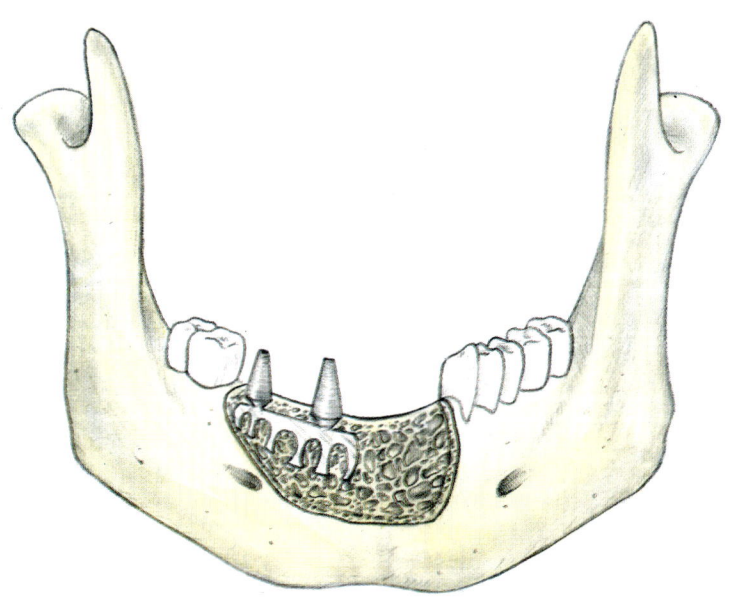

Fig. 70

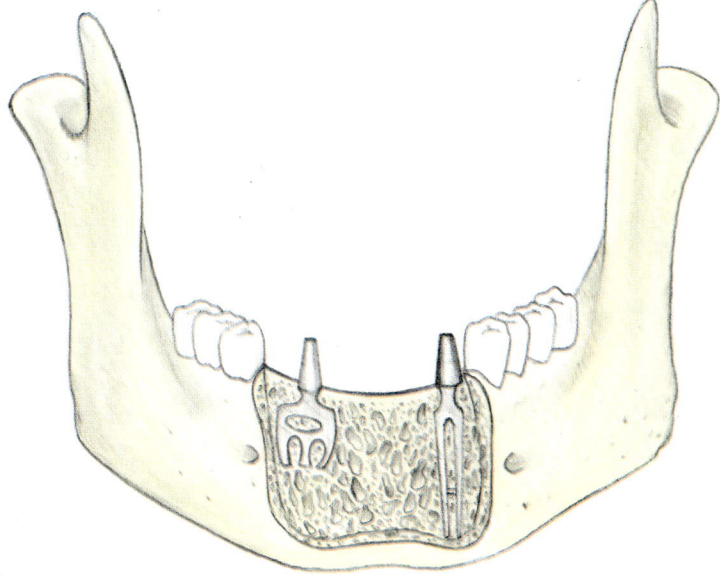

Fig. 71

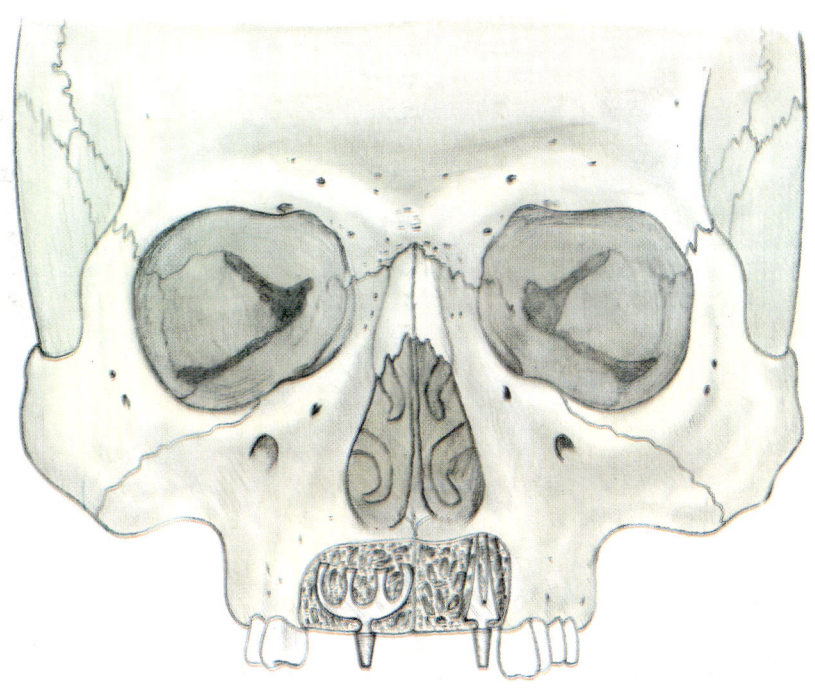

Fig. 72

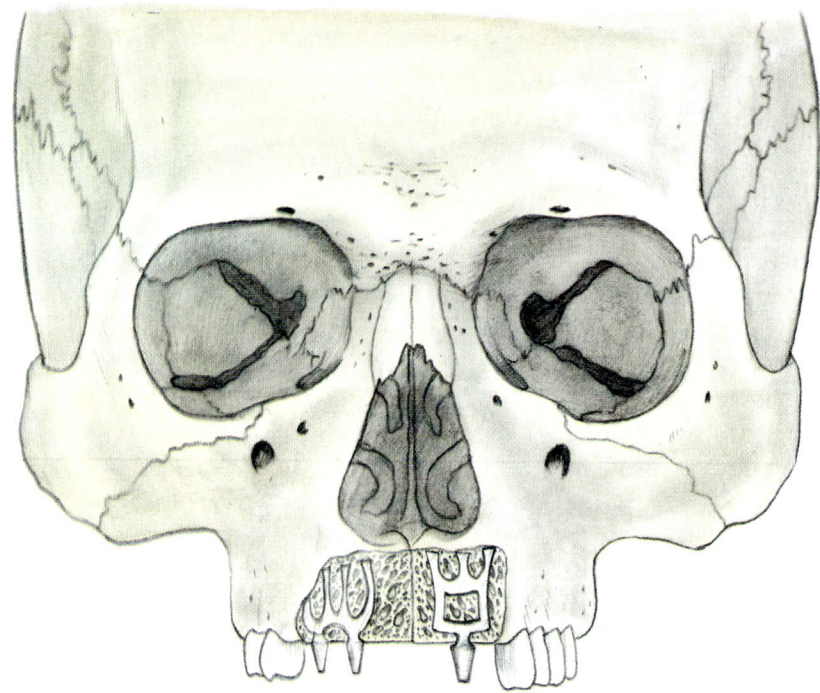

Fig. 73

6. Operative Procedure

6.1 STERILIZATION AND ANESTHESIA

An implant operation is a kind of oral surgery. The operative field should be sterilized according to the ordinary methods of sterilization.

The operation involves stripping a comparatively wide region of mucosa and forming a channel for the implant blade in the alveolar bone. Hence an anesthetic is always required. The amount used is more than twice that used in ordinary tooth extraction. Usually topical swelling will occur as a side effect of the increased anesthetic. But this should not be considered problematic as swelling is also a natural effect of stripping the mucosa.

Infiltration anesthesia should always be used; avoid block anesthesia.

If block anesthesia is applied to the mandibular foramen, the mandibular canal is also anesthetized. Consequently, even if the blade accidentally intruded into the mandibular canal during the operation, the patient would experience no pain. The accident would go unnoticed unless caught by the operator himself. Infiltration anesthesia, in contrast, does not anesthetize the mandibular canal; the patient can inform the operator of his pain, should the blade accidentally injure the canal.

Many dental offices have piping for nitrous oxide gas, that is, the so-called laughing gas. For the patient who is sensitive, this gas anesthesia might be helpful when applied together with infiltration anesthesia.

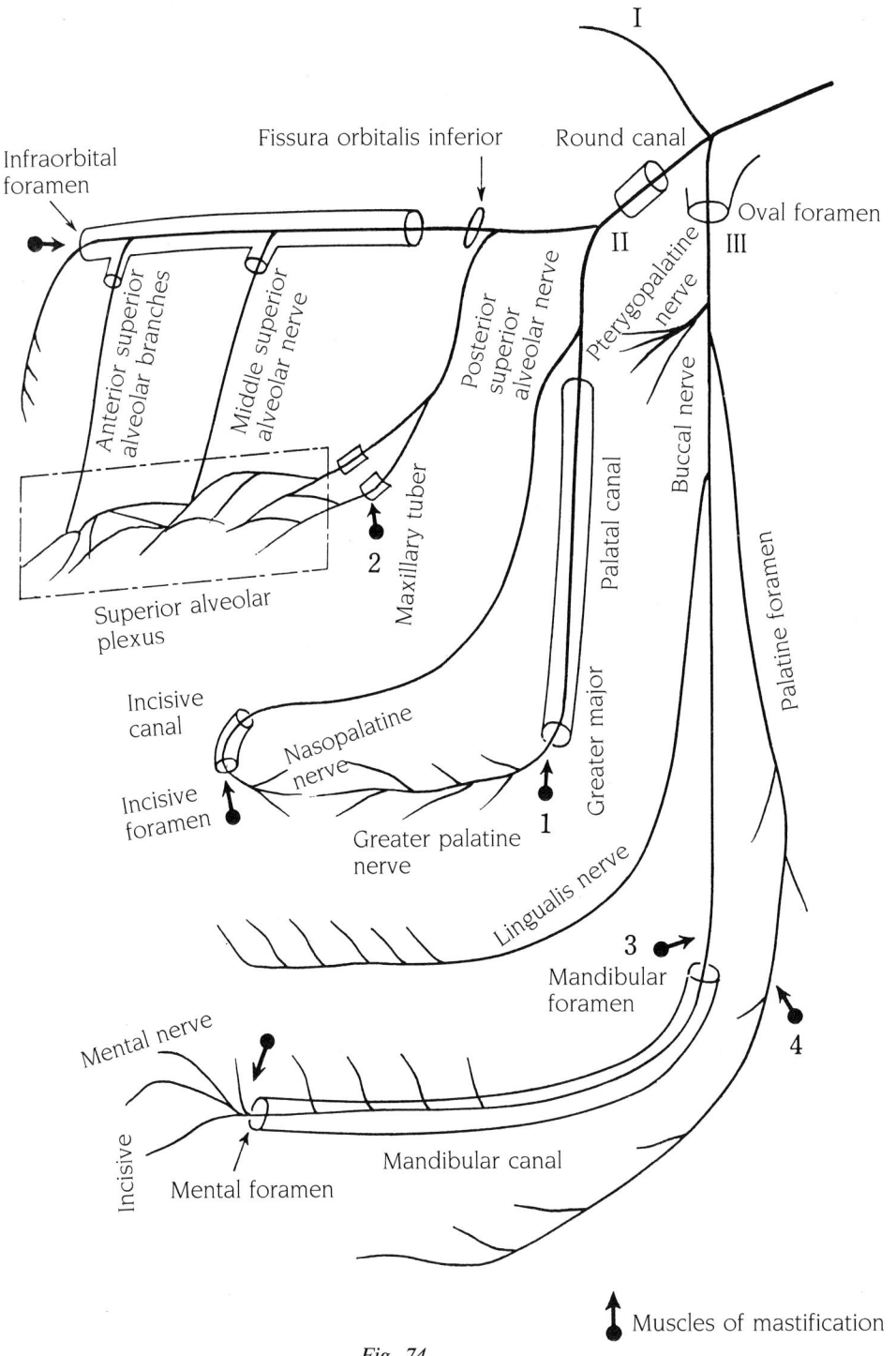

I

Infraorbital
foramen

Fissura orbitalis inferior

Round canal

Oval foramen

II

III

Anterior superior
alveolar branches

Middle superior
alveolar nerve

Posterior
superior
alveolar nerve

Pterygopalatine
nerve

Buccal nerve

Palatine foramen

Maxillary tuber

2

Superior alveolar
plexus

Palatal canal

Incisive
canal

Nasopalatine
nerve

Greater major

Incisive
foramen

Greater palatine
nerve

1

Lingualis nerve

3

Mandibular
foramen

4

Mental nerve

Incisive

Mandibular canal

Mental foramen

Muscles of mastification

Fig. 74

Fig. 75

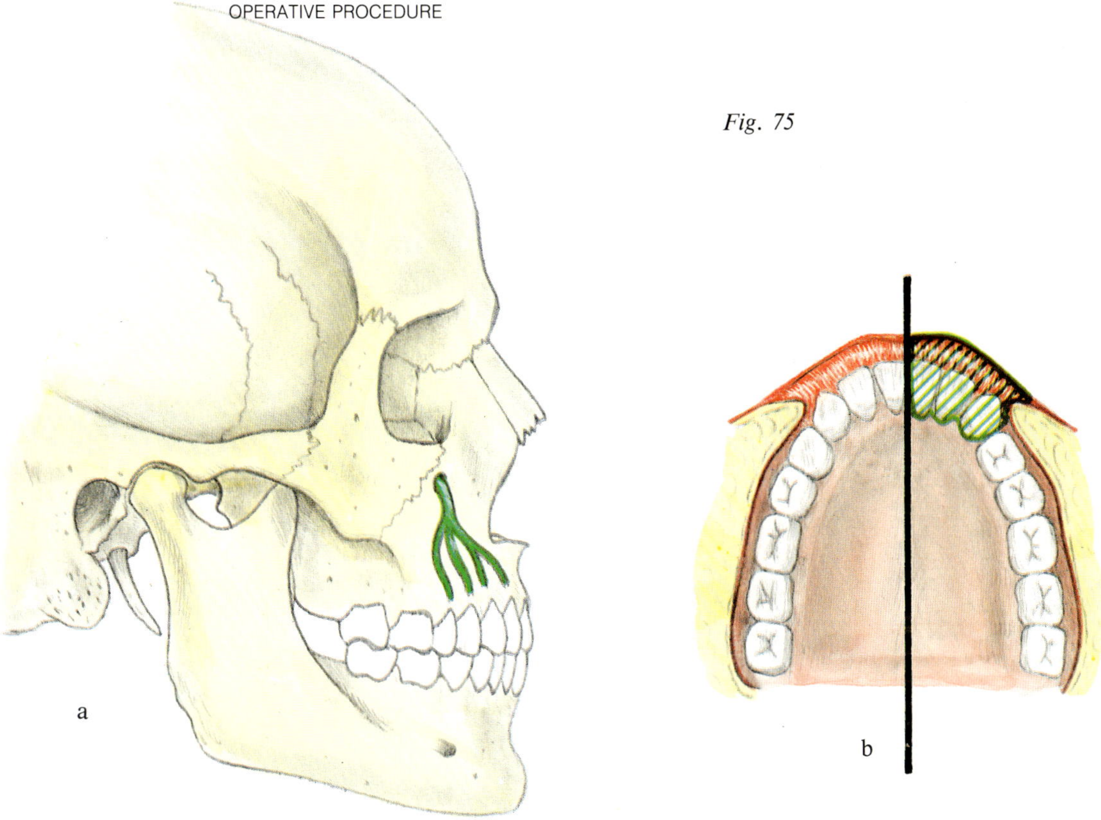

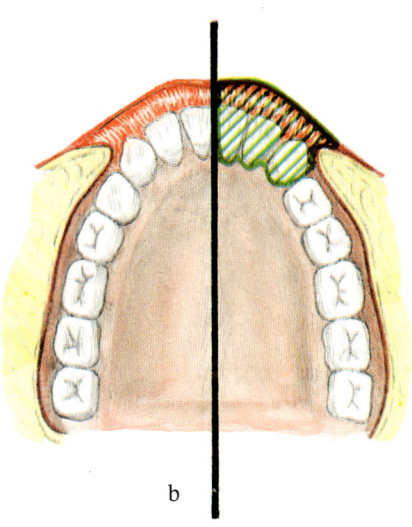

a

b

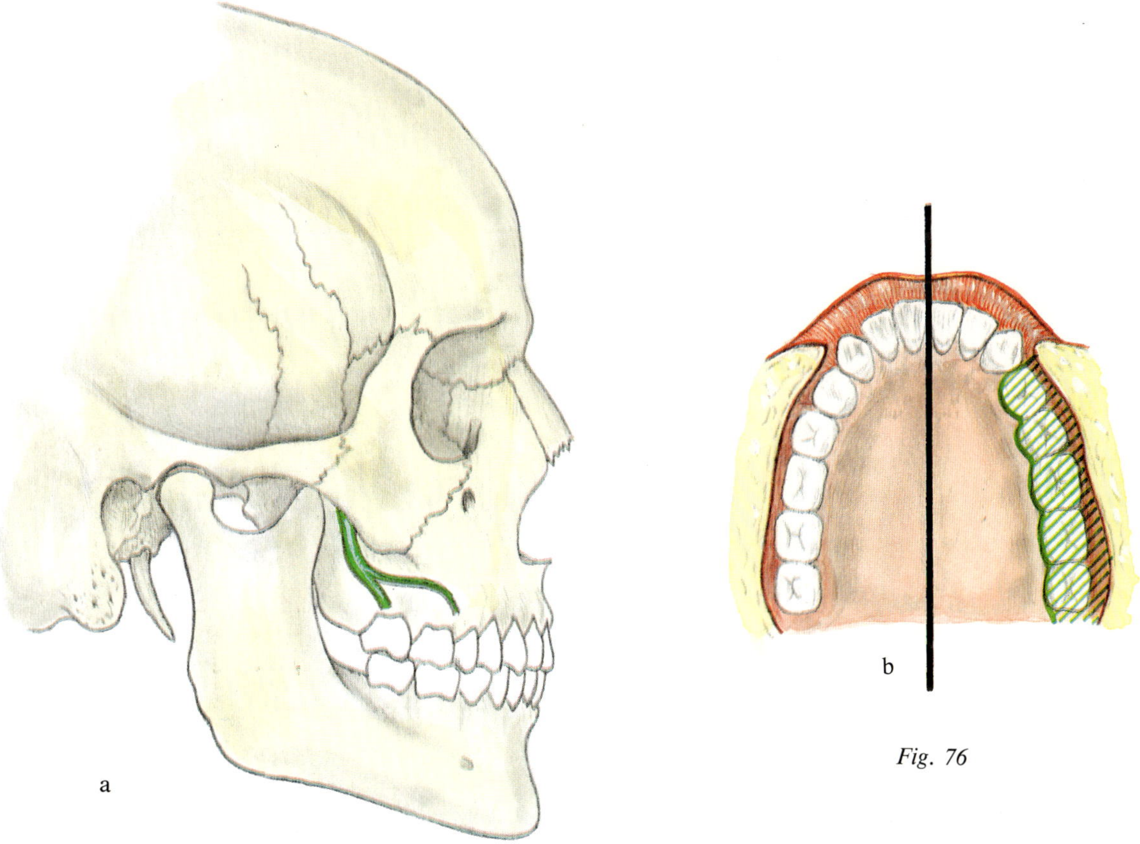

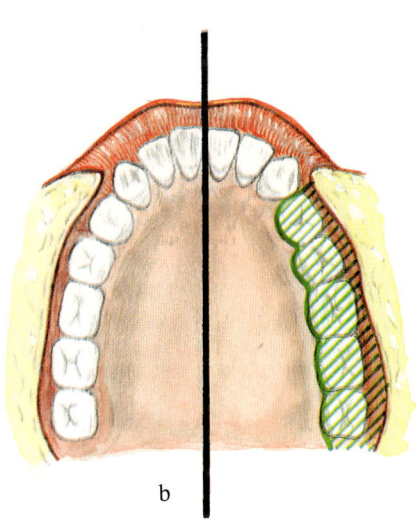

a

b

Fig. 76

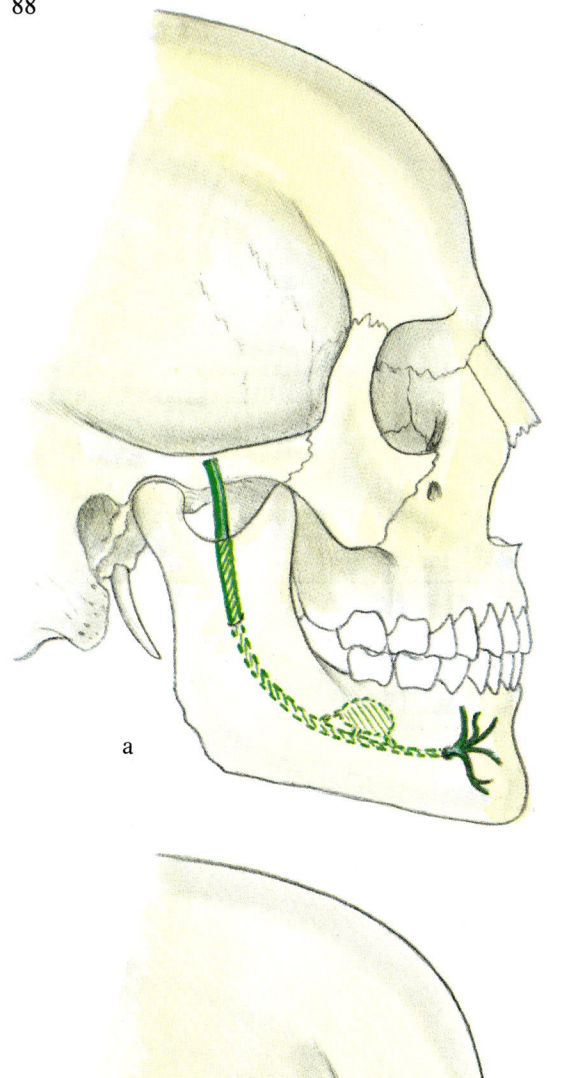

a

Fig. 77

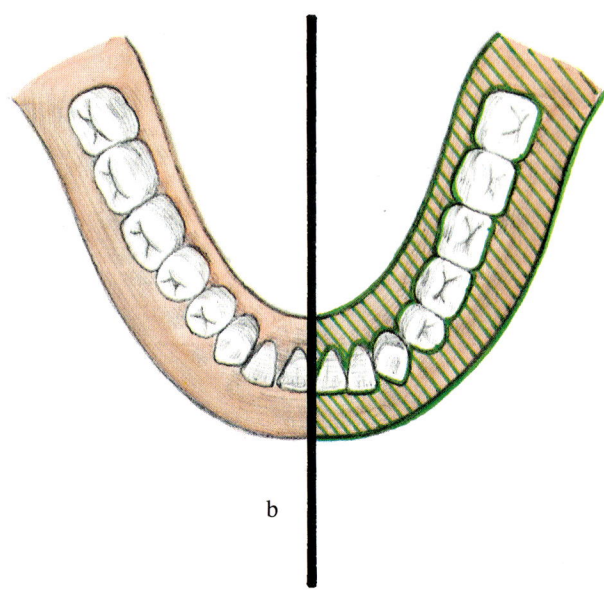

b

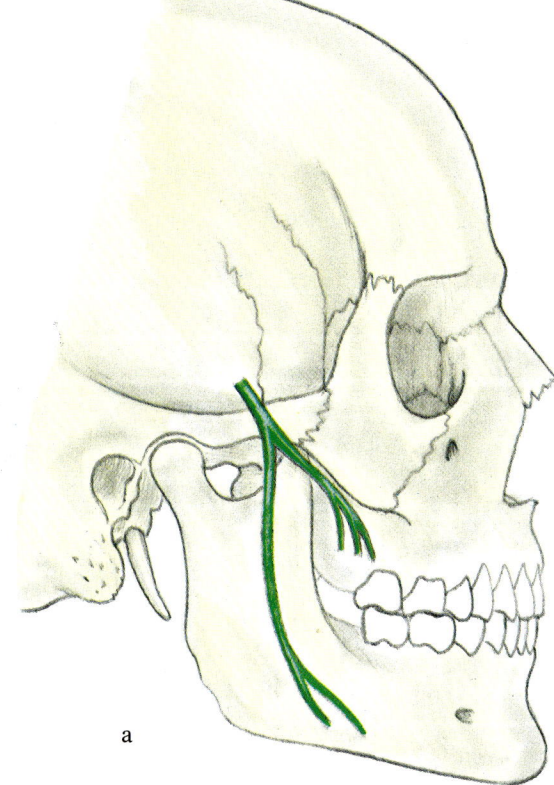

a

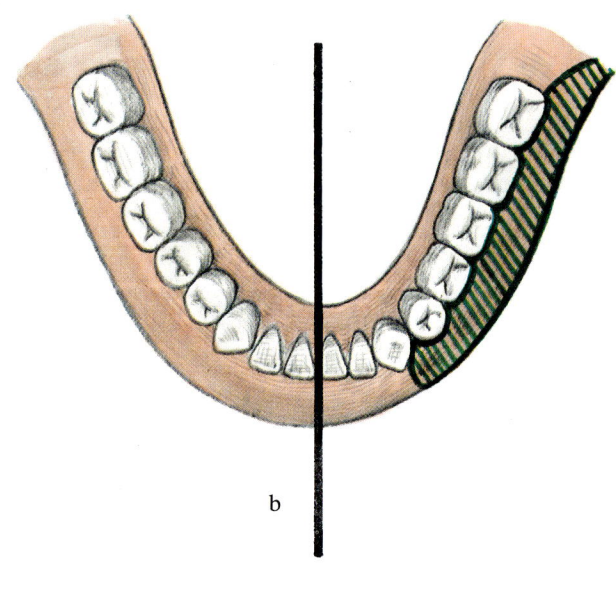

b

Fig. 78

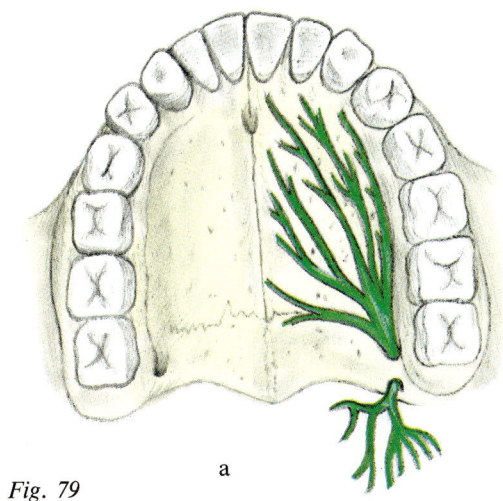
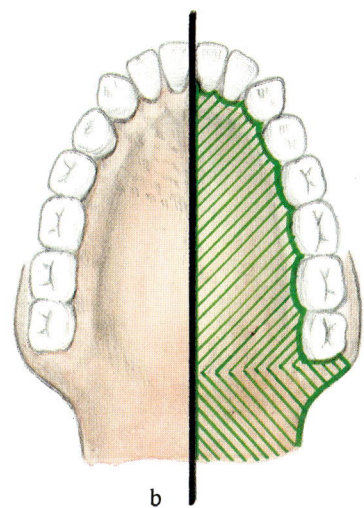

Fig. 79   a   b

6.2 INCISION

Make an incision line in the gingiva directly over the center of the alveolar crest where the blade is to be inserted.

For the mandibular gingiva, the incision line is preferably made a little to the lingual side, particularly in the molar region. An incision line made in the buccal side could cause trouble after suturing or later, in designing the superstructure.

Incise the gingiva down to the bone with a sharp scalpel to where the pointed end of the scalpel reaches the periosteum of the alveolar bone. Incision should always be in a distal to mesial direction.

Incomplete incision makes it difficult to strip the mucosa and sometimes will require redoing. Repeated incisions might cause secondary wounds resulting in unsatisfactory healing. Thus it is important to incise deep enough to reach the periosteum throughout the incision line.

Fig. 80

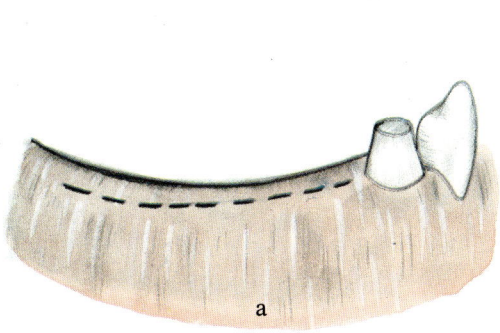
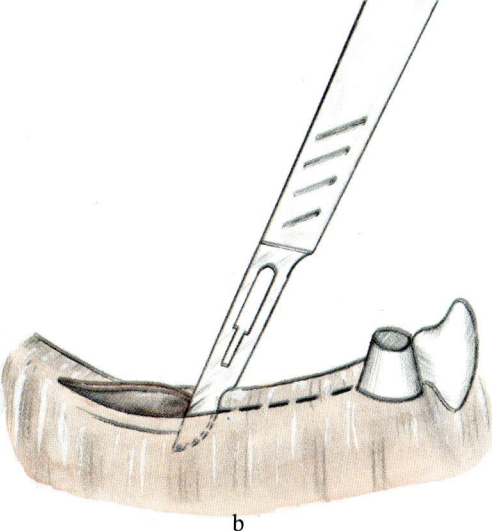

a   b

6.3 STRIPPING ORAL MUCOSA

Strip oral mucosa by inserting an elevator in the incision line. The convex side of the elevator must face the mucosal membrane, the concave side the alveolar bone surface. The elevator, if inserted in reverse, may perforate or injure the membrane.

In general, strip the mucosa widely in the intended region for blade insertion, exposing the alveolar bone.

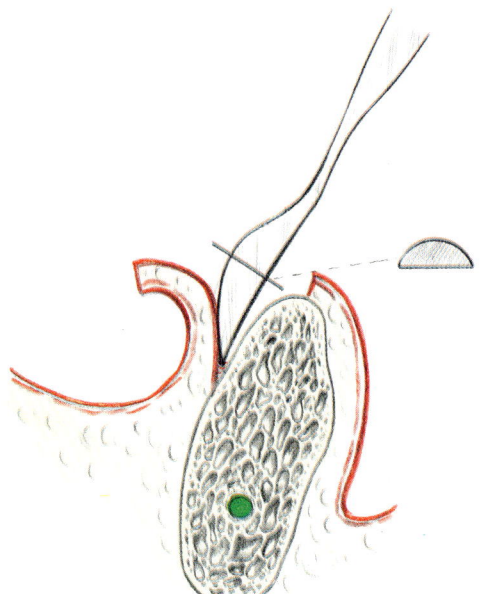

Fig. 81

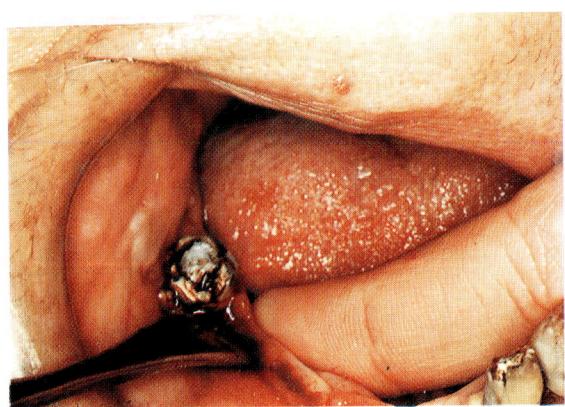

Fig. 82

6.3.1 Maxillary anterior region

In this region, strip the mucosa of the buccogingival border in the mucosal plane. Strip the mucosa to the bottom end of the anterior septum nasi in the facial cutis plane.

For implant blade insertion in this region, a channel is prepared parallel to the buccal side of the alveolar bone. The oral mucosa of buccal side should therefore be stripped wide enough. Otherwise, the buccal side of the alveolar bone cannot serve as an effective guide line for the channel. Besides, during malleting the alveolar bone must be firmly pressed from the buccal side by the assistant operator.

When stripping mucosa horizontally from left to right in the mesial region, in addition to the horizontal incision line, a cross incision is required, in view of the flexibility of the mucosal membrane. This cross incision can be made on either side of the frenulum labii superioris. Cross incision elsewhere is to be avoided. The mucosa on the palatine side of the anterior teeth region should also be stripped wide enough to the nasal palatal nerve and the incisive foramen.

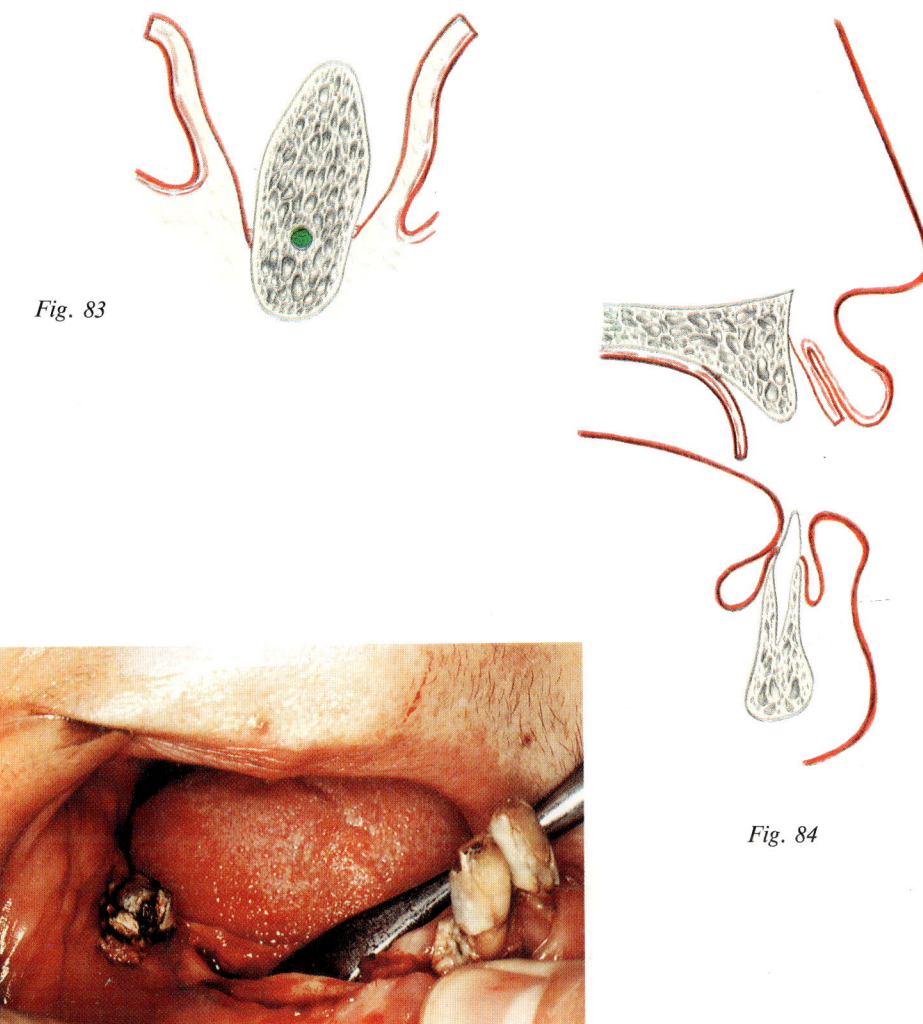

Fig. 83

Fig. 84

Fig. 85

6.3.2 Maxillary molar region

In cases without molar teeth 6 7 8 or fully edentulous maxillary, incision and mucosa stripping are performed from the posterior alveolar crest, 1 mm to the maxillary posterior wall from the junction of maxillary bone with the pterygoid process of the sphenoid bone.

The alveolar bone in this region of the maxillary posterior molars 6 7 8 is comparatively thick. The implant blade is easily inserted.

Strip the buccal side of the mucosa to the buccogingival angle or to the junction of the maxillary bone and the molar arch. On the palatine side, strip approximately 190 mm of the palatine mucosa. Care must be taken to avoid cutting the palatine nerves.

Expose the alveolar bone of the maxillary molar area completely, especially the posterior wall of the maxillary bone. The inserted blade could partly come out in this area.

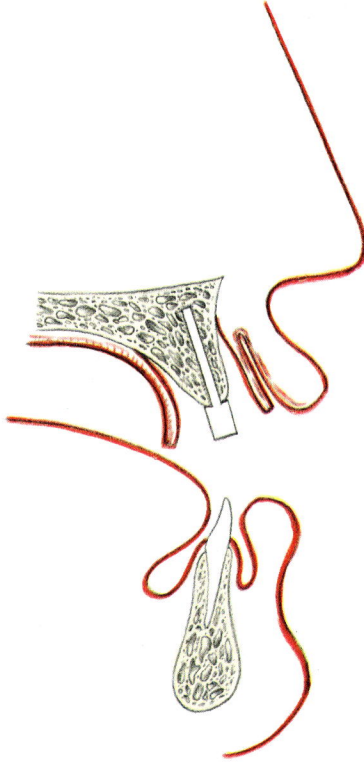

Fig. 86

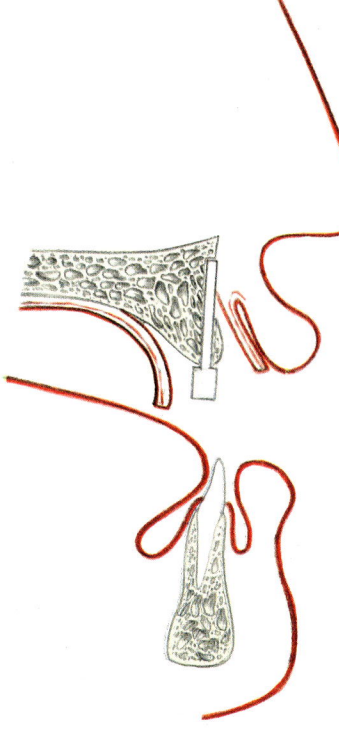

Fig. 87

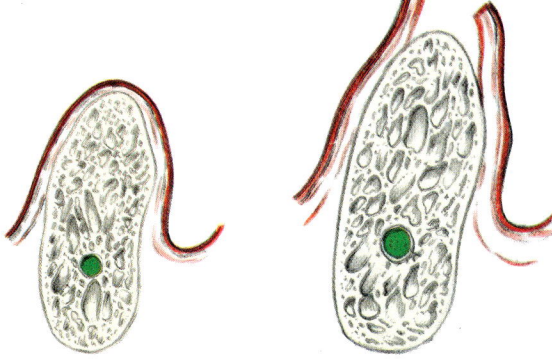

Fig. 88

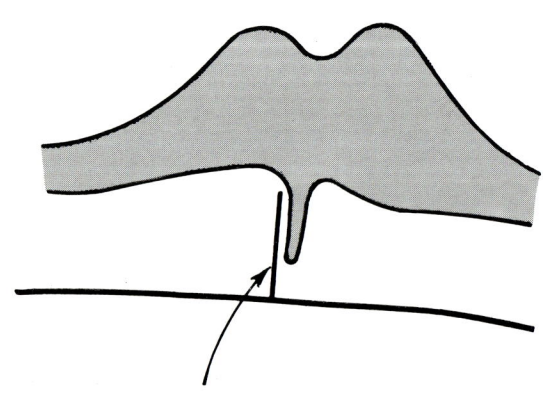

Fig. 89

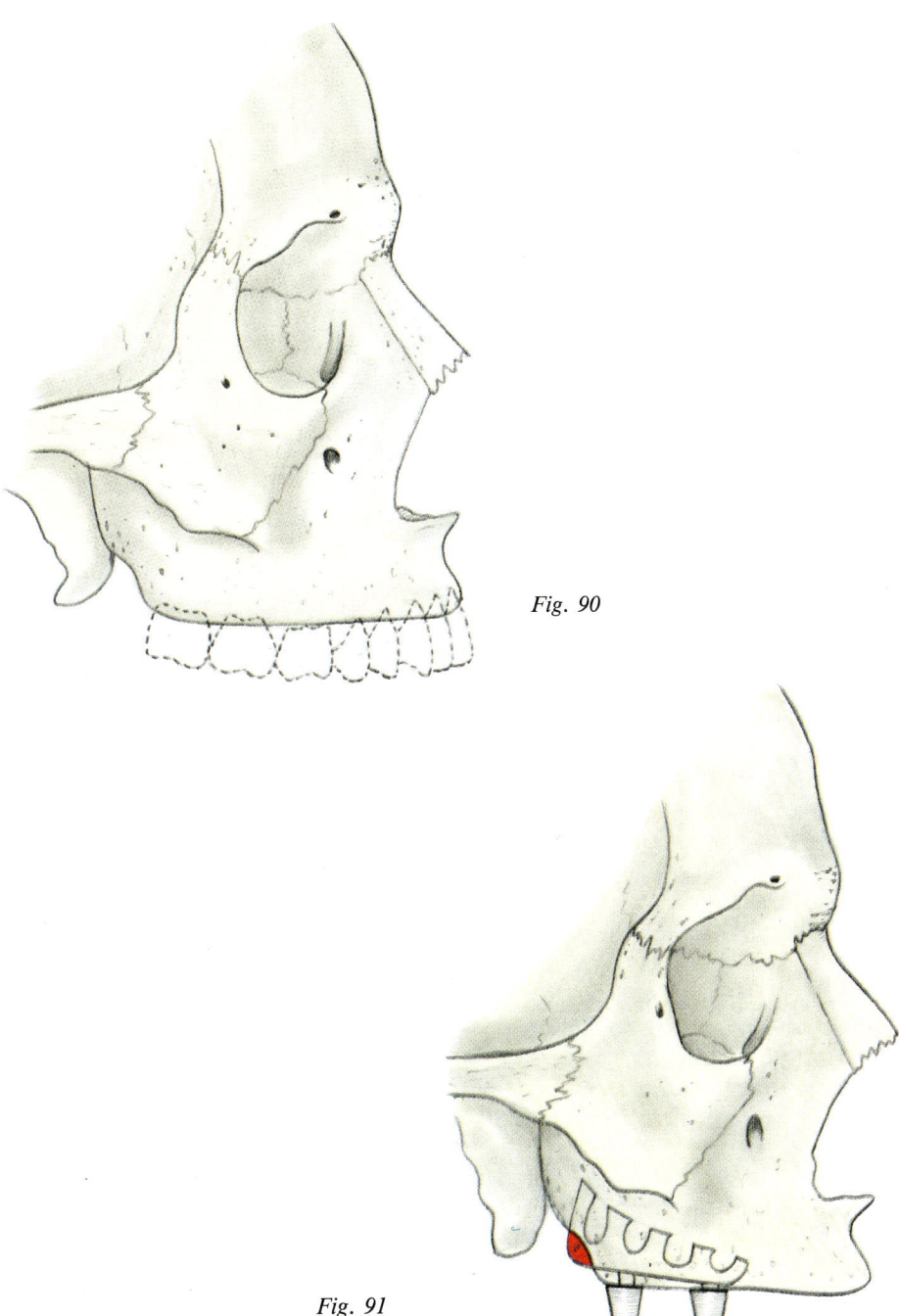

Fig. 90

Fig. 91

6.3.3 Maxillary bones

The fully stripped palatine mucosa should be sutured so that it does not move.

Patient who are of advanced age or have worn dentures for a long time will often have much more resorbed alveolar bone than had been visually estimated before stripping the mucosa. This is particularly true of the anterior 8 8 where the alveolar bone sometimes has the shape of a knife edge (Fig. 92).

An endosteal blade implant therefore becomes impossible; the operator must now use a subperiosteal implant. It will be necessary to take an impression of all or part of the maxillary bone region. To meet variable situations like this, one wide stripping of the mucosa is recommended.

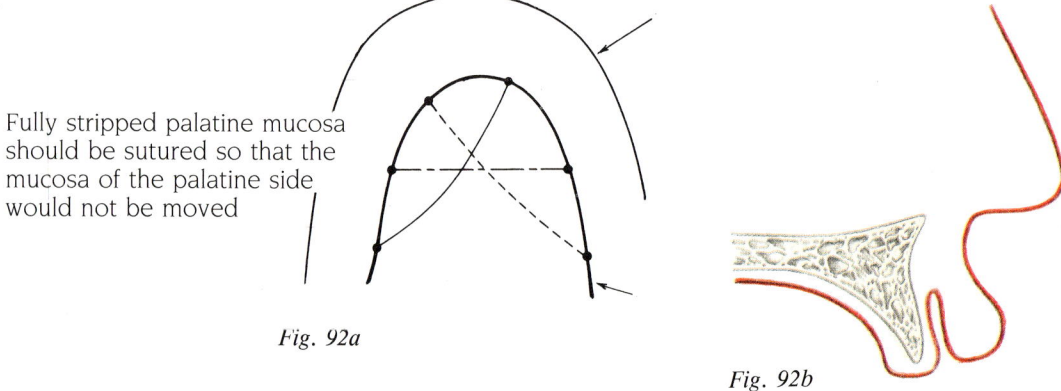

Fully stripped palatine mucosa should be sutured so that the mucosa of the palatine side would not be moved

Fig. 92a

Fig. 92b

6.3.4 Mandibular bone

Because of the shape of the mandibular bone, the oral mucosa of the lingual side should be retracted as far as the oral base. The body of the mandible is usually sloped to the buccal side in the basal region and the center of the mandible comes to the buccal side in the oral cavity.

The soft tissues of the lingual side of the oral mucosa must be completely separated from the bone. The protuberance of linea mylohyoidea appears first, followed by the protuberance of sulcus mylohyoideus; then the mandible slopes down to the buccal side.

The implant channel in the mandibular molar region generally parallels the lingual side; the mandibular surface must be clearly exposed, by complete separation of the mucosa. Correct channel preparation is thus achieved by ensuring that the exposed mandible is visualized.

When inserting blade in the mandible tilting sharply to the buccal side, the mucosa must be stripped as far as to the base of the cavity on the lingual side. Otherwise, accidental penetration of the blade into this region cannot be noticed during the operation. Unfortunately, this might occur sometimes, due to two factors: (1) excessive narrowness of the stripped mucosa, and (2) insertion in the wrong direction as a result of emphasizing occlusal balance with the corresponding tooth.

6.3.5 Mandibular mental foramen region

In stripping the mucosa from the periosteal tissue in the mandibular mental foramen, care must be taken not to injure or cut the mandibular nervous tissues emerging from the mental foramen.

Soft tissues must be slowly retracted and separated from the bone surface, exposing carefully the area around the mental foramen. Nervous tissues are comparatively flexible and will not be cut if retracted gently with a periosteal elevator. Thus, if rough stripping is avoided, injury of nervous tissues will be unlikely.

The purpose of exposing the mental foramen is to estimate the location of the mandibular canal which runs at the same level as the mental

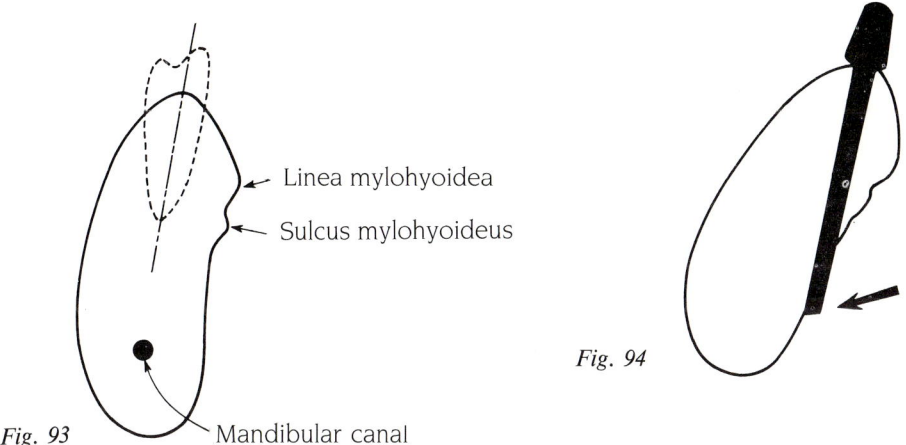

Fig. 93

Linea mylohyoidea

Sulcus mylohyoideus

Mandibular canal

Fig. 94

foramen. No blade or frame should ever be inserted in the mental foramen region of the mandibular alveolar bone.

6.3.6 Mandibular mesial region

In stripping the lingual side, be careful not to injure the frenulum linguae, as a functional disorder of the tongue could result. Soft tissue must be stripped horizontally as far as the linea mylohyoidea in the molar region, and vertically to the superior region of the spinae mentalis. A cross incision at the frenulum labi inferioris facilitates clear exposure of the bone for the same reason as has been explained in the section on the maxillary bone. A cross incision is recommended when the stripping area is wide and covers the entire mandibular region and for superiosteal implant operations in particular. In contrast it will not be needed for partial stripping in endosteal blade implants.

Usually, for endosteal blade implants in the anterior mandibular region, mucosa stripping is limited to exposing the alveolar crest. Mucosa separation for subperiosteal implants will be discussed in Chapter 8.

As shown in Figure 95, resorption of alveolar bone progresses buccolingually at first. The main purpose of mucosa stripping in endosteal blade

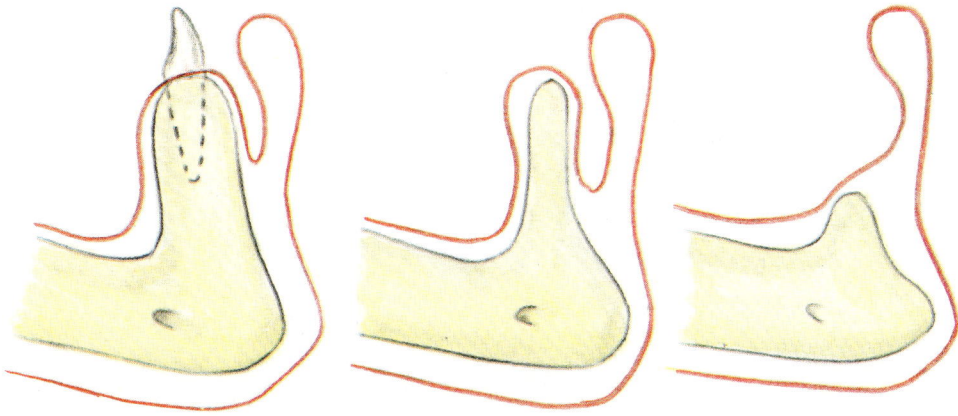

Fig. 95

insertion is to confirm the buccolingual thickness of the alveolar bone and to inspect the direction for the inserted blade. When the oral mucosa is stripped in the entire mandibular region, the stripped mucosa should be fixed temporarily by suturing, using the method explained in the maxillary case.

6.4 SURFACE TREATMENT OF ALVEOLAR BONE

When the surface of the alveolar bone is exposed, it will not always be found to be flat. In fact, it will often be rough like pumice. This is because in the process of resorption of the alveolar bone after dentition the bone surface is usually resorbed unevenly.

This unevenness is, of course, undesirable for purposes of blade insertion. The surface should therefore be flattened and smoothed. A bone bur should not be used as it could dig a ditch in the bone, particularly if the operator is insufficiently experienced. Rasping the surface smooth with a

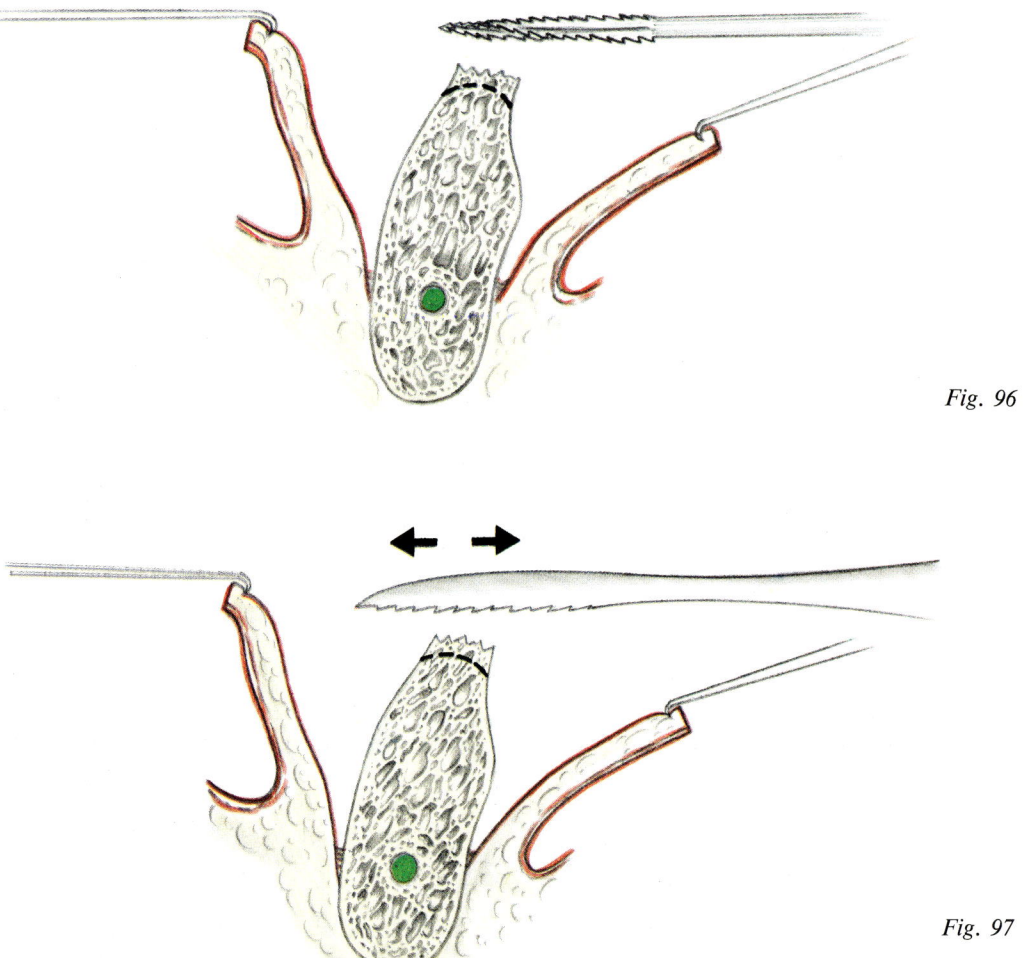

Fig. 96

Fig. 97

raspatory, such as the Otobe-type raspatory, is recommended instead. The shaping and trimming rongeurs supplied by Implants International are not so practical; an ordinary surgical bone-raspatory is much better for this purpose.

After flattening the surface, the channel is prepared by using the bur. Furthermore, close contact between the safety stop and the alveolar bone is obtained only when the surface of the bone is smooth, so that the blade can be inserted up to the desired depth (Fig. 98).

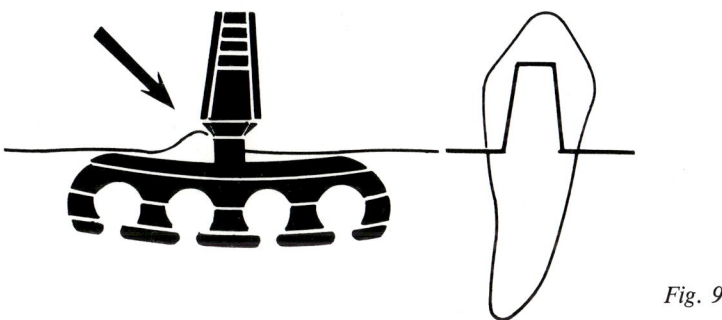

Fig. 98

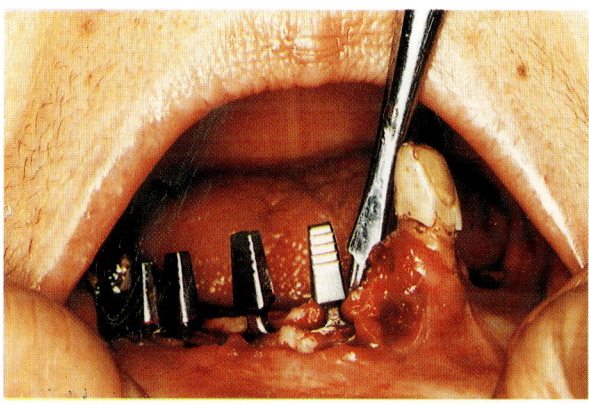

Fig. 99

6.5 CHANNEL PREPARATION

6.5.0 The most important and most difficult procedure in the blade implant operation is the preparation of the channel. It is important that the operator be relaxed when performing this procedure. Excessive tension should be avoided. Making a groove in the exposed alveolar bone parallel to its contour requires great concentration. Remember, concentration and excitement are quite different. Operators are advised to perform deep breathing exercises if they feel excited or terse prior to performing surgery. A short break during the operation for the purpose of relaxing is not inappropriate. Small errors made in the first stage of the operation can sometimes be compensated for in the following stages if the operator is able to stay calm.

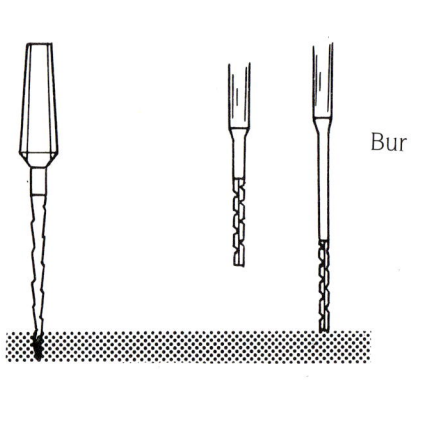

Bur

Fig. 100

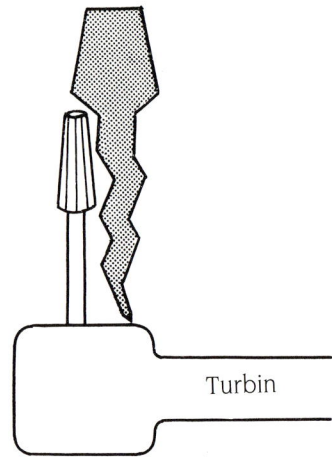

Turbin

Fig. 101

6.5.1 Measure the exact height of the implant blade from the end of the foot to the safety stop. Set the tapering fissure bur at the same height as the turbine. Use metal check to fix the bur for keeping the height constant. This effectively eliminates the possibility of boring too deep a groove. The water cooler of the bur protects the bone surface from the heat generated by friction.

6.5.2 Fit the blade on the exposed alveolar bone, determining the intended channel line on the buccolingual center region of the alveolar crest. Marking with a marker pencil is helpful.

The channel must be 2 mm longer mesiodistally at both ends. Too long a channel line is quite useless.

In the channel preparation procedure, there are several rules that must always be followed:

In the maxillary anterior region, the channel line is kept approximately parallel to the buccal side of the alveolar bone.

In the maxillary molar region, the channel line is kept parallel to the buccal side of the alveolar bone.

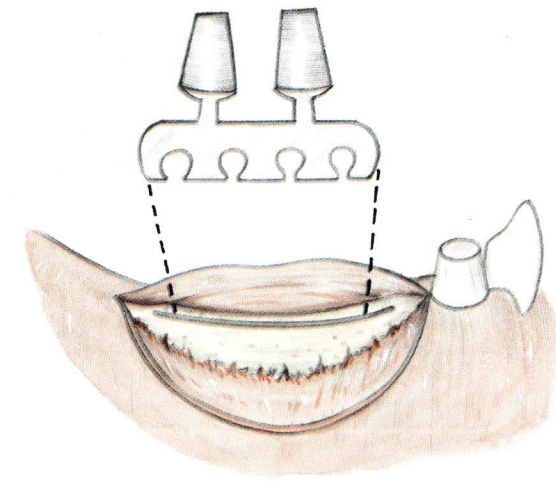

Fig. 102

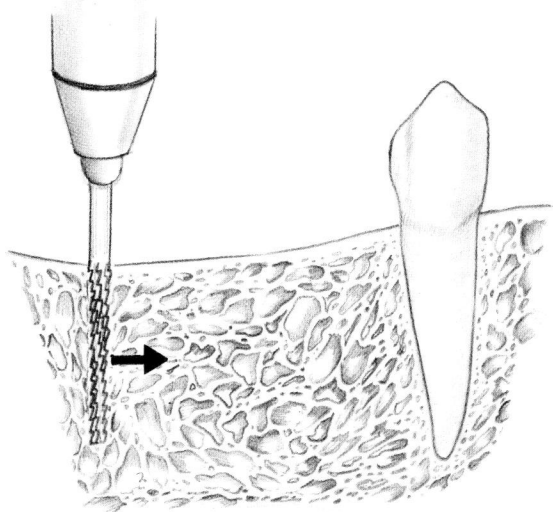

Fig. 103

In the mandible, the channel line is kept parallel to the lingual side of the alveolar bone.

Parallelism is determined independently of the direction of the remaining teeth. The channel line is liable to be misconstructed if the calculations are based on the occlusal relation to the corresponding teeth of the opposite jaw. As a result the blade edge might penetrate and be exposed in the buccal side of the alveolar bone.

6.5.3 Always make the groove in a distal to mesial direction. Avoid making a zigzagging channel. Osseous tissues are not all equally hard; care must therefore be taken to fix the handpiece firmly at first and hold the turbine tight.

The buccolingual width of the channel should not exceed that of the blade. A channel that is too wide can easily result from going back and forth with the bur. The channel bur should always be used in a distal to mesial direction repeatedly if necessary. Making a channel into which the blade fits exactly will mean the future stability of the implant.

Always use the bur in a distal to mesial direction; do not stop midway; do not shuttle.

Using a deep gauge can be helpful for the inexperienced operator. It insures that the channel is made to the exact depth desired. And while measuring with the gauge, the operator can also feel any bone chip that has been left in the channel because of the uneven density of osseous tissues, and remove the chips from the channel. For the expert operator, this depth gauge is not necessary. He can feel with the bur instead of a gauge and drive out chips with a water gun operated by his assistant.

Use water unsparingly throughout the process of forming the channel. Clean the inside of the channel removing all chips and debris.

As mentioned the channel must not be made too wide buccolingually. A channel that is slightly longer anteroposteriorly than the length of the blade will usually not cause any problems. In contrast a wide channel cannot hold the blade. The blade will be moved and loosened by external pressures during impression taking, intaking food, fitting and removing temporary splint unless it has been firmly tapped into a channel that is just the right width. Moreover the operation site heals better, that is, ossification is more effective in a light channel than in a wide channel (Fig. 104).

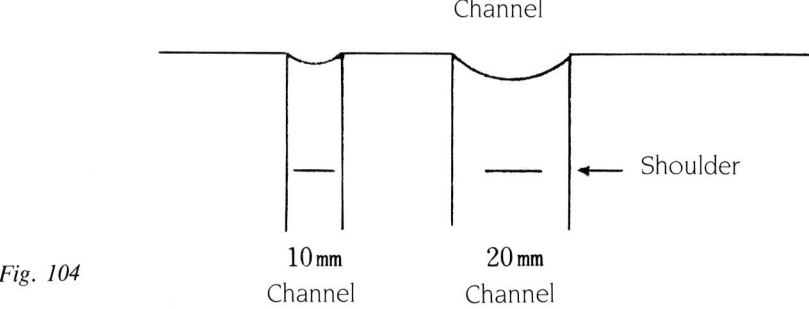

Fig. 104

Recently Morita Co. published the Japanese version of a clinical manual for the implant operation. The pamphlet, however, features an erroneous method of channel preparation. This is the method of channel formation by connecting previously made dots. If this method is used the channel will be wider than necessary at the dots and may lie in the wrong direction buccolingually. Dr. Linkow has repeatedly warned me against forming channels by such a method.

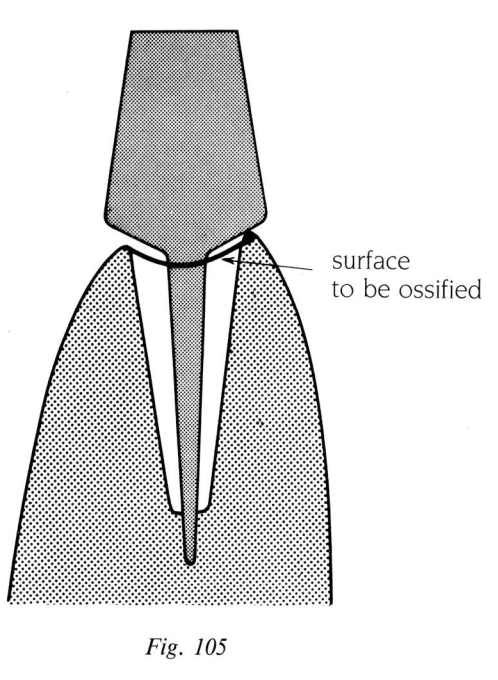

Fig. 105

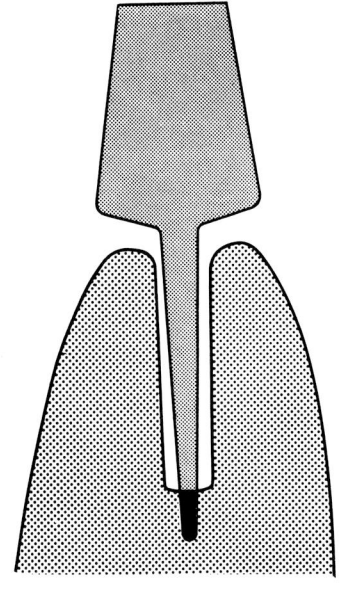

Fig. 106

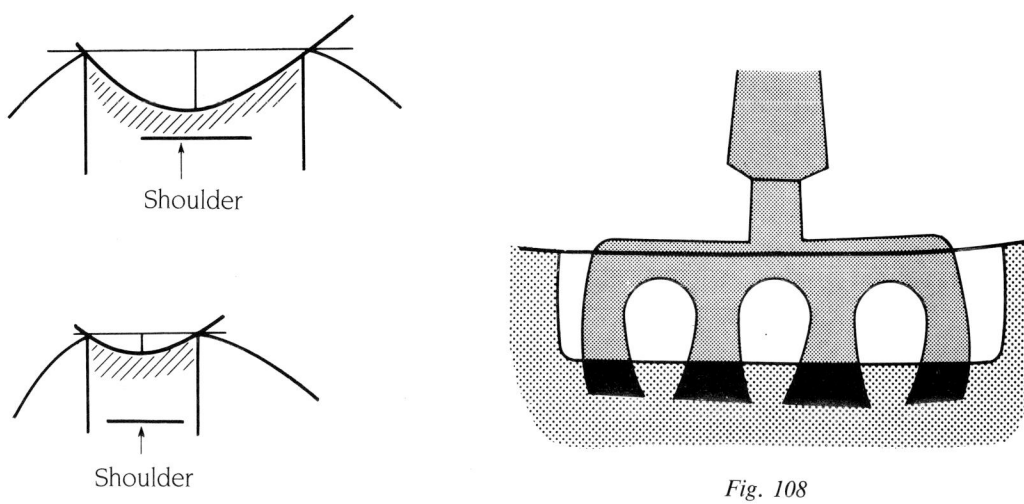

Shoulder

Shoulder

Fig. 107

Fig. 108

6.6 FITTING AND ADJUSTING OF BLADE

6.6.1 With a pair of pliers, adjust the blade so that it has the same curve buccolingually as the prepared channel. Unless this adjustment is made, the blade cannot fit the channel exactly. The blade body is bent gradually, with the pliers holding both ends, until it has the same curve as the channel line (Fig. 109).

6.6.2 Fit the adjusted blade to the channel. Inspect the fit carefully in terms of both length and depth.

6.6.3 Attach the blade to an inserting instrument such as the Otobe inserting instrument. The advantage of this instrument is that it enables the operator to mallet the blade precisely to the desired depth; and prevents him from malleting too deep.

Fit the blade in the channel and tap lightly with a mallet. Trial fitting needs no hard malleting. If any resistance is felt before the blade is inserted to the intended depth, stop malleting. Remove the blade and inspect the channel. Modification of the channel is usually required. The bottom end of the instrument, indicated by arrows, contacts on the surface of the alveolar bone. The blade cannot go deeper into the channel.

After the blade has been inserted to the desired depth, remove the instrument leaving the blade in place.

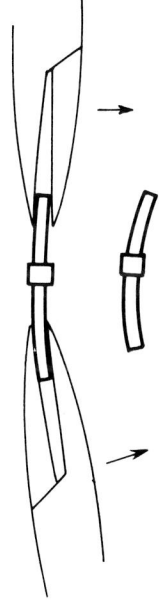

Fig. 109

6.6.4 The next step is adjusting the direction of the head to the direction of the remaining teeth. Decide how far the blade head is to be bent mediodistally and buccolingually, to place it parallel to the remaining teeth. When two or more blades are inserted, inspect and adjust the direction of each, keeping them parallel to one another. Scraping the blade head after insertion, particularly after the final malleting, is an undesirable way of ad-

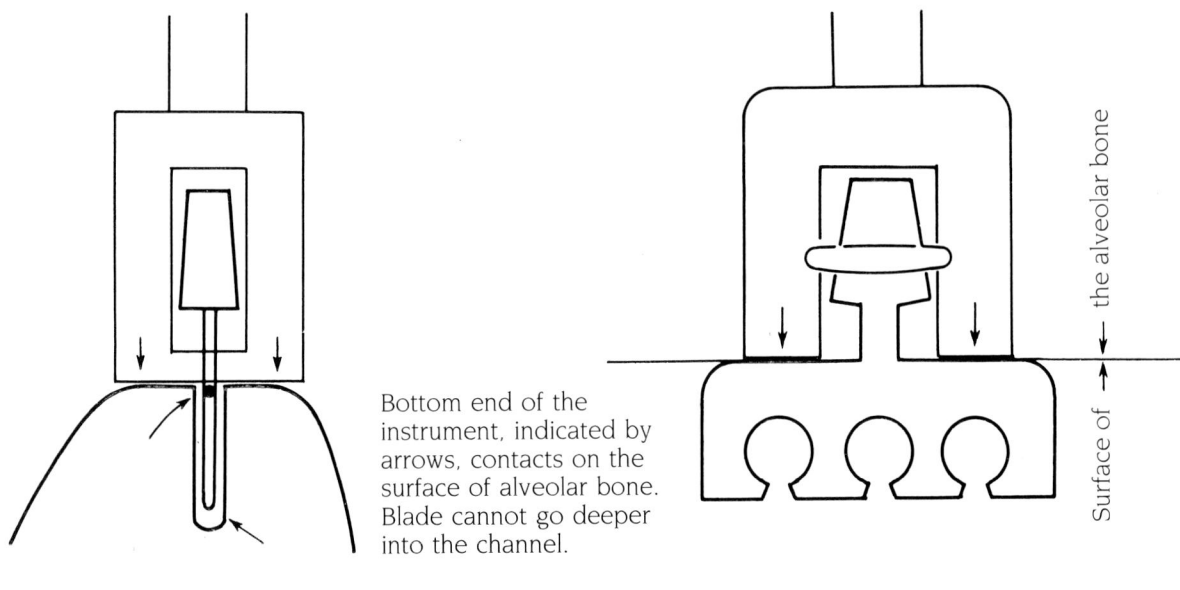

Bottom end of the
instrument, indicated by
arrows, contacts on the
surface of alveolar bone.
Blade cannot go deeper
into the channel.

Fig. 110   *Fig. 111*

justing direction; it requires a lot from the patient. Instead the blade should be removed from the channel and bent at the neck with two pliers, as
illustrated in figure 110.

   An implant blade that is made of good material can be bent without
breaking, unless subject to repeated bending. If a blade breaks in the bending procedure, replace it with a new one and try again. Adjust carefully
until the desired head direction is obtained.

   A general purpose inserting instrument is not appropriate for trial fitting of the blade. With such an instrument the blade might be malleted too
far into the channel. It is better, therefore, to use an inserting instrument
especially designed for the purpose.

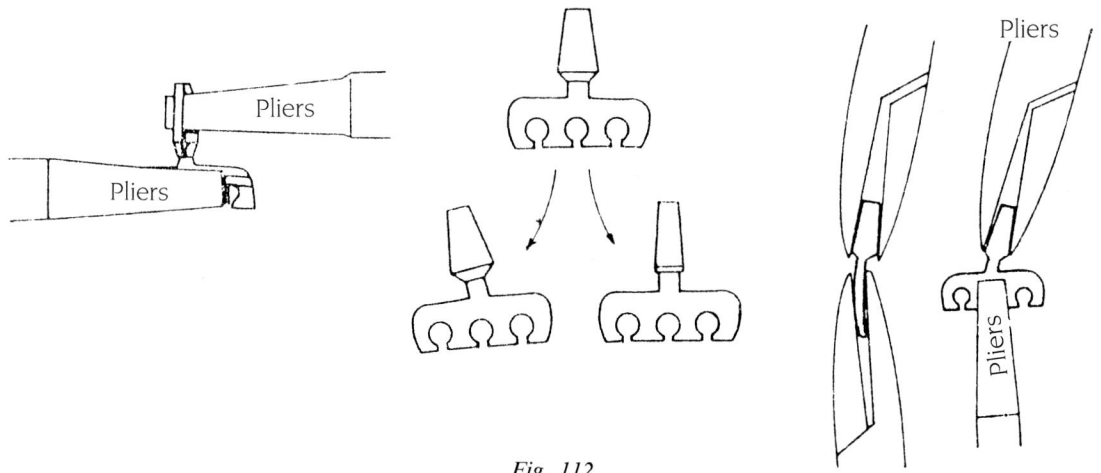

Fig. 112

6.7 USAGE OF REMOVER

During the trial fitting stage, the blade is frequently inserted and removed from the channel. In removing the blade, it is better to use a special remover.

Even after temporary insertion, the blade is held quite firmly in the bone. Removing the blade, therefore, will require a certain amount of force. It also requires carefulness. A blade that is carelessly removed could fall into the oral cavity and could event be swallowed by the patient. Similarly, if excess force is used, the blade might fly up and the sharp end of the remover accidentally injure the patient's oral cavity or face.

Handle the remover in the right way; (1) Insert the angled top end of the remover under the bottom end of the head of the safety stop; (2) Hold both the head and the top of the remover together with your thumb and index finger; then (3) Remove the blade upward with great care.

These are the basic steps for safe removal of the blade A left, as illustrated in Figures 113 and 114.

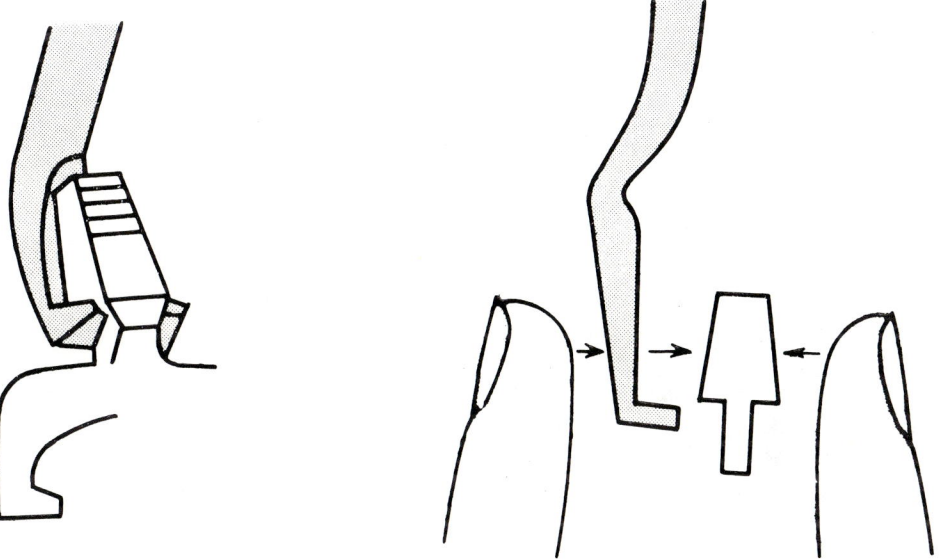

Fig. 113   *Fig. 114*

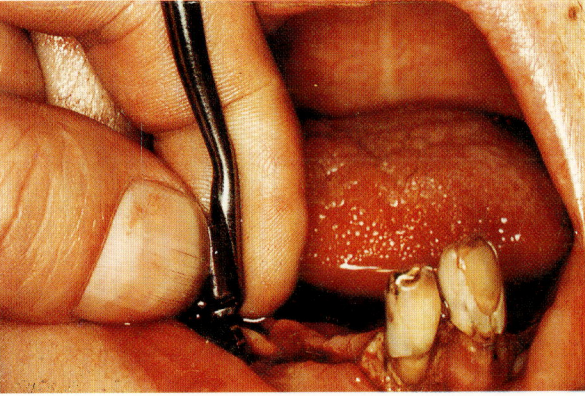

Fig. 115

6.8. MALLETING

In an endosteal blade implant, the following rule is a must: *Fix the blade in the alveolar bone 1 to 2 mm deep by malleting.*

There are no exceptions to this rule.

However, do not mallet hard at the beginning and do not tap the blade in all at once. At first, tap the blade lightly, leaving at least 2 mm space before the final tapping. Adjust the direction of the blade head to the remaining teeth if necessary.

If the blade was inserted easily into the channel up to the safety stop in the trial fit, it will not be able to function effectively after the final insertion. This is the result of too deep a channel. Replacement with a larger size blade is required. The inserted blade should not move when touched by fingers; it should bear occlusal pressure repeatedly exerted. It takes a long time before the implant site is ossified and the blade is supported firmly. Like the injury site caused by tooth extraction, an implant site takes 3-6 months to heal completely.

Avoid using too much force in the final malleting of the blade. Excessive force could crush the osseous tissue in the channel. The mandibular bone should be held tightly by an assistant operator while the blade is malleted into the mandible to prevent excessive pressure on the mandibular joint.

Do not use a hard material such as a wooden board to support the mandible during malleting, as the shock may fracture it. That the best shock absorber is simply the assistant operator palm has been clinically proved (Fig. 116).

When the blade is inserted in the thinner regions of the alveolar bone, particularly in the anterior maxillary region, the assistant operator should keep a finger pressed tightly against the buccal side of the exposed surface bone throughout the malleting procedure.

In an anterior maxillary implant, with the blade head angled at the neck, malleting exerts stronger pressure on the buccal side of the alveolar bone than on the lingual side. This could cause fracture of the bone on the buccal side, which would have serious adverse consequences for the patient, distorting the shape of his face. Further, no effective denture could then be designed for this region of the fractured alveolar bone.

In the maxillary molar region, particularly near the maxillary sinus base, if the alveolar bone is thin, there is some danger that malleting with excessive force will fracture the bone. In the worst case, the edge of the blade could penetrate the bone and the maxillary sinus.

In general, maxillary bones are constructed of less hard and more spongy osseous tissues. This makes it more difficult to insert the blade and to insert it in such a way that it will be supported and function at length.

Blades should not be inserted into the maxilla until the operator has acquired enough knowledge of and experience with implantology. Keep in mind the difference between maxillary bones and mandibular bones in terms of the osseous tissues.

If the blade can be easily moved after the final malleting, simply remove it and stop the implant. The operation has failed as the result of an error in forming the channel or selecting the blade or both. On the other hand, never try to remove a blade once it is properly malleted as far as the safety stop in the intended place.

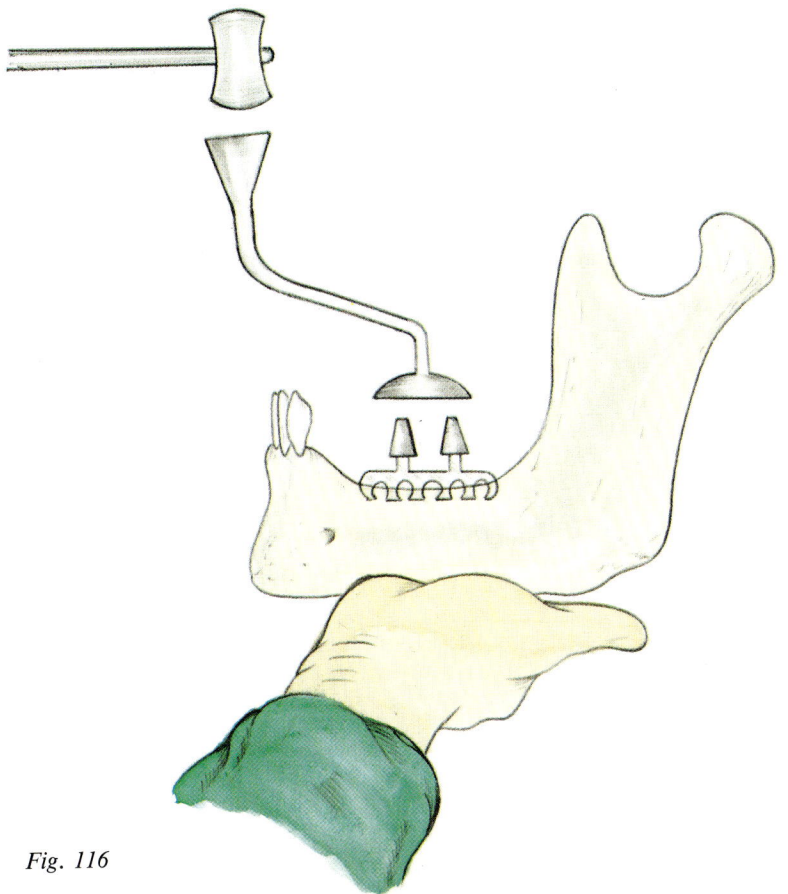

Fig. 116

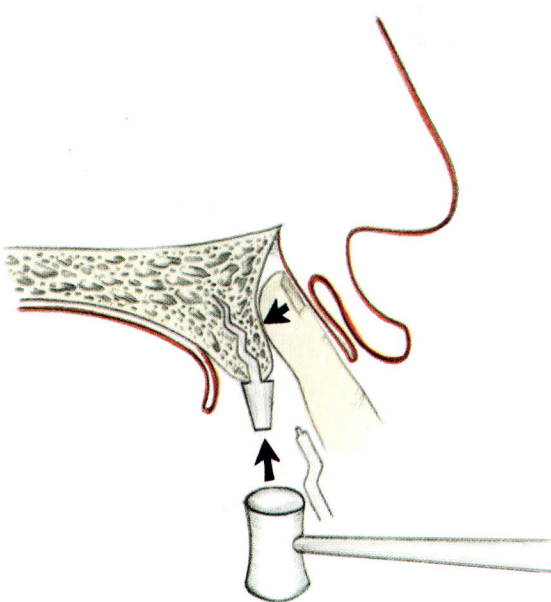

Fig. 117

A nail that has been removed from a wooden board can be hammered back into the same spot and still serve the intended function. With an implant blade and alveolar bone, however, the situation is somewhat different. Sometimes the operator may find that the blade inserting is eccentric or uneven, that is, that either the mesial or the distal portion has been inserted deeper than the other. In this case, mallet the blade again. For a single head, apply the inserting instrument at the upper shoulder of the blade. Care must be exercised in malleting not to touch the instrument edge against the bone. Malleting the sharp edge of the instrument into the alveolar bone could fracture the bone.

If a double-head blade is used, apply the inserting instrument for single-head blades on the upper shoulder of the blade, while the assistant operator uses a finger to support the lower shoulder, as illustrated in figure 118. When the shoulder line of the blade parallels the alveolar bone surface, the final malleting can be done using the inserting instrument for double-head blades.

Mallet the blade until its safety stop is close to the alveolar bone surface; at this point malleting is completed.

If any space is left between the safety stop and the alveolar bone, the ossified region above the blade shoulder is limited, which means that the blade has less supporting capacity.

As mentioned before, there are too many radiograms showing blade implant cases with an exposed shoulder or a space left under the safety stop. Such implants can be considered failures.

When tapped lightly with a metallic material, a completely inserted blade produces a dry, metallic tone.

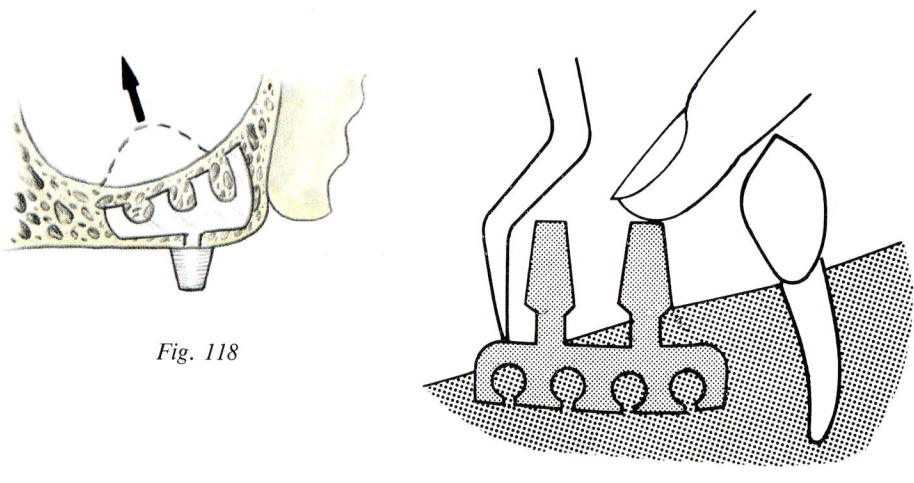

Fig. 118

Fig. 119

This provides a helpful indication that the insertion is over and further malleting is unnecessary. Thus, use of a special metallic mallet, instead of a wooden one, is recommended. After malleting, tap the blade head with the grip end of the mallet, or with another metallic object such as a pincer or a mirror grip, listening carefully to the tone.

It is worth repeating here that if a properly designed inserting instru-

ment such as the Otobe implant instrument is used together with a mallet,
the blade will stop when the safety stop contacts the bone. The error of
inserting the blade too deep is thus eliminated.

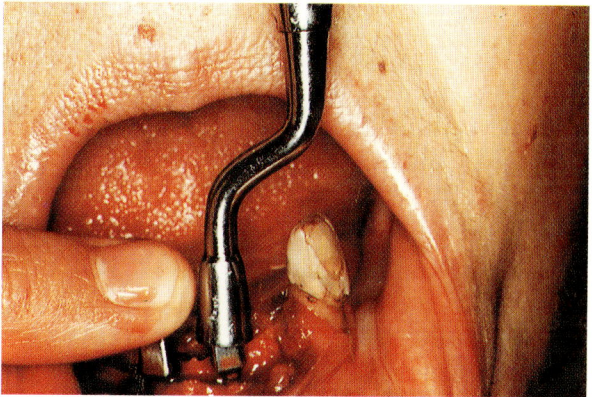

Fig. 120

6.9 USE OF TISSUE PUNCH

After the malleting is over and the blade is in place, try to fit the stripped mucosa to the blade head before closing the incised edges. If any slack
or fold is found, the mucosa around the head should be cut with a tissue
punch and the edges then closed by suturing. If no slack is noticeable, there
is no need for trimming.

When a double-head blade is used, it is generally advisable to trim the
membrane a little bit on both the buccal and lingual sides for easy suturing
and rapid healing. Be conservative in the amount of trimming done and do
not try to trim the membrane with ordinary surgical scissors. Always use a
tissue punch for clear trimming and easy suturing.

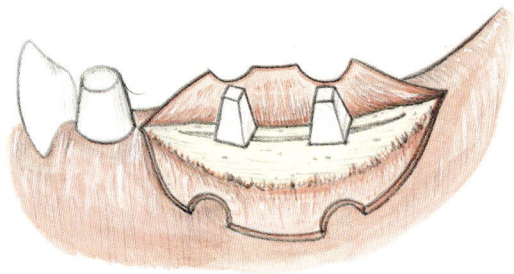

Fig. 121

6.10 SUTURE

On competition of the blade insertion procedures the stripped membrane is closed by suturing, which is performed according to the rules and
techniques of ordinary surgical suture. Since the oral mucosa is stripped

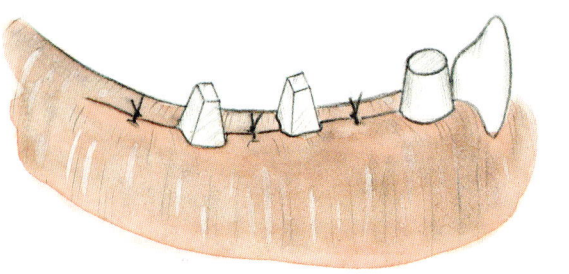

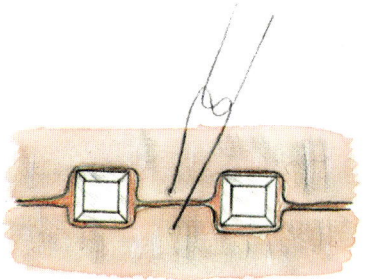

Fig. 122   *Fig. 123*

widely start suture from the point, keeping a certain distance from the incision line for best results.

The oral membrane is rather thin and tears easily; suture carefully, usually in a distal to mesial direction.

As illustrated in Figure 124, in the distal area the suturing point is distal on the buccal side, mesial on the lingual side; in the mesial area, the suturing point is mesial on the buccal side and distal on the lingual side.

Follow any surgical suturing method. In the example in Figure 125 the following steps are involved:

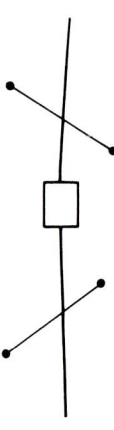

(1) A is the end of the stitch with the needle, B is the other end of the stitch. The remaining thread, about 5 cm in length, is held by the assistant operator.
(2) Remove the needle from the needle holder; wind the stitch around the needle holder twice.
(3) Catch B with the needle holder.
(4) Pull B first, then pull A to make a knot.

Fig. 124

Using a needle holder is advisable, particularily when the area to be sutured is in the back of the oral cavity near the throat. If the operator has no needle holder, both his hands must be placed deep in the oral cavity. Although often done, this takes too much time and energy.

6.11 IMPRESSION TAKING

Take an impression immediately following the suture. This is a general rule of Linkow and one with which I fully concur.

About six hours after the operation, topical swelling is observed in the operative site of the oral mucosa. This swelling lasts for 6 days. Obviously impression taking should be avoided during this period, as an exact impression cannot be obtained.

Taking an impression immediately after the suture has two advantages:

(1) An exact impression is obtained before swelling begins in the operation site.
(2) The period to final completion of the prosthesis is shortened. Fitting the final prosthesis is crucial to the patient, for regaining the occlusion and fixing implant blade in the bone. Therefore, the earlier the completion is, the more favorable the prognosis.

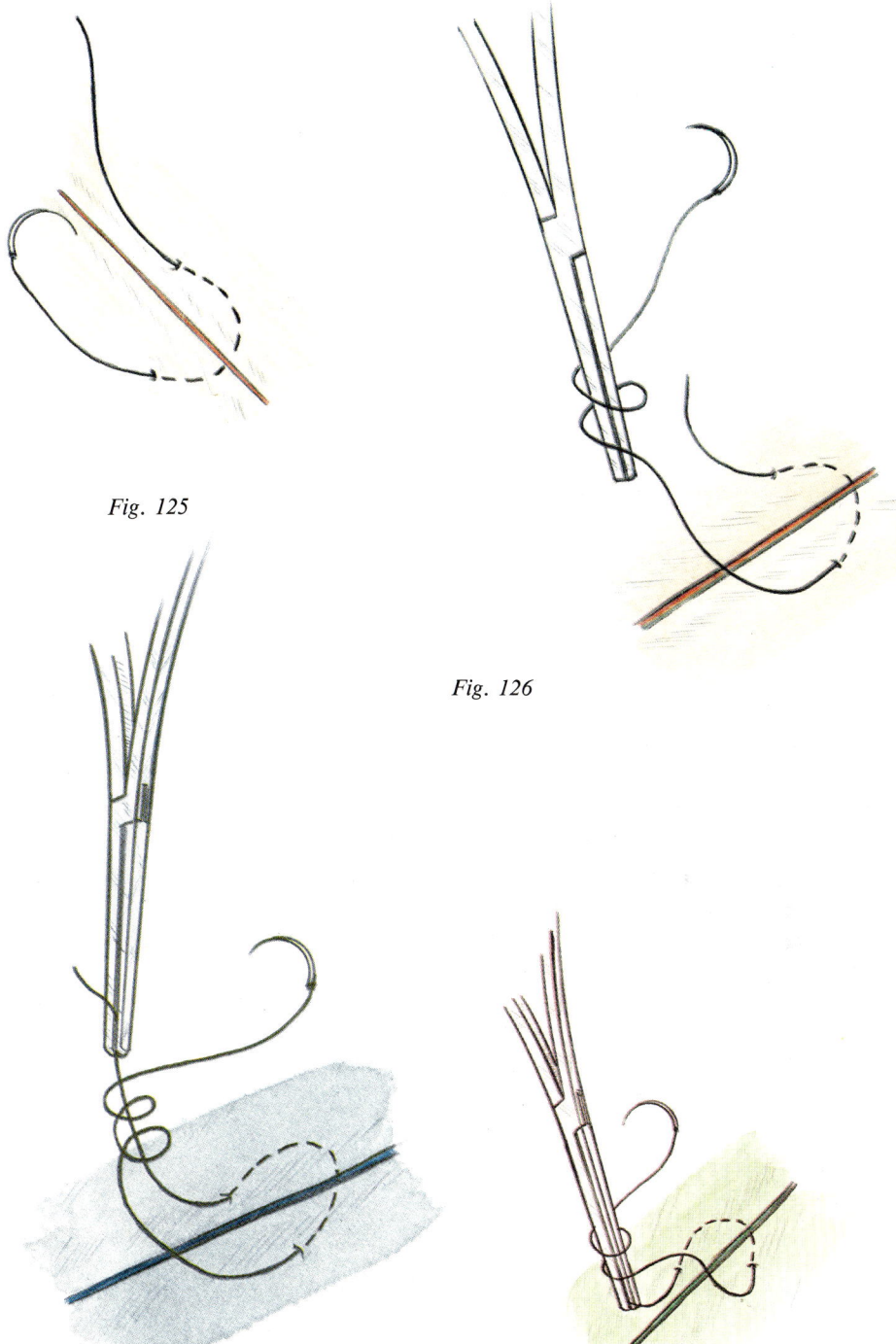

Fig. 125

Fig. 126

Fig. 127

Fig. 128

However, immediate impression taking also has several disadvantages:

(1) When the operation takes a long time, both the patient and the operator are tired.
(2) Bleeding in the operation site may cause foam in the impression phase.
(3) Impression materials may go too deep into the operation site.
(4) Sutured membrane may tear during impression taking.

Judy argues that impression taking should wait until 10 days after the operation. However, delayed impression taking also has its disadvantages, particularly when the sutured membrane is not healing well and needs resuturing. Above all, it delays the completion date.

I therefore agree with Linkow from the clinical point of view. The reason is simple: both the patient and the operator would like to complete the final prosthesis as quickly as possible.

As for the impression material, gelatine and hydrocolloid are to be avoided. Hot gelatine on the exposed bone surface may have unfavorable effects. Linkow now uses input supplied by Vicom, although one of his old case records shows he had once used hydrocolloid as an impression material.

Before you take the impression, press the operated field well with a sterilized gauze to eliminate any dead space. Do not leave any impression material in the operative site, especially between the oral mucosa and the alveolar bone. Impression material left in the organic tissues would cause lasting pain in the region; also the alveolar bone is resorbed there.

When a patient complains of pain considerably after the operation, this is possibly caused by impression material carelessly left in the operation site.

6.12 POSTOPERATIVE RADIOGRAPH

After the blade is inserted, the operator *MUST* take a pantoradiogram of the operation field. Although this was once not acknowledged, it has now become the standard practice.

The purpose of the postoperative radiograph is clear: to verify the location of the implant blade that has just been inserted. Thus a radiogram

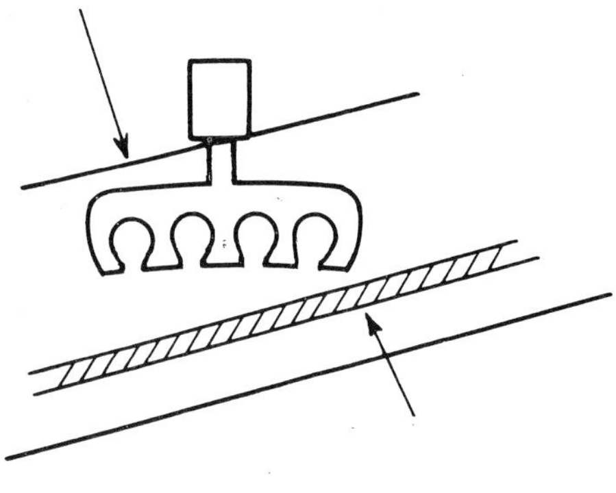

Fig. 129

can sometimes warn the operator that the blade has been inserted too near the mandibular canal or that the edge of the blade has penetrated the bone and entered the maxillary sinus, etc. In the diagnostic process, variations in magnification ratio and deformation of the radiogram must be compensated for postoperatively; however, the radiogram judges the result of the operation much more objectively than could any human eye. In Figure 129, for example, we can see that the mesial shoulder of the blade is too near to the alveolar bone surface and the distal foot of the blade is almost touching the mandibular canal. This would not be perceptible from an outside view of the exposed blade head.

6.13 MEDICATION

6.13.1 Anodyne
Generally speaking, an endosteal blade implant operation, that is, stripping the oral mucosa and inserting an implant blade in the alveolar bone, gives the patient no serious postoperative pain as the alveolar bone has no nervous tissue. The pain felt comes mainly from the oral mucosa; in any given case it is comparable to that the patient would feel after the extraction of a tooth in the same region. For example, the pain caused by an implant operation for lost teeth 7 6 5 is similar in degree to that caused by the extraction of teeth 7 6 5 or 7 6.

The wound and stitches cause pain when they are touched by the tongue; this is prevented by putting a temporary splint on the blade head.

Patients often are subconsciously anxious and afraid of experiencing postoperative pain. To curb this anxiety and relieve any possible pain, an anodyne should be prescribed to the patient.

6.13.2 Antibiotic medicine
Secondary infections in the operative field are the responsability of the operator. When they occur the pain, of course, lasts longer. To prevent possible suppuration, antibiotic medicine should be prescribed.

6.13.3 Anti-inflammatory enzyme
Together with the antibiotics, an anti-inflammatory enzyme should be prescribed.

6.13.4 Tonic and hematinic
If the operation covers a large part of the oral cavity, or several blades are inserted at once, the operation time is quite long, the region of stripped oral mucosa is large and a considerable loss may be involved. Several days after his operation, a patient once complained to me that, although the operation itself had been nothing, he still felt giddy. Exhaustion and weakness caused by a long operation and loss of blood had left him giddy.

Difficulty in taking normal food after the operation naturally results in poor nutrition. Prescription of a tonic and a hematinic is therefore recommended.

6.14 MISCELLANEOUS

With an implant operation, think more in terms of postoperative swelling than post-operative pain.

Stripping the oral mucosa produces topical swelling. Implants in the posterior molar region of the mandible result in swelling of the lymphatic glands in the larynx and difficult swallowing.

The operator must anticipate these after-operative effects. Medicine should be prescribed and regulated according to the needs of individual patients. After the operation the patient should be told to expect some minor temporary pain and swelling. However, any emphasis on these factors before the operation should be avoided, as the patient might be dissuaded from undergoing the operation.

7. Endosteal Blade Implant (4): Clinical Tips and Suggestions

7.1 IMPORTANCE OF DIAGNOSIS

7.1.0 General

In any dental treatment, the operator must have accurate knowledge of the patient's condition through exact diagnosis. Performing an implant without such knowledge is very dangerous and should be avoided. They say that research provides the facts, the basis on which to act. Similarly diagnosis provides the plans on the basis of which to operate.

7.1.1 General examination

(1) Quantitative analysis of sugar in the urine: at very least the quantitative analysis of sugar in the urine of the patient should be performed by the operator himself. This analysis is easily done using testing paper. However healthy he appears, a patient who has glycosuria is not to be operated.

(2) Heart disease: examination for heart disease is indispensable. An implant operation involves bleeding and pain, and often postoperative exhaustion.

The psychological shock of the operation, including fear of pain, bleeding, injection, anesthesia, etc. might cause the condition to worsen. Implantologists must be aware of all these factors.

The full-scale examination of the heart is complicated and requires special equipment. Implantologists should therefore entrust this examination to others but should themselves at least measure the patient's blood pressure.

7.1.2 Pantoradiograph

The significance of radiographic diagnosis, particularly of the pantoradiograph, has already been discussed in previous chapters.

A typical failed operation may involve an implant blade of the wrong size, which, inserted in the anterior maxillary region, has penetrated the alveolar bone near the nasal fossa base exposing the blade edge in the nasal fossa. Such failures are caused primarily by poor diagnosis on the part of the operator, who has neglected to exactly measure the thickness of the alveolar bone in the region by interpreting the pantoradiogram. The operator's rough estimate results in his selecting too large a blade, and the insertion of this blade results in the penetration. Given the current state of implantology, failures of this kind are unnecessary and must be completely eliminated.

The amount of osseous tissue in the alveolar bone of the relevant area should also be carefully confirmed by interpreting the radiogram. An implant that is inserted in a bone with an insufficient amount of osseous tissue will soon loosen and the blade must be removed. After removal of the blade, the bone in the implant site is badly damaged. Moreover a loosened blade sometimes causes fracture of the bone buccolingually in both sides of the implant channel, and fractured pieces of bone remain in the membrane. As a result the patient suffers great pain. Fractured alveolar bone is rapidly resorbed and the alveolar crest soon disappears, leaving a flat, alveolar base. No kind of denture can be fitted here.

In short, before an implant operation is performed, a pantoradiogram of the intended operative field must be interpreted carefully for an exact diagnosis and a correct operative plan.

7.1.3 Denture

Patients who wear dentures should be asked for how many years they have done so. Implants are usually impossible for patients who have used dentures for more than 5 five years. The friction from the dental plate greatly accelerates the resorption of the alveolar bone (see Chapter 3).

7.1.4 Remaining alveolar bone

The question of whether alveolar bone still remains in the maxillomandibular bones is critically important. A general rule is that implants should be undertaken only in areas where a sufficient amount of alveolar bone remains. Inspect the inside of the oral cavity carefully. The following must be checked:

(1) Is the eminence of the alveolar bone found in the lost tooth region?
(2) Is there enough room mesiodistally for inserting the implant blade?
(3) What is the occlusal relationship to the corresponding tooth?
(4) Does alveolar bone exist?
(5) Is there enough space for occlusion?

All remaining teeth should be checked carefully for caries and pyorrhea. Treatment of any defective teeth must precede the operation implant. The stability of the remaining teeth should also similarly be checked. By pressing the oral mucosa hard with his fingers and questioning the patient as to whether he feels pain, the operator can estimate the location of the mental foramen. This information will prove very helpful in performing the operation.

7.2 IMPORTANCE OF CHANNEL PREPARATION

7.2.1 Location of the channel

Before inserting an implant blade, the channel for the blade is made on the surface of the alveolar bone with a special bur.

Using a study model, the operator must select the most appropriate blade for the individual patient; an arbitrary selection would result in failure.

The blade is to be located so that occlusal pressure will be properly dispersed considering the relative position of the supposing tooth. No irregular occlusion pressure should be exerted to the blade.

Before forming the channel, draw a draft line on the bone and attempt a trial fit of the blade. The channel should be made on the highest portion of the alveolar bone, namely, on the alveolar crest. If the crest is not flat but forms acute angles on both sides, it must be planned with a bone raspatory or bur before the channel is made.

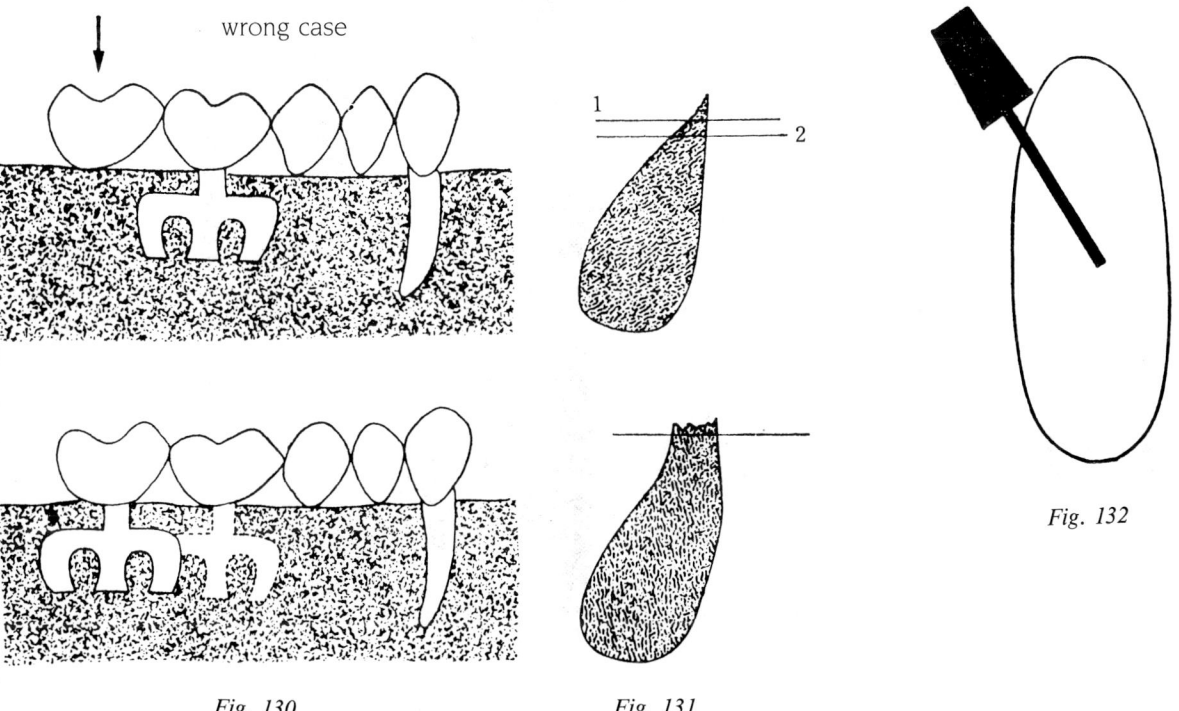

wrong case

Fig. 130   Fig. 131   Fig. 132

Avoid making the channel on the crest edge: only one side of the blade inserted on the crest edge can come into contact with the bone surface. Select the place in the alveolar crest where both the buccal and lingual sides of the safety stop can come into contact with the surface of the bone.

The channel should be slightly longer than the widest antero-posterior part of the blade. This length can be determined by fitting the blade during the channel-forming procedure.

Channel formation should start at the most distal point and proceed in a mesial direction. This is a general rule of channel formation. It is wrong to start from the center and then extend the channel in both distal and mesial directions.

Implantologists must always carefully consider the entire procedure of the implant operations including the final stage of prosthesis fabrication. The durability of the implant depends on the structure of the prosthesis as well as the implant blade itself.

These are the initial steps in channel formation. First, the distal position of the blade head and the distal end of the channel are determined. The portion of alveolar bone to be used in the alveolar crest is flat; when found unflat, it must be flattened before forming channel. Then channel formation begins from the distal end in a mesial direction.

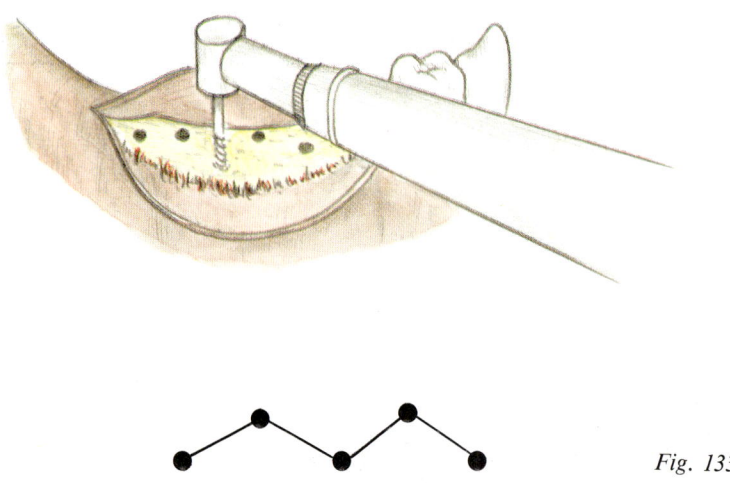

Fig. 133

7.2.2 Avoid zigzag lines

In making the channel avoid zigzagging. As already mentioned, a manual published by Implants International unfortunately advises an erroneous method of channel formation. According to the manual, the channel is to be formed by connecting previous dots (Fig. 133). This method is clearly disadvantageous in that it is conducive to zigzagging the channel. Both Linkow and I disapprove of this method.

Amending or modifying a zigzag line into a linear or compound curve involves making the channel wider buccolingually than is necessary. In short there should be no zigzag lines in channel formation.

Channel preparation is the first step of the operation. Errors made at this stage become amplified and affect all subsequent procedures. Avoid broken channel lines such as those in the upper half of Figure 134.

External pressure exerted on the blade will not be evenly distributed at a bend in the channel. Any implant, particularly a blade implant, must be inserted so as to distribute occlusal pressure effectively and evenly without it exceeding the holding capacity of the blade or the remaining teeth.

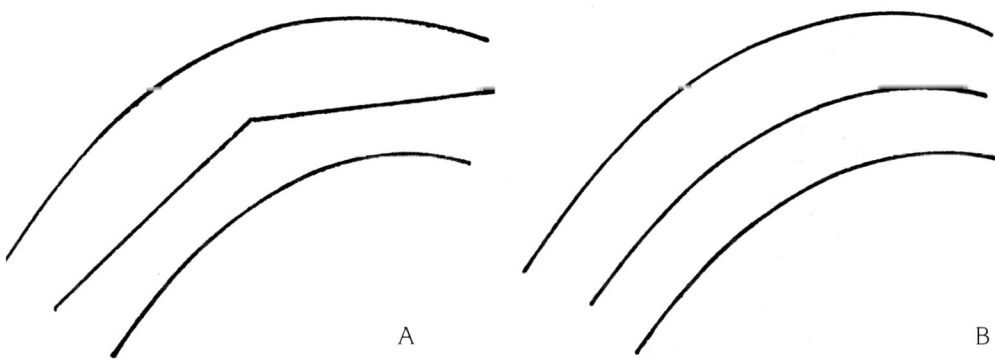

A   B

Fig. 134

7.2.3 Width of the channel

The channel should not be any wider buccolingually than necessary; it should be as near as possible to the width of the blade. In making the channel, avoid back-and-forth movement, as this may result in widening the channel.

In most dental treatment, for instance, crown formation involves buccolingual reciprocating scraping with the bur driven by a dental turbine. Not surprisingly, in making the implant channel the operator is apt to use the reciprocating method. It is important to always follow the general rule of *distal to mesial*. I have found through clinical experiences that this is easily done by using a tilted bur as illustrated in Figure 136 (1). The surface of the alveolar bone is formed of hard osseous tissues and the bur can sometimes be flipped up out of the channel when it hits the hardest portion of the bone. A tilted bur, however, does not come out of the intended channel line and, consequently, can make a clean and sharp channel.

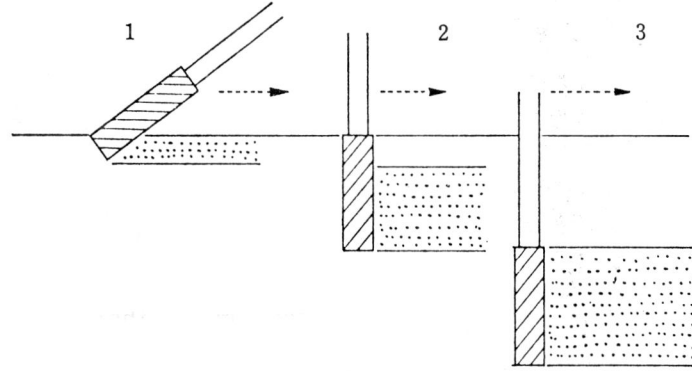

Fig. 135

Do not make the channel wider buccolingually than the width of the bur used in the earlier stage. After forming the channel to the intended depth, enlarge it buccolingually to fit the width of the blade. This is the most effective way of not making the channel wider than is necessary.

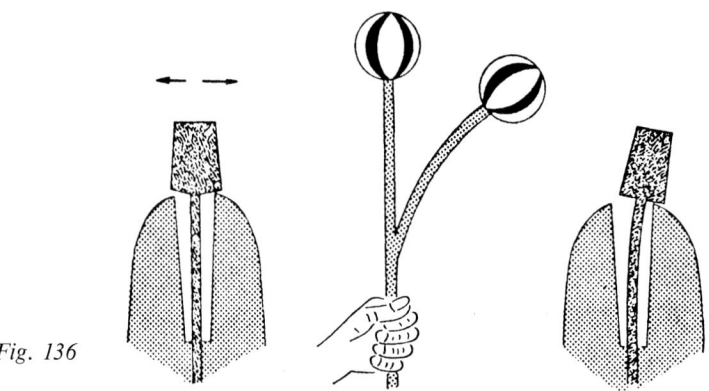

Fig. 136

An excessively wide channel is the major factor in most failed blade implants. The buccolingual looseness in the surface of the alveolar bone caused by the wider channel hinders favorable ossification and finally the blade comes loose. Generally, the wider the channel is, the fewer the hard osseous tissues that form on the blade shoulder.

Even after ossification is completed, a too wide channel is sometimes discernible in the form of a open ditch. This is, of course, highly undesirable.

7.2.4 Correct depth

The depth of the channel should be exactly the same as the length of the blade body, that is, excluding the length of the neck. The 2 mm length of the neck is left for malleting the blade into the bone. Malleting should tap the blade into the bone, bringing the safety stop close to the bone surface.

If the channel is too thin, the blade needs additional malleting. The blade may not go any further after too much malleting because of the resistance of the osseous matrix and the fact that the blade edge has become blunt. Crushed bone tissues caused by too much malleting lead to the decomposition of the affected portion of the alveolar bone.

If, on the contrary, the channel is too deep, malleting will not have the effect of tapping the blade edge into the bone. The inserted blade is then held only buccolingually; it is moved mesiodistally by the excertion of external pressure.

A Japanese implantologist once reported a case of a "no malleting" blade insertion. The channel was simply 2 mm deeper than the length of the blade body and placed in the channel without any malleting. An implant blade could never be held in place by this method. It must first be fixed temporarily to the bone by malleting if the blade is to be held firmly in place by ossification firmly.

It is no coincidence that in any kit of implant instruments, several mallets are always included and clinical experience shows this to be necessary.

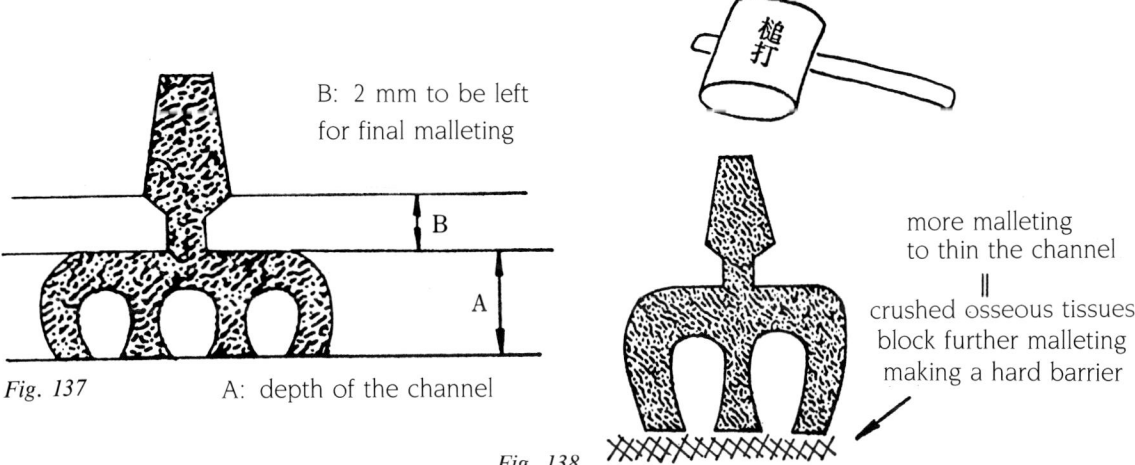

B: 2 mm to be left
for final malleting

B

A

Fig. 137　　A: depth of the channel

more malleting
to thin the channel
‖
crushed osseous tissues
block further malleting
making a hard barrier

Fig. 138

7.2.5 Heat

Heat generated by the friction between the bur and the bone burns the osseous tissues in the channel. Once burned, the bone loses its natural flexibility. It is important to water well, to cool down the channel whenever the bur is used. This watering procedure is usually performed by the assistant operator.

Burned osseous tissue is degenerated tissue and thus adversely affects the durability of the blade.

7.3 IMPORTANCE OF MALLETING

7.3.0 General

Malleting has a function of paramount importance in the implant blade operation. It usually takes 3-6 months until the full process is completed, that is, until ossification holds the implant blade firmly and the final prosthesis is attached.

Until ossification is completed, the blade must be fixed in the channel by other means. This is achieved by malleting the blade 2 mm deep into the alveolar bone. In addition a temporary bridge denture is put in immediately after the blade insertion and a final bridge denture is fabricated and fitted to the blade head as soon as possible.

The main function of this first bridge denture is to hold the blade temporarily; Then, it is replaced with the second higher quality bridge denture after the blade is completely fixed in the alveolar bone. In other words, malleting is simply the first step of temporary blade fixing. Long term holding capacity cannot be obtained by malleting; rather, the blade is fixed and held by the ossified tissues in the alveolar bone. It is important to correct the common misunderstanding that the implant blade is fixed in the bone by malleting. The evidence of the contrary is readily apparent. A patient once told me that, although he could bite anything 6 months after the operation, he had still felt considerable anxiety when biting. In the case of this patient, the ossification was completed, that is, the implant was finished 6 months after the actual operation.

7.3.1 Insufficient malleting

For fitting purposes mallet the blade lightly; if it stops at the blade shoulder, the depth of the channel is suitable. Then mallet again harder until the safety stop of the blade comes into contact with the alveolar bone surface. Do not stop malleting before this point, no matter how firmly the blade seems to be held in the bone. The safety stop of the blade *must* contact with the alveolar bone surface. This is indispensable for the full functioning of the blade.

If the blade will not go in any further but there is still dead space above the bone surface, although malleting has been repeated two or three times, and a metallic tone has been heard, stop malleting. Remove the blade from the channel and dig the channel deeper before malleting again. The dry metallic tone is a signal to stop malleting; learn to recognize and use this tone as a helpful indicator.

7.3.2 Violent malleting

Do not mallet with excessive force when the blade is not going in. Such malleting causes patient discomfort and exhaustion. If the assistant operator is not holding the patient's jaw firmly, excessively forceful malleting might crush the jaw at that point. In addition the blade edge will crush the osseous tissues instead of penetrating them. Crushed tissues set up a barricade in the bone and then decompose. It actually happened that the mandible of a patient was fractured during an implant operation and that the jaws of several others have been injured not insignificantly.

7.3.3 No malleting insertion

When the implant blade is inserted in the channel without any malleting, or when the inserted blade is easily moved by a finger, the channel has been formed too deep. The only solution is to use a larger blade assuming that such a substitution is the particular case.

7.4 OPERATIVE TIPS

7.4.0 General

Before closing this last chapter on blade implants, I would like to summarize the suggestions I have given concerning implant blade insertion.

7.4.1 The area of lost teeth 7 6 or 7 6 5 (and 6 7) in the mandibular bone is the easiest for the beginning operator to work. The operator should perform implant only in this region until he has mastered the basic implant techniques, at least five cases.

Avoid blade implants in maxillary bone. The weak construction of this bone makes it extremely difficult even for expert operators to perform blade implants with successful results.

7.4.2 Avoid performing an implant immediately after an extraction as there is some danger of fracturing the buccal side of the alveolar bone. There should be at least a 2 month interval between the extraction and the implant. Inexpert operators in particular should follow this rule.

7.4.3 Be as relaxed an possible while performing the operation. This is of course difficult at first. I remember vividly watching an operation performed by a beginning operator. After the suture of the oral mucosa, not the patient but the operator fainted.

It is important to be fully confident so that the operation will be successful. If anxious about a case, it is a good idea to ask a senior expert for help as a guest assistant operator. However, avoid inviting an observer or visitor before feeling fully confident about the basic technique. Beginners are apt to experience greater stress in the presence of observers. There are many psychological reasons for this. But regardless of the reasons, stress and excitement can have as powerful an adverse effect on the operation as can anxiety and fear.

An operator who finds himself overly excited and nervous during an operation, must try to relax in his own way, whether by taking several deep breaths or humming his favorite tune.

7.4.4 Be careful in talking to the assistant and/or observer during the operation. Under the local anesthesia the patient is aware of all that is said. It is important not to arouse or increase any anxiety and fear the patient may feel. Observers should remain silent during the operation. Discussion of the case can be conducted afterward.

7.4.5 A sufficient amount of anesthetic should be applied. If the patient complains of pain during the operation, apply another injection. Keep in mind, however, that additional anesthetics work rather slowly after the stripping of the mucosa. Sufficient application of the anesthetic initially is therefore advisable. In offices with piping for gas, nitrous oxide can also be helpful.

7.4.6 To prevent secondary infection, the patient should not be allowed to gargle. After sterilization and anesthetization this should be explained to the patient and the gargling cup removed from the unit.

7.4.7 An implant operation involves exposing a considerably large area of the alveolar bone. Care must therefore be taken to protect the bone. To prevent drying, which can be quite harmful to the bone, the bone surface should be covered with sterilized gauze dipped in a saline solution.

In a subperiosteal implant operation, an impression is taken on the surface of the alveolar bone. Covered with the impression material the bone is shut off from the air and naturally becomes dry. Thus, the bone should be moistened after the impression has been taken; this also serves to wash out any remaining impression material.

7.4.8 When the channel is being formed in the alveolar bone, friction between the bone bur and the bone produces heat. Strong heat applied locally to the bone can naturally burn it. Generally, a bone that is burnt does not regenerate; the burnt portion of alveolar bone does not ossify. Thus it is important to wet the alveolar bone well when making a channel in the exposed surface. Water from the turbine unit might be insufficient; ask the assistant operator to water with a water gun.

7.4.9 Blades can be modified, by cutting and planing, if they are found too large for the patient. Care must be taken not to scrape the shoulder portion of the blade. Beginners sometimes make the head too short; this mistake should be avoided. After suturing, the head would disappear in the gingiva due to its being too short. Electrolytic abrasion should be applied to the modified blade, which must be cleaned and sterilized before insertion.

7.4.10 After the channel is formed, do not try to insert the blade immediately. Stop malleting when the blade shoulder is at the level of the alveolar bone surface and check the location of the blade head relative to the remaining teeth. If the blade is not parallel, designing and fitting the final prosthesis becomes extremely difficult and the blade may loosen.

7.4.11 A blade that has been inserted in the alveolar bone by malleting cannot be moved easily with a finger or occlusion. If it does move, the insertion is incomplete. The blade should be removed and reinserted after modification, which is usually required in the channel site. In a channel that holds a loosened blade, ossification does not proceed normally because the blade crushes osteoblasts or cuts the osseous tissue whenever it moves in the channel. The blade should be checked immediately after insertion by pushing it with a finger or two to see if it moves easily or not. If the blade is still loose and easily movable after a certain period of time, the implant is a failure. Remove the blade and operate again.

7.4.12 The inserted blade does not cause pain in the alveolar bone but only in the soft tissues such as the incised stripped oral mucosa. If the patient complains of any pain after the soft tissues, such as the oral mucosa, in the operation site have healed, there must be a specific reason. Examine the patient carefully to ascertain the cause.

7.4.13 Most failures are attributable to the operator's errors, misdiagnosis, inexpert surgical procedures, imcomplete blade insertion, and so forth. Rarely is a failure attributable to the blade itself.
    Usually failures are found early, within 1-3 months of the operation.

7.4.14 The implant blade must be malleted 2 mm deep into the alveolar bone. Otherwise the blade will not be fixed effectively and will eventually loosen and fall out. On the other hand, if the depth is more than 2 mm, the blade edge will crush the osseous tissues of the alveolar bone. Excessively forceful malleting may injure or even fracture the bone around the blade. Crushed or injured osseous tissues may lead to a failed operation.

7.4.15 The patient's mandible should be held firmly by the assistant operator while the blade is being malleted into the alveolar bone. If it is not properly held, the operator cannot mallet effectively, since the mandible which has no support would be moved under the pressure of the malleting.
    As the mandibular joint is outside the anesthetized zone, the patient would experience pain. Further, with excessively hard malleting the mandibular joint might be dislocated or injured. The assistant operator should hold the lower jaw of the patient firmly to prevent such accidents.

7.4.16 Generally speaking, blade implants should not be applied to fully edentulous maxillary bone. I have made four such attempts and in each case the result was not satisfactory. All were finally solved by applying another method of implantation, namely, subperiosteal implants.

A failed blade implant means a damaged alveolar bone. It can also be psychologically damaging to the patient. In the maxillary bone implant operations should be performed only where there is an exact diagnosis and success is certain.

7.4.17 A failed implant operation can be corrected only by another implant operation. The implantologist must therefore have the convincement that implantology is the best approach to the treatment of lost teeth.

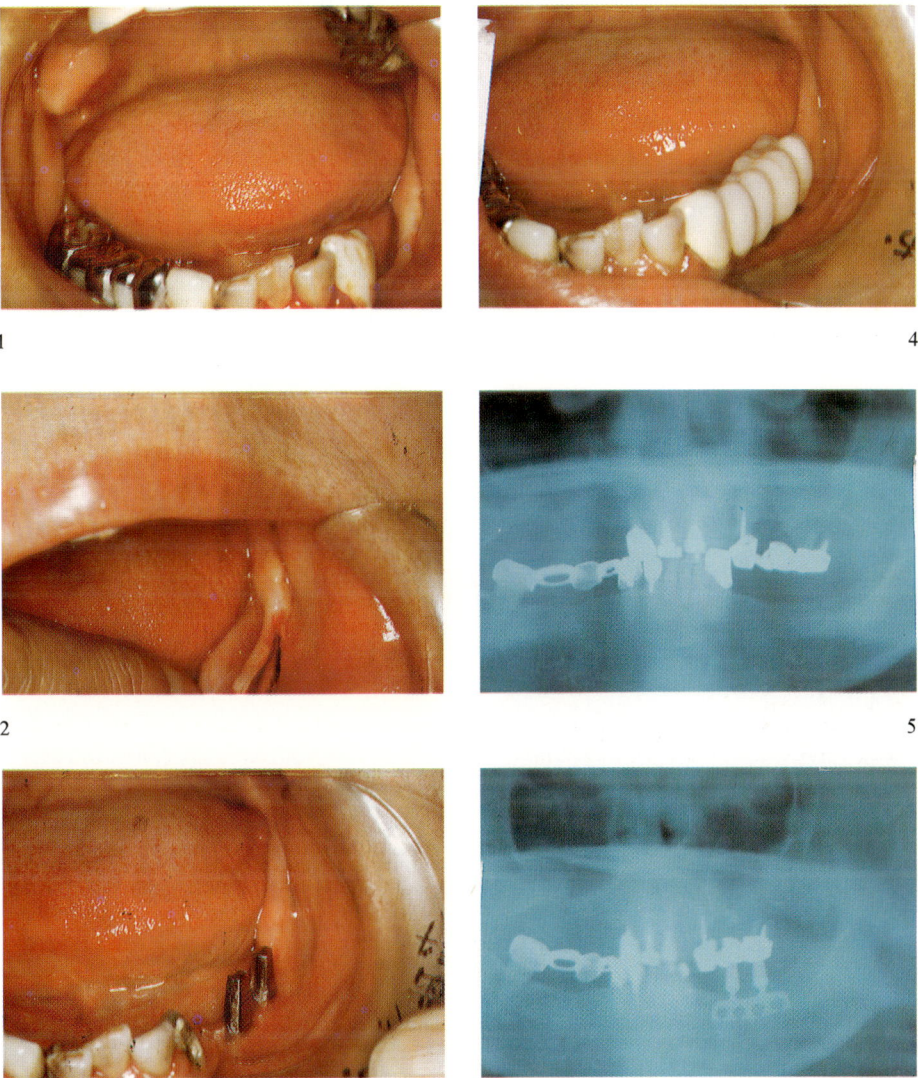

Case 1
1. Preoperative photo.
2. Channel preparation.
3. One week after implant insertion.
4. Superstructure is cemented.
5. Preoperative panorama X-ray.
6. Postoperative panorama X-ray.

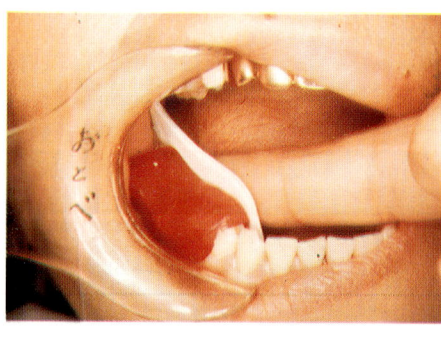

1

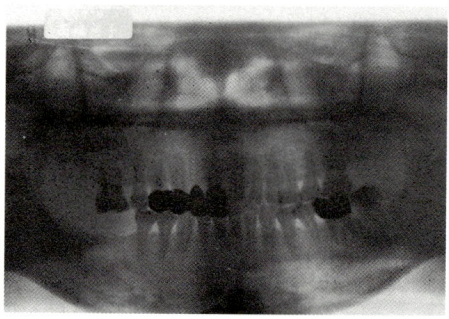

2

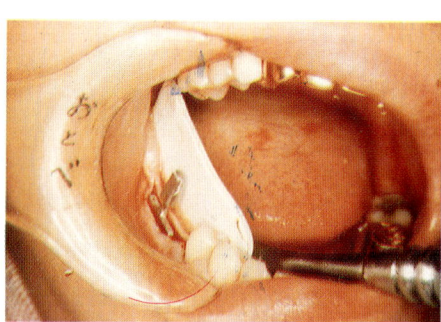

3

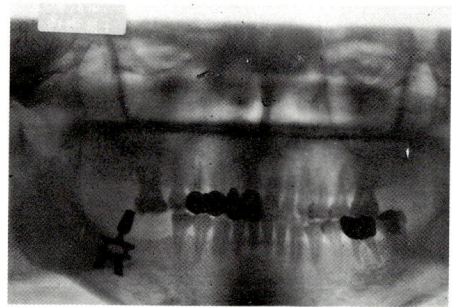

4

Case 2
1. Showing method of implant without pantoma X-ray appliance.
2. Channel deepened step by step; preventing possible danger.
3. Pantoma X-ray photo before the operation.
4. Pantoma X-ray photo after the operation showing the blade inserted near the mandibular canal. Otobe's original blade having the mark of Tonii: Tonii is the Japanese traditional symbol of shrine on a happy place; it means, therefore, praying for happy result of the operation as well as everlasting health of the patient.

Case 3
1. Oral cavity before operation.
2. Forming abutment for remaining teeth before operation.
3. Applying temporary denture.
4. Stripping mucosa.
5. Channel preparation of the blade.
6. Blade inserted.
7. Implant bridge in oral cavity: operation site cured up completely.
8. Bridge now applied.   →

Case 3

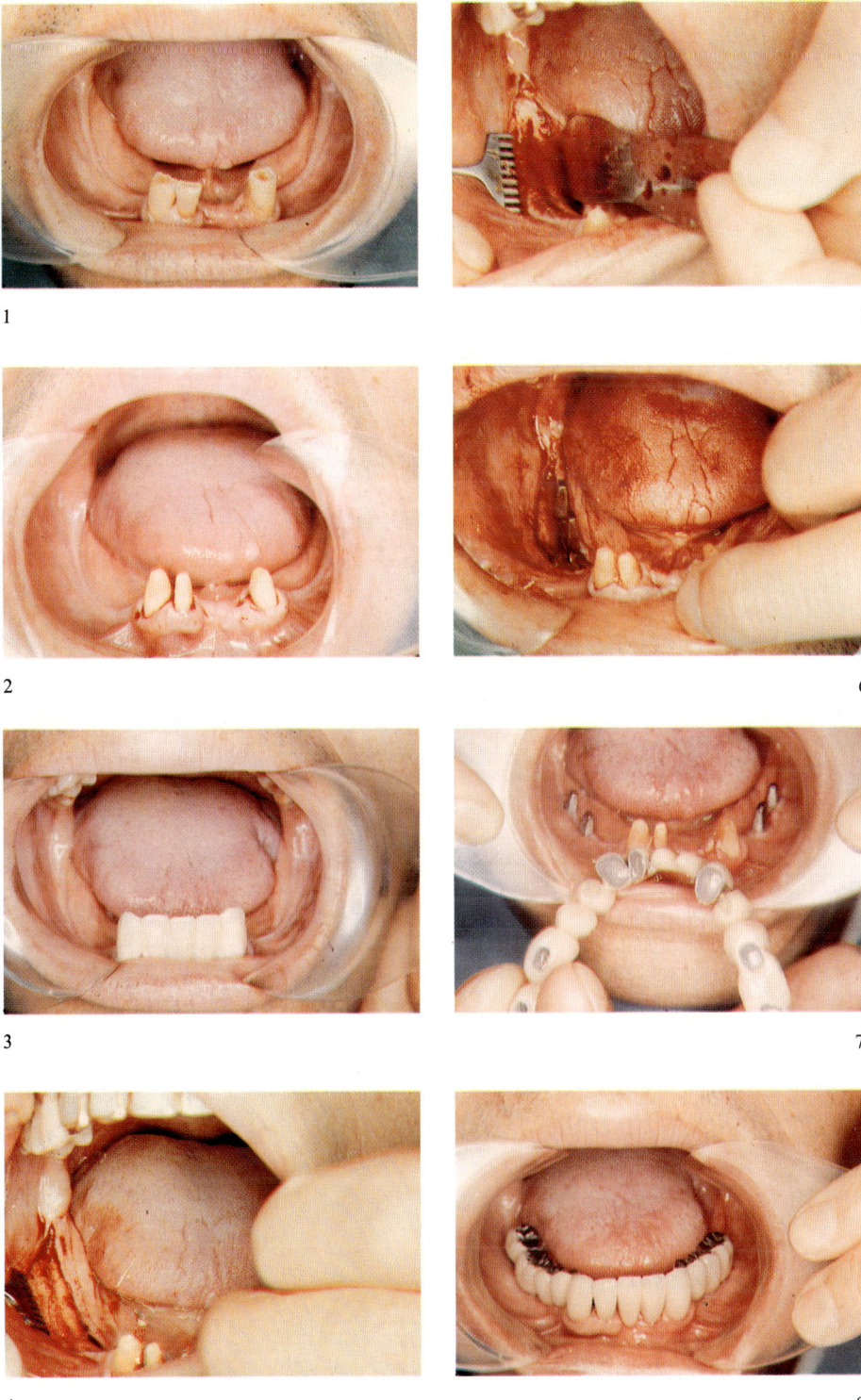

1

2

3

4

5

6

7

8

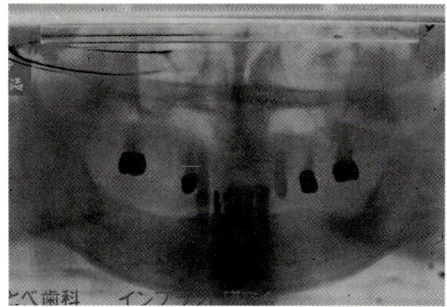

1

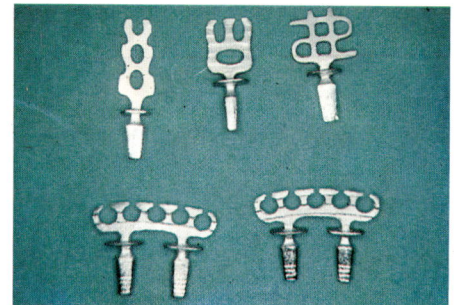

2

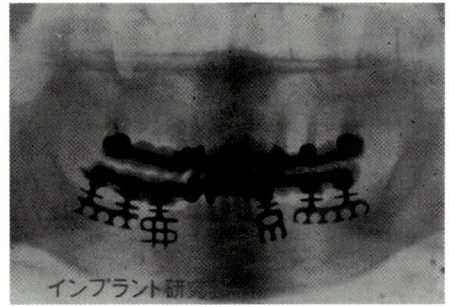

3

Case 4
1. Pantoma photo before the operation.
2. Otobe's original blade: blade having the mark «s» inserted. Several years have passed without problems.
3. Pantoma photo after the operation.

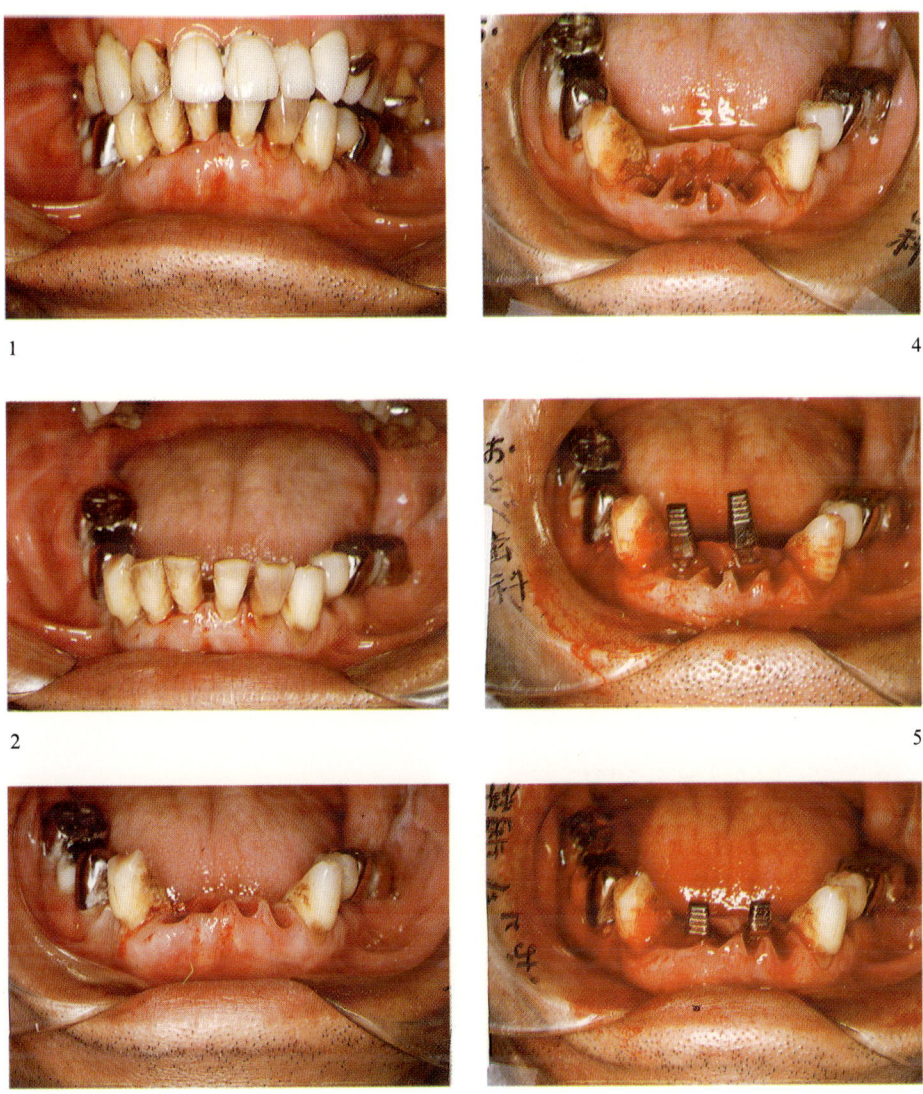

1

2

3

4

5

6

Case 5 (a)
1. Preoperative photo. Occlusion of upper and lower teeth.
2. Mandibular front teeth before extraction.
3. After extraction.
4. Site of extracted teeth.
5. Inserting blade in extracted hole.
6. Blade inserted.

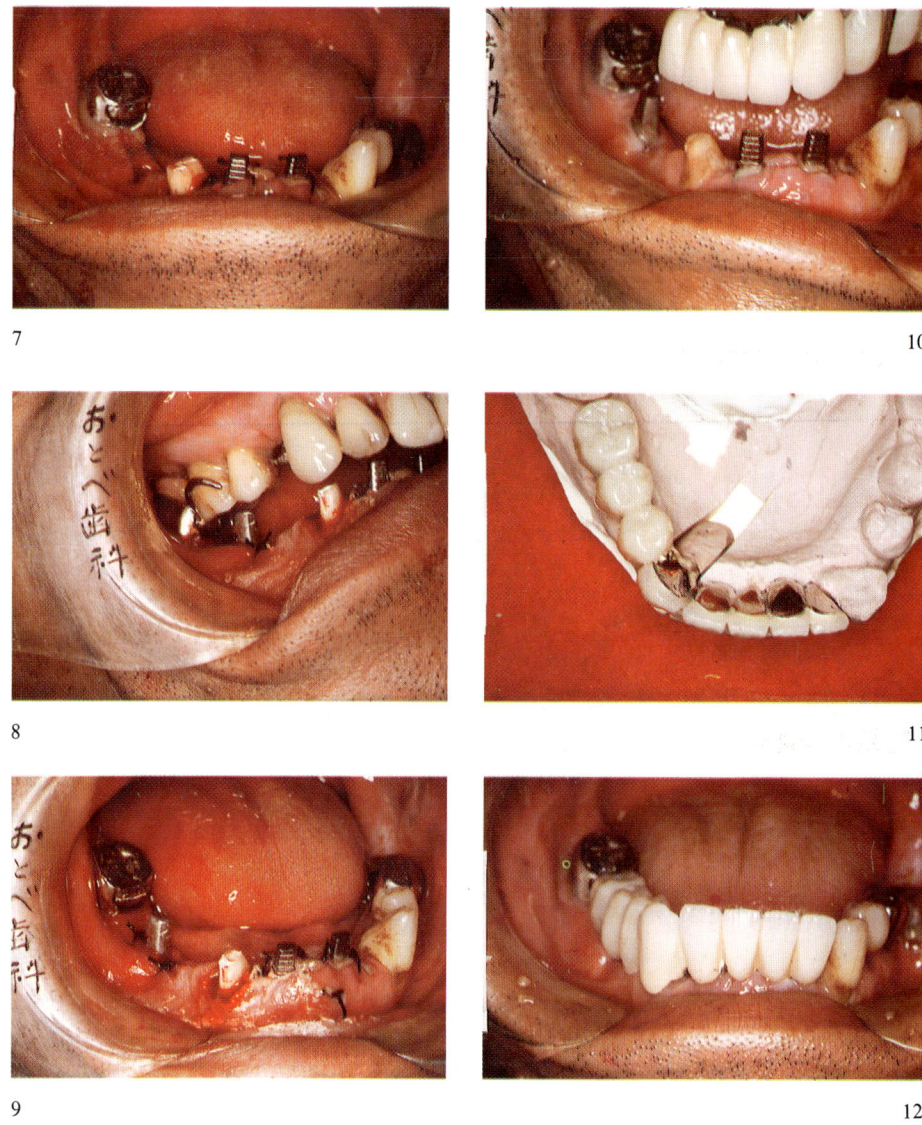

7

10

8

11

9

12

Case 5 (b)
7. Pre-molar teeth are extracted.
8. Blade inserted in the right side.
9. Blade inserted in the right side.
10. One week after the operation.
11. Superstructure.
12. Superstructure is cemented.

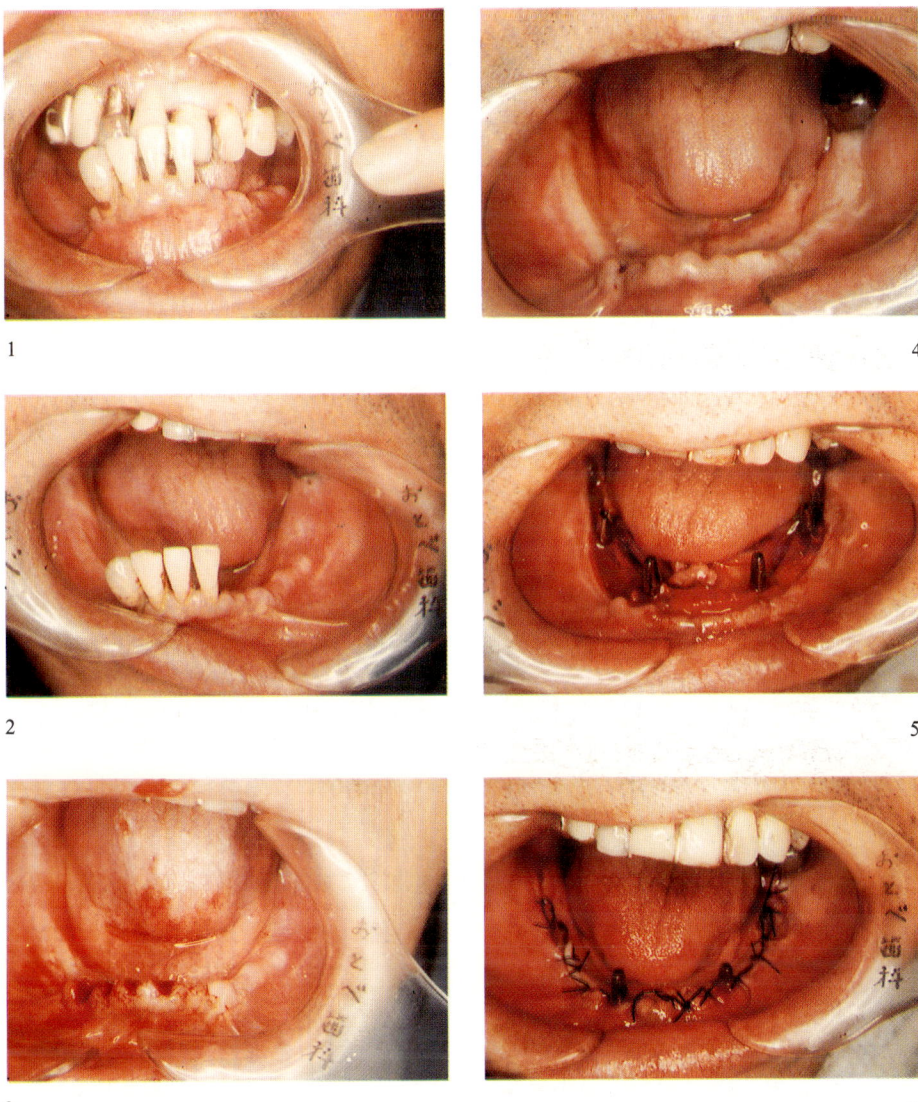

1

4

2

5

3

6

Case 6 (a)
1. Oral cavity before operation: mandibular front tooth to be extracted.
2. Mandible before operation.
3. Teeth extracted.
4. Cured site of extraction.
5. Stripping mucosa; 4 blades inserted.
6. Just sutured.

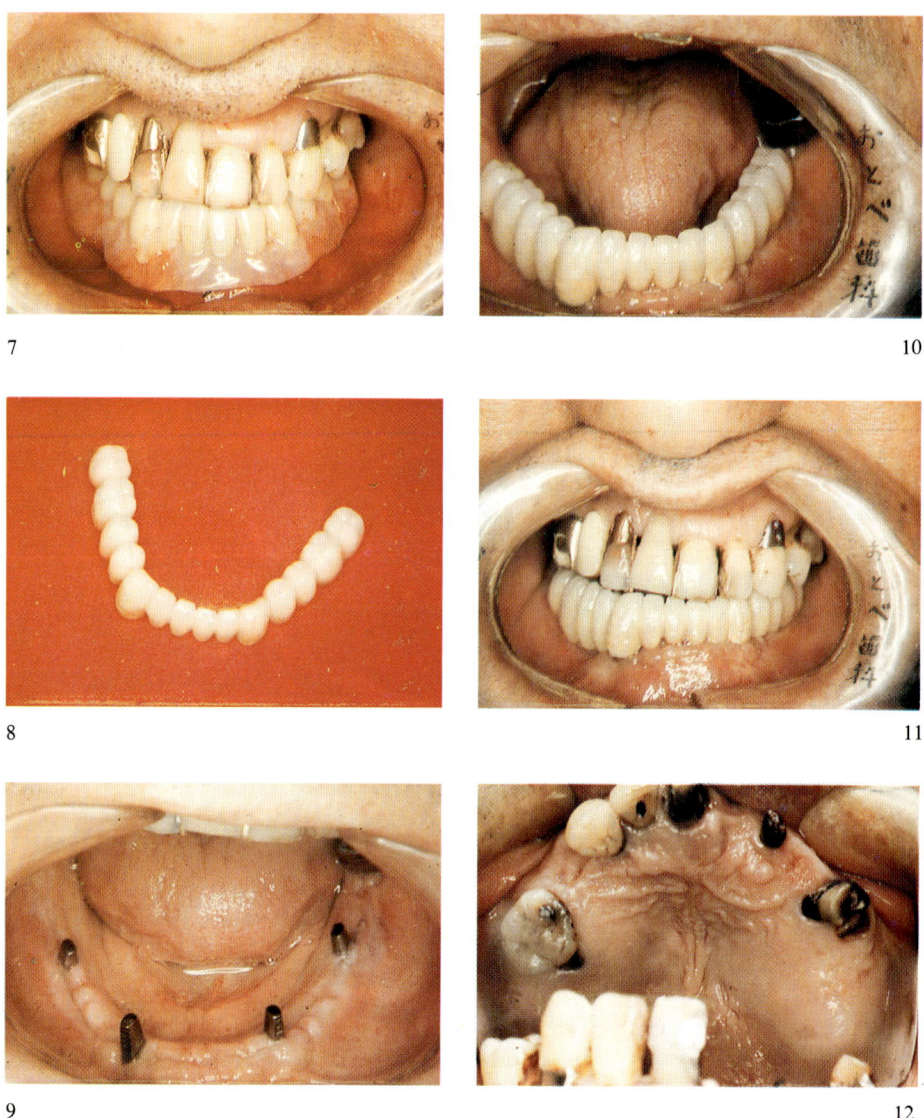

7

10

8

11

9

12

Case 6 (b)

7. Temporary denture applied: temporary denture to be prepared before operation; denture to be applied immediately after the operation.
8. This is a porcelain bridge.
9. Oral cavity 10 days after the operation.
10. Porcelain bridge cemented.
11. Mandibular implant 3 years after the operation; maxillary bone to be operated subperiosteal implant.
12. Bridge removed.

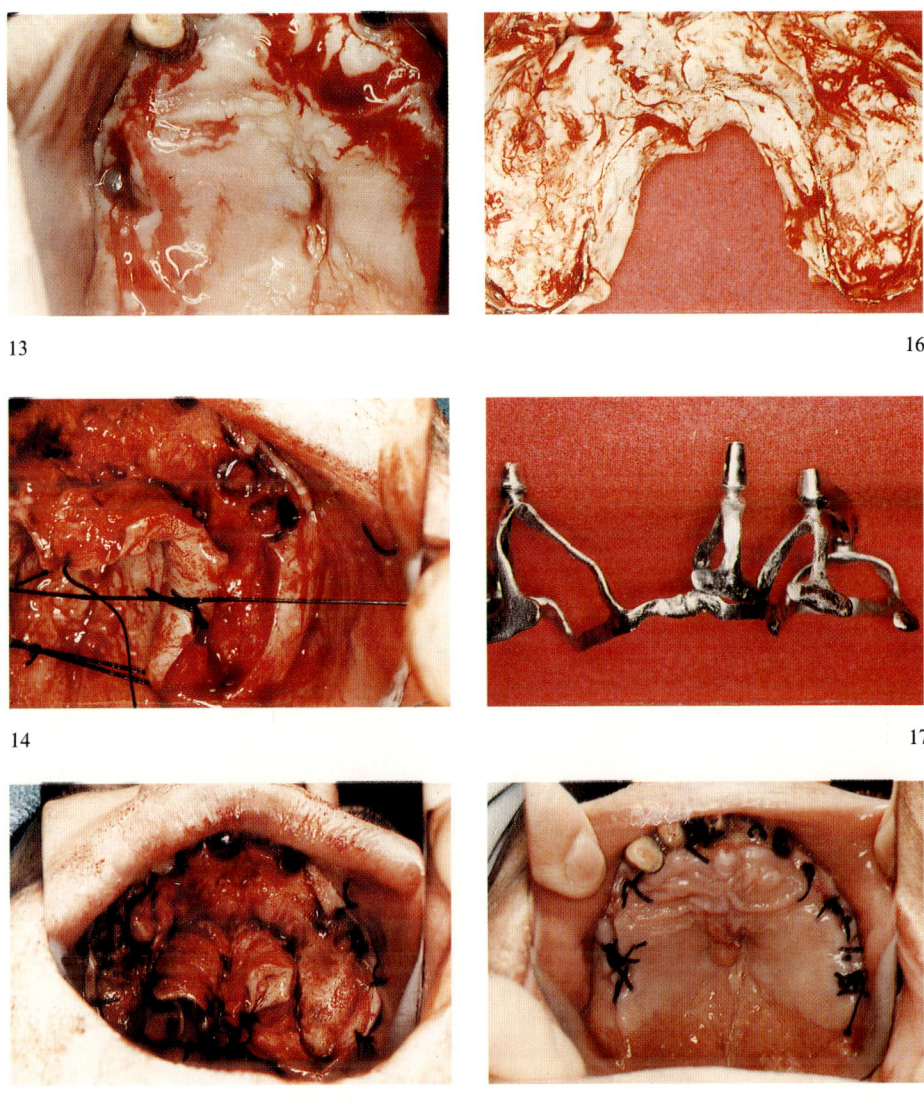

13

16

14

17

15

18

Case 6 (c)
13. Incising maxilla.
14. Stripping maxillary mucosa; maxillary bone exposed.
15. Stripping maxillary mucosa; maxillary bone exposed.
16. Impression taking of maxillary bone (the so-called bone bite).
17. Substructure.
18. One week after the first operation, reincise and expose maxillary bone again.

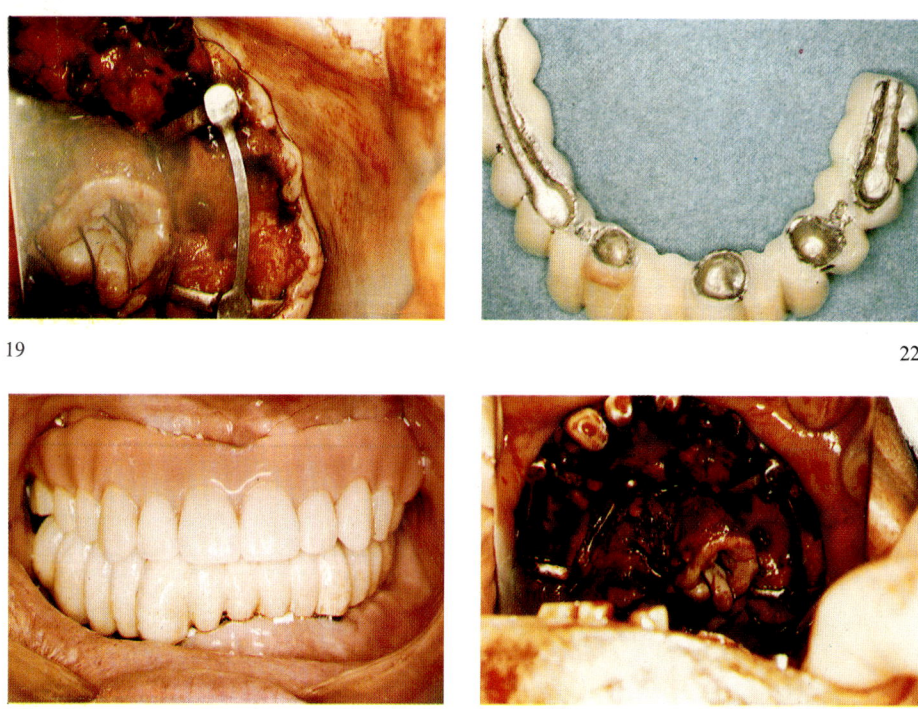

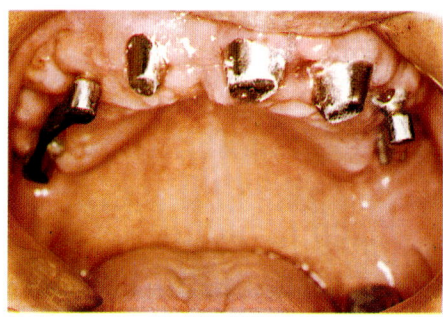

Case 6 (d)
19. Fitting substructure to maxillary.
20. Fitting substructure to maxillary bone.
21. Ten days after the operation.
22. Porcelain ceramic bridge.
23. Applying temporary denture.

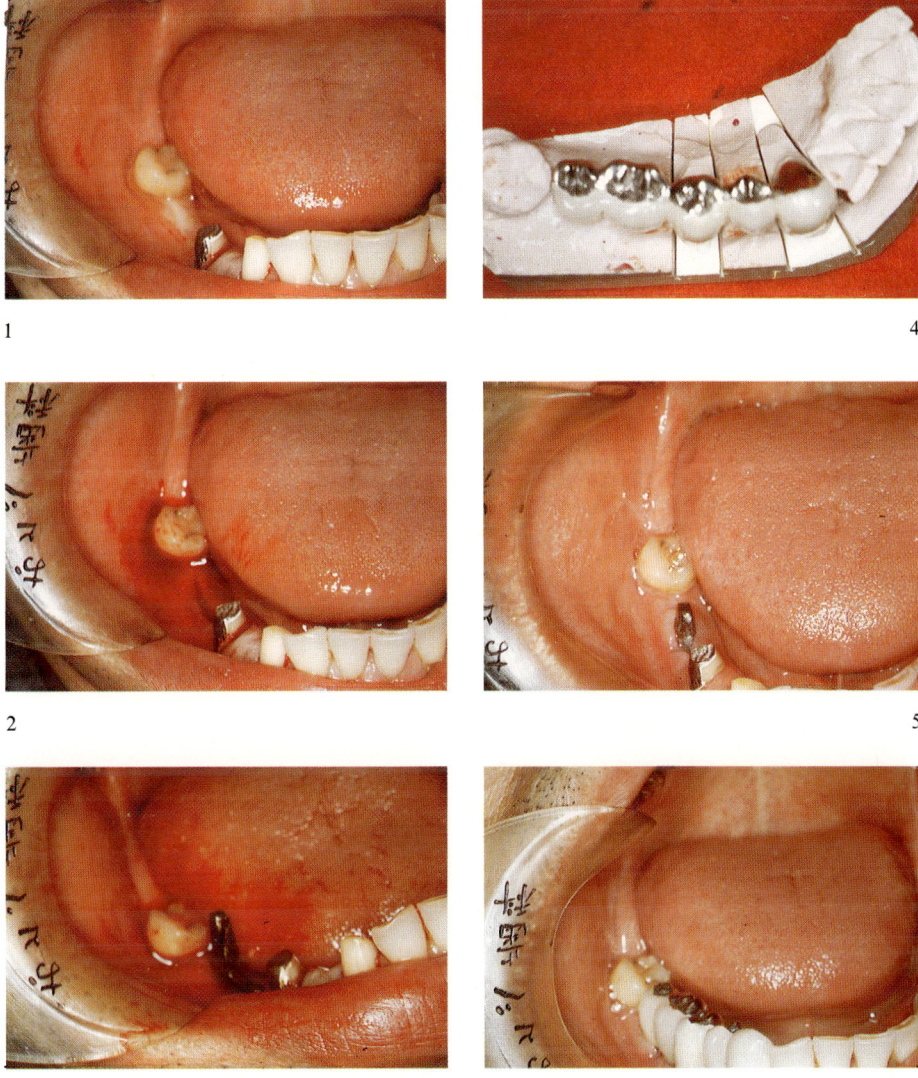

Case 7
1. Forming abutment before operation.
2. Incision.
3. Inserting blade.
4. Bridge.
5. Ten days after the operation.
6. Bridge cemented.

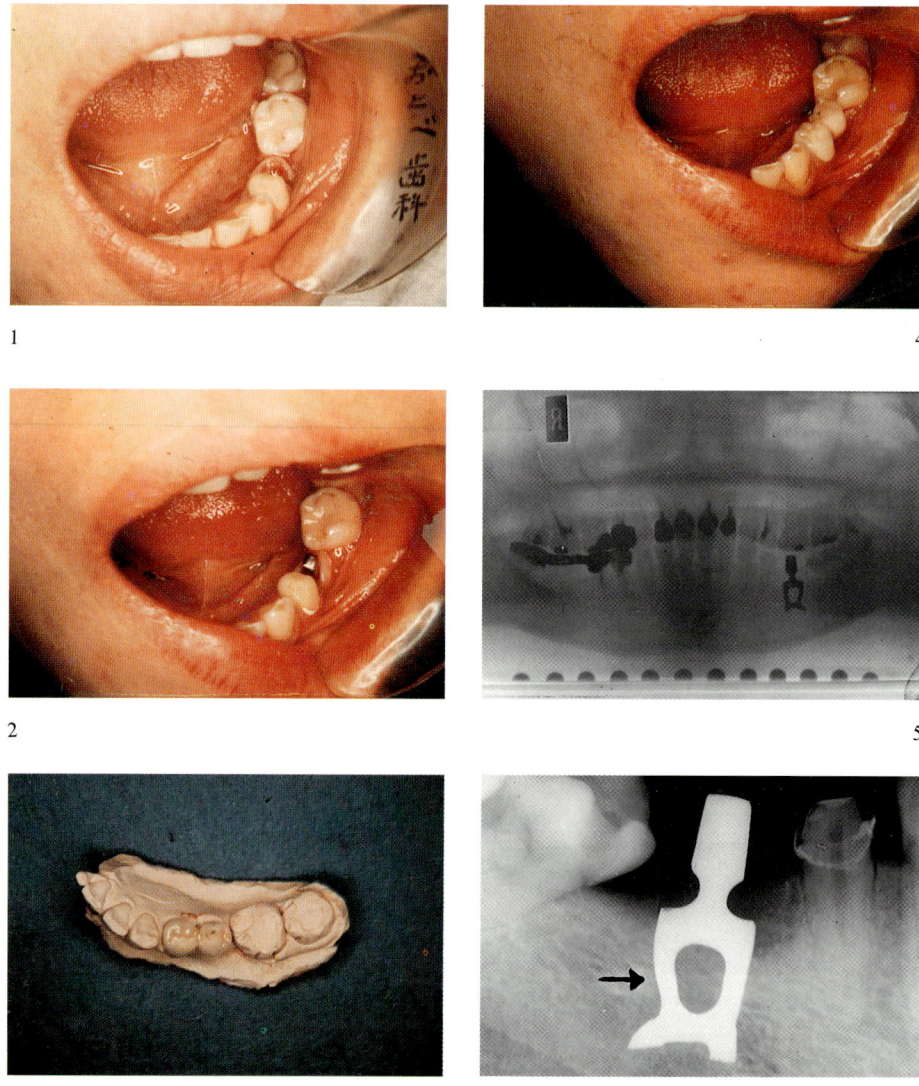

1

2

3

4

5

6

Case 8
1. Site of extracted tooth.
2. Operation site cured up in a week.
3. Model and bridge.
4. Cementing bridge.
5. Pantoma X-ray photo after the operation.
6. Dental X-ray film: Otobe's original blade having the shape after the peninsula of Italy.
   Ten years have passed after the insertion and with no trouble.

Part 4

Subperiosteal Implant

8. Subperiosteal Implant

8.1 PROBLEMS IN CLINICAL APPLICATION

Several problems arise in the clinical application of subperiosteal implants. They can be summarized in the following:

1. Unless the operator has full knowledge of oral anatomy and extensive experience in oral surgery, he or she will not be able to operate with confidence.
2. Taking an impression of the alveolar bone surface is much more difficult than taking an impression for ordinary dental treatment. At the same time, perfect accuracy is required, since a suitable substructure cannot be made from an imperfect impression.
3. The design of the substructure must also take occlusal balance into account.
4. From the point of the view of the patient, because two or more operations are required, greater pain is inevitable.

For these reasons, subperiosteal implants have been considered much more difficult than endosteal implants, and most implantologists appear to avoid their use. However, it is important that this situation be rectified. Implantologists should study and master not only endosteal implants, but also subperiosteal implants. As already discussed, there is a significant number of cases where only the latter type of implant will be suitable. To cope with all cases confidently and correctly, the implantologist must be able to perform subperiosteal implant procedures.

8.1.2 Cases of failed blade implant application

Before entering into the main subject, subperiosteal implant, let us take a short look at several cases of failed blade implant (sapphire implant) application.

1. Occlusal pressure and strength of the blade. When the occlusal pressure is stronger than the blade, the holding function of the alveolar bone cannot bear the occlusion pressure transmitted through

the implanted blade. To circumvent this, make the buccolingual diameter of the occlusal surface as small as possible, not exceeding
70% at most. Use a blade with as large a size as possible for stability.

2. Insufficient binding property of the cement. When the binding
property of the cement fixing the superstructure to the implanted
blade is inadequate, there results a disconnection or dropping off
of the cement. This happens mainly between the remaining natural
teeth and artificial teeth supported by an implanted blade, the so-
called implant bridge. About 80% of blade implant failure is traceable to the cement. This is an unavoidable drawback of the implant
bridge, trying to combine a natural tooth and a blade-supported artificial tooth.

With occlusal pressure the natural tooth sinks, while the artificial tooth and blade stand still. Repeated sinking of the natural
tooth results in cement dropping.

3. Occlusion of upper and lower alveolar arcs. In general dentistry,
occlusion simply means the relation of the upper and lower rows of
teeth when in functional contact with the activity of the mandible.
In implantology, however, occlusion refers to the alveolar arcs as

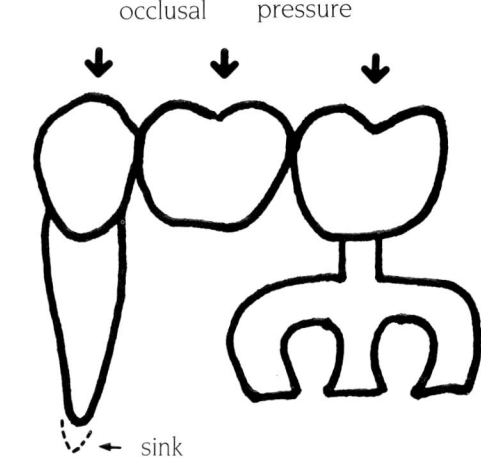

Fig. 139

well. The maxillary alveolar arc is smaller than the mandibular arc,
and the mandibular bone projects noticeably in the front-teeth
part. These observations are very important for carrying out a subperiosteal implant operation successfully.

The maxillary alveolar arc is smaller in size than the mandibular
alveolar arc.

The mandibular bone projects noticeably in the front-teeth part.

8.1.3 Maxillary bone

The maxillary bone is easily resorbed by various stimuli, including
dentures; the quality of osseous tissue is usually limited. It is therefore difficult to apply subperiosteal implant to maxillary bone. The difficulty is
less in applying subperiosteal implants to mandibular bone.

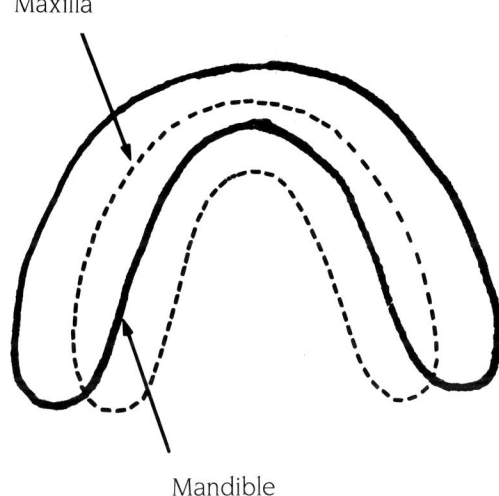

Maxilla

Mandible

Fig. 140

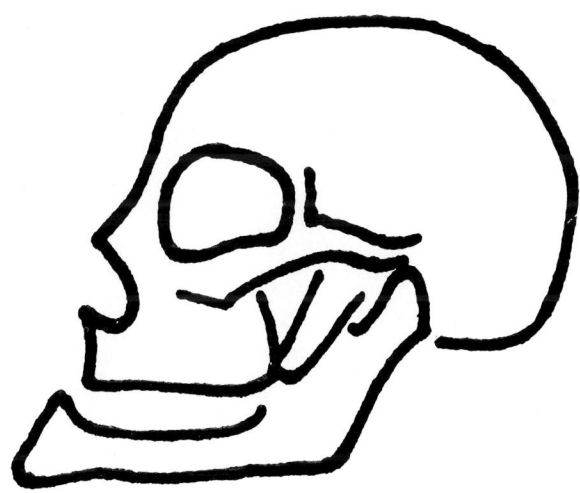

Fig. 141

Let us now consider the difficulty of performing maxillary subperiosteal implants on a step-by-step basis.

1. The osseous tissue of maxillary bone is spongy: it is not compact, but highly porous.
2. Because this tissue is spongy, it is liable to break into tiny pieces under minimal pressure; these bone pieces are then resorbed and disappear.
3. Unlike the mandibular bone surface, which is formed of cortical bone, the maxillary bone surface has no cortical bone. Particularly from the alveolar crest to the central palate, the surface of the bone is spongy, cratered and rough.
4. The spongy bone is easily resorbed as a result of friction or other external stimuli. Thus, for example, when occlusion presses the denture base, it may cause resorption of spongy bone. Consequently, gaps arise between the denture base and the mucosa; finally, the denture may fall out.
5. The sinus is too close to the bone surface. That is, there is a very limited quantity of osseous tissue between the sinus and the bone surface.
6. Strong occlusal pressure exerted on the maxillary bone is supported by only two points, the nasal spine and the pterygoid extension.
7. The palatal bone is extremely thin and is formed of spongy tissue. Therefore, it cannot resist strong occlusal pressure.
8. The maxillary bone bordering the molar arch has a smooth surface and looks as hard as cortical bone. It is, however, extremely thin and easily resorbed under pressure.

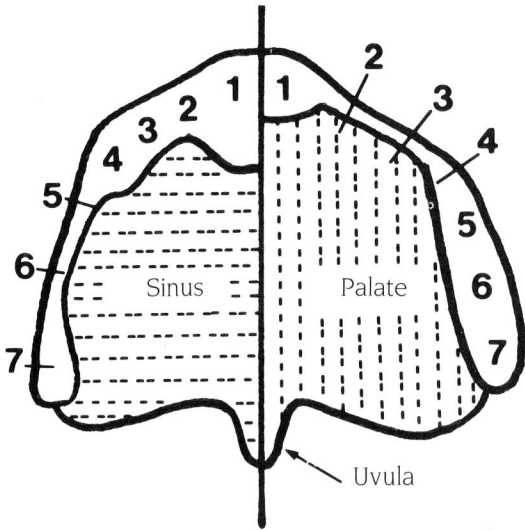

Fig. 142

As mentioned, one of the crucial factors in subperiosteal implants is accurate judgment of the quantity of remaining bone tissue. This judgment is the basis of substructure design.

The left side of Figure 142 shows the depth of the alveolar bone from its surface to the sinus, and thus indicates the quantity of remaining bone. The right side shows the width of the buccal-palatine alveolar crest. According to the figure, the width of region 6 is the thinnest. Applying an endosteal implant in this region is practically impossible due to the danger of perforating the sinus.

In the palate, regions 2 and 3 buccal-palatally are the thinniest. It would be difficult to prepare a channel for blade implants in these regions.

Where there is much resorbed maxillary bone, endosteal implants cannot be applied and subperiosteal implants are indicated.

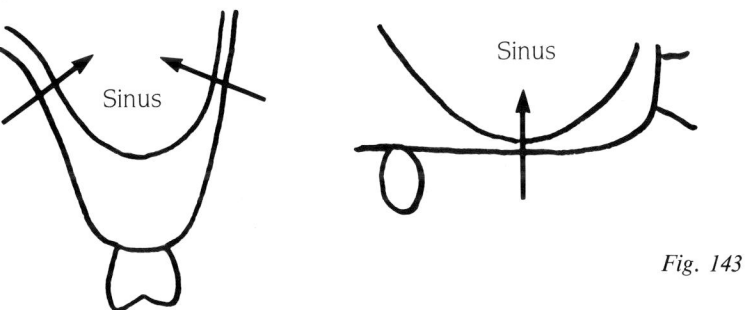

Fig. 143

The arrows in Figure 143 show areas of possible perforation of the sinus.

As revealed in the preceding discussion, there are several areas in which the maxillary bone is most hard and solid, so that strong occlusion pressure can be effectively received and dispersed. These areas include the following:

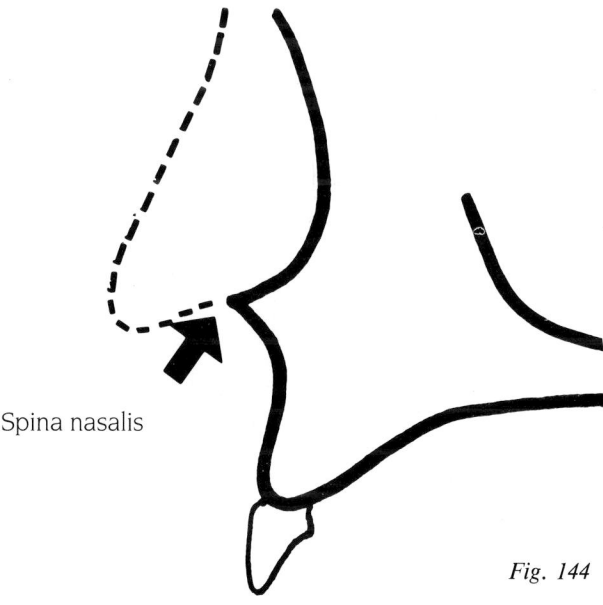

Spina nasalis

Fig. 144

1. The nasal spine, which is located below the nasal cavity, on the buccal median.
2. The area around the incisive canal opening, that is, the opening of the nasopalatine nerves. Here the nasal septum and maxillary bone are firmly sutured together.

Here, the maxillary bone is sutured to the nasal septum and connected to the bottom of the cranium. Pressures can be supported effectively, even strong occlusal pressures.

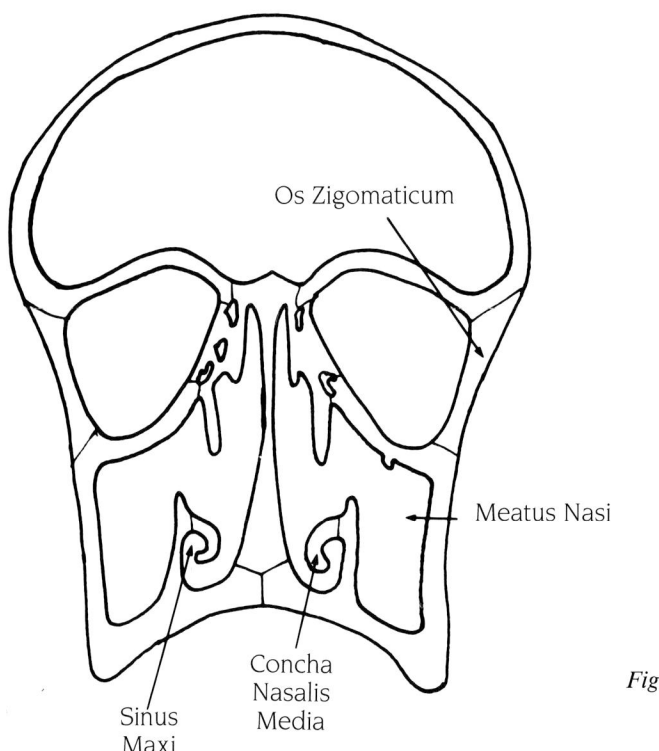

Fig. 145

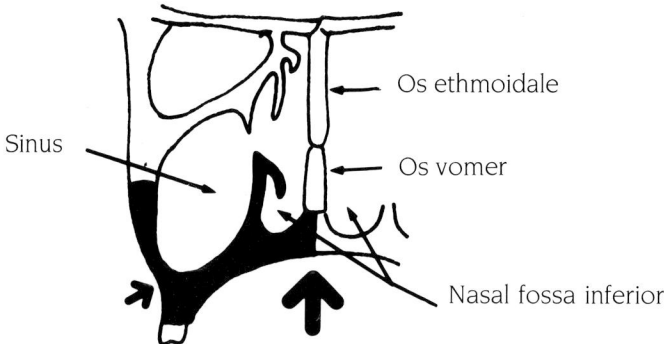

Fig. 146

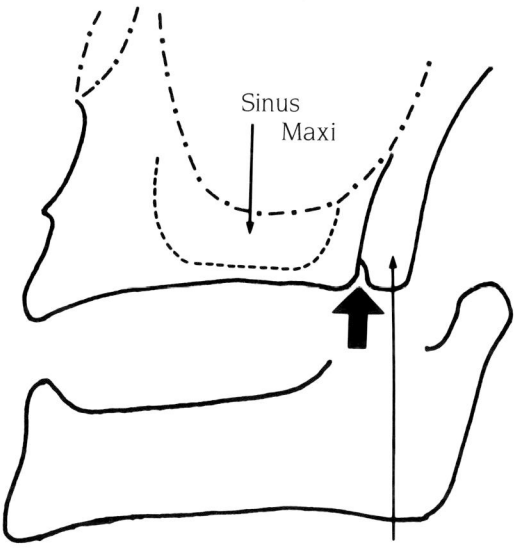

Hamulus Pterygoideus   *Fig. 147*

3. The symphysis of the posterior wall of the maxillary bone and the pterygoid extension is approximately 10 mm long. This is also a suitable region to receive and disperse strong occlusal pressure.
4. In the region where the maxillary bone borders the molar arch, the surface of the bone is wide and flat, resembling the surface of cortical bone. As already noted, however, this region is located too close to the sinus, and the thickness of bone is not sufficient to bear high pressure, such as occlusal pressure. There is the possibility that

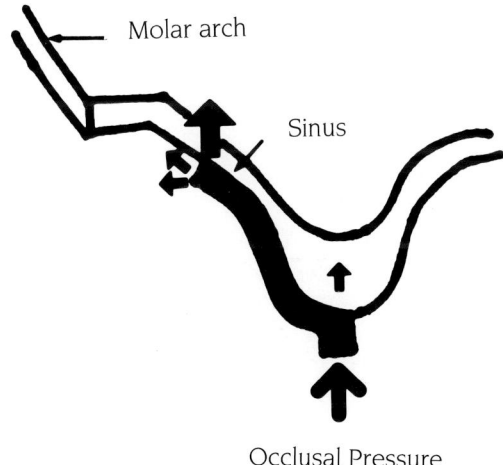

Occlusal Pressure

Fig. 148

the sinus could be perforated. It should be noted that subperiosteal implant failures are caused by unexpected resorption of the bone in this region.

Making a peripheral border or strut of the substructure may result in perforation of the sinus.

N --- Spina nasalis   S --- Sinus

A --- Arcus zygomaticus

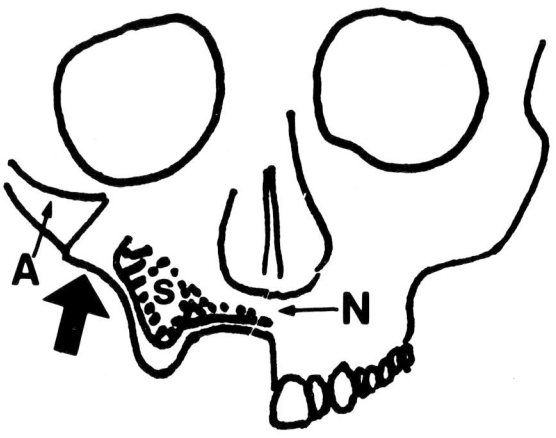

Fig. 149

5. The region of the maxillary bone just in front of the suture, with the molar arch, is very hard and usually thick enough; this is also the part where occlusal pressure is exerted perpendicularly.

Figure 149 shows the suture region of the maxillary bone and molar arch. The arrow indicates where the peripheral border is to be placed and strong occlusal pressure is dispersed.

8.2 DIAGNOSIS

One of the motives for careful diagnosis is to prevent incorrect or excessive treatment. Unfortunately, implants are sometimes performed when ordinary conservative treatment would have sufficed. I am aware of one case at least where a subperiosteal implant was performed when an endosteal implant would have been appropriate.

8.2.1 Principles of diagnosis

There are several guiding principles for diagnosis in implantology:
1. An endosteal implant is selected when sufficient osseous tissue is found.
2. A subperiosteal implant is indicated when the amount of osseous tissues found is insufficient for an endosteal implant.
3. An implant should be applied only when it is really necessary.
4. Do not implant immediately after an extraction unless absolutely necessary.

    To disregard any of these principles in applying an implant is unwise and potentially very dangerous.

8.2.2 Check points of diagnosis

As with an endosteal implant, the dental and medical records of the patient should be carefully checked and the patient questioned in detail. Questions should include the following:

1. How long have you been edentulous? How many years have you been wearing your full denture?
2. How many times have you replaced or readjusted your denture base?
3. Have you ever suffered from glycosuria in the past? Do you at present suffer from glycosuria?
4. Why and how were your teeth extracted?
   a) Was the extraction due to pyorrhea alveolaris?
   b) Was the extraction due to leaving decayed, untreated teeth?
5. Have you ever suffered from heart disease? Is your blood pressure normal?
6. Have you ever suffered from anemia? Are you suffering from anemia now?

Each of these questions is considered in detail below.

8.2.2.1 How long a full denture has been worn

When a full denture is worn, the occlusal pressure is transmitted to the alveolar bone through the oral mucosa. The alveolar bone consequently becomes involuted and resorbed. In contrast, inner stimuli are not associated with resorption. Excessively strong stimuli may, of course, seriously damage the tooth root. Moderate and regular stimuli will accelerate the metabolism of the alveolar bone and are indispensable to keeping bone healthy.

The denture base will vibrate slightly under occlusal pressure whenever the wearer eats or speaks. No denture designer, however expert, can prevent this microvibration. Although small at first, the vibrations are harmful to the alveolar bone surface. Repeated vibration of the denture base causes resorption of the bone and the vibrations increase as resorption progresses. Thus, we have a vicious circle in which the alveolar bone shrinks rapidly. In view of this process the first question to ask patients is how long have they been wearing a full denture. A reply of 5 years should make the operator aware of a possible need for a subperiosteal implant.

In my experience, it is after about 5 years that most patients find their full dentures inefficient and uncomfortable, and hence begin looking for a dependable alternative. By then resorption has caused the denture base to loosen to a point where the denture may easily and frequently fall out. It is necessary then to either rebase the denture, which is troublesome, or replace it, which is expensive.

An endosteal implant, of course, prevents the resorption of the bone by providing stimuli to the bone through the implanted blade, pin or button.

8.2.2.2 How many times the denture has been readjusted

As explained in the preceding subsection, if the denture of the patient has been rebased because the alveolar bone has been resorbed, an endosteal implant may not be possible.

8.2.2.3 The patient and glycosuria

With a patient who has suffered from glycosuria, it is necessary to be extremely cautious about performing any form of surgery, including an implantological operation. The prognosis and recuperation after the initial operation are usually less favorable if the patient is diabetic. The patient's physician should be contacted and the operation performed when the patient's blood sugar is as low as possible.

Typically, the problems are the following. The recovery after the suturing may be slow and resuturing may even be necessary. Moreover, the suturing material may become coated with a tartarlike substance two or three days after the operation. The incised wound may also become coated with this tartarlike substance; sometimes the coating is as deep as the alveolar bone surface. Due to the tartar coat, the alveolar bone surface may become exposed. This coating progresses with increasing rapidity and a wide area of the alveolar bone is finally exposed, so that there is a paucity of mucosa. If the coating comes to the abutment of the substructure, the abutment must be cleaned carefully before the superstructure is fitted. The cleaning process is not a simple one, however, and the abutment may become recoated within a week.

8.2.2.4 When and how the teeth were extracted

The condition of the patient's alveolar bone will depend largely on the condition of the teeth when they were extracted. In order to disperse occlusal pressure effectively, the root of the tooth ideally should be two times longer than the crown (Fig. 150).

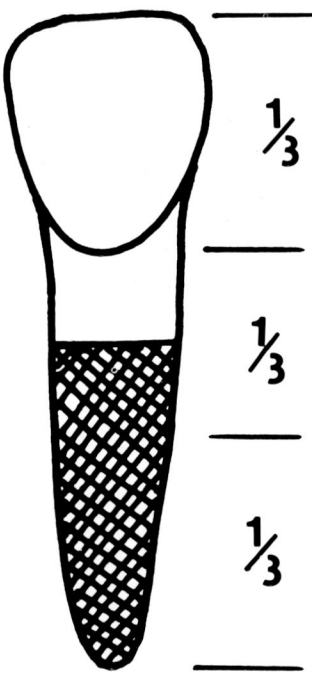

Fig. 150

The direction and diameter of the natural tooth root varies among individuals according to the direction and intensity of the occlusal pressure exerted on the tooth. The stronger the occlusal pressure, the greater the diameter of the tooth root. The tooth root curves in accordance with the direction in which the occlusal pressure is exerted on the tooth. When the occlusal pressure is exerted vertically, the tooth root is almost straight (Fig. 151). When the occlusal pressure is exerted diagonally, the root curves to withstand and disperse the pressure effectively.

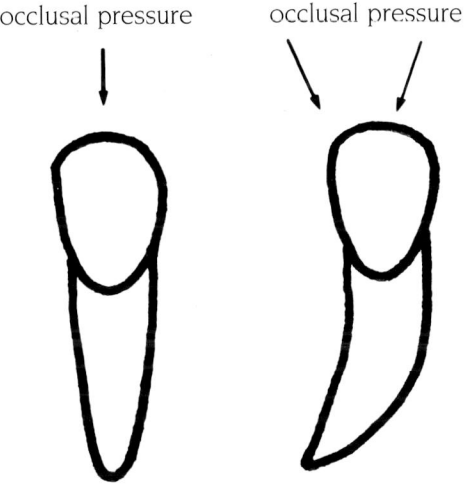

Fig. 151

8.2.2.5 *Pyorrhea alveolaris*

In pyorrhea alveolaris, the alveolar bone is resorbed and shrinks, exposing the upper part of the tooth root. The exposed root is a sign that occlusal pressure is no longer balanced and the capacity of the alveolar bone to hold teeth in place is diminished. Once begun, this process accelerates rapidly. The lost balance causes vibration of the tooth; this, in turn, damages the alveolar bone. Thus, there again arises a vicious circle, which continues until the tooth eventually falls out. In the case where damage has progressed to the cusp of the tooth root, the tooth is easily extracted: fingertips will suffice, or even the slight pressure of the injection of the

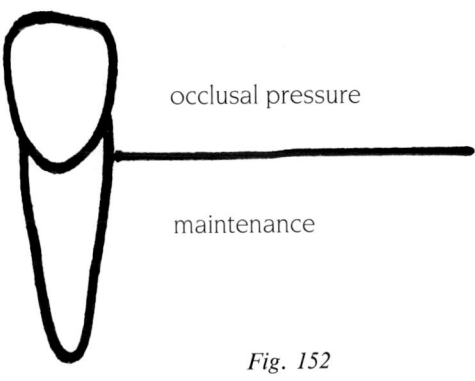

Fig. 152

anesthetic. The recess of the extracted tooth will heal within a day or two. This is an extreme case, of course, but in general very little alveolar bone remains when a tooth is extracted following pyorrhea alveolaris.

Before the damage reaches the root cusp, vibration of the tooth causes pain. Extracting the tooth at this early stage may have the merit of preventing extreme resorption of the alveolar bone. I do not mean, of course, that a decayed tooth must always be extracted as soon as possible. Rather, from the viewpoint of protecting the alveolar bone, it is not always correct to try to preserve a tooth that is affected by pyorrhea alveolaris as long as possible. I extract a tooth only if more than one-half of the root is exposed. In such cases the process has progressed too far for the tooth to be held in the alveolar bone, and the alveolar bone itself should be protected.

Whether a sufficient quantity of osseous tissue still remains in the alveolar bone, it naturally affects the condition of the mucosa covering the bone. This is the key factor separating successful and unsuccessful subperiosteal implant operations, for reasons that will be explained in more detail later.

With pyorrhea alveolaris the resorption of mandibular bone will alter progress to the point where pantomoradiograms show an unbelievably thin mandible, which looks as if it could be fractured with just a little external pressure.

As for the maxillary bone, in certain cases it will consist of only the bottom of the maxillary sinus and nothing more. There are also cases in which even the osseous tissue at the bottom of the maxillary sinus will have already been resorbed and disappeared; it is closed with soft tissue, a kind of cartilage, instead.

The cases above, needless to say, present the most severe difficulties in designing maxillary and mandibular denture bases, as well as performing an implant procedure.

Questioning the patient about the condition of the extracted tooth turns out to be very important here. This questioning should be carried on in a careful and effective manner, because it might yield information relevant to the diagnosis.

Here let us consider the case of the patient who has suffered from pyorrhea alveolaris or from glycosuria. Inspection of the patient's oral cavity sometimes reveals a large quantity of tartar coating on both the remaining natural teeth and the denture base. Generally speaking, the degree of tartar coating depends largely on the density and viscosity of the patient's saliva. Thus, it is important to note when patients have saliva of a high density and viscosity. In such cases, the post of the implant might easily become coated by tartar. Postoperative coating of the implant head and surrounding parts of the blade is of course undesirable, for not only is it unsanitary, but it may also shorten the life span of the implant.

Cleaning up and removing tartar around the implant head at least once a year is highly recommended. The implantologist should follow the patients and instruct them in proper care.

It is my conviction that an implant must be properly cared for by the wearer in the same way that he or she cared for the natural teeth. Of course, the implanted blade, pin or button, and the substructure are not natural but artificial and are generally composed of biometal or ceramic. They nonetheless require daily care, preferably each morning after getting up and each night before going to bed. In fact, an implant that is not properly cared for may be affected by pyorrhea alveolaris. An implant should never be coated by tartar.

The durability of an implant depends largely on the attitude and habits of the wearer. If daily cleaning is neglected, regardless of how accurate the design and how skillful the operation, the implant may last no longer than two or three years. There have been cases in which the substructure implanted in the mandibular bone was found coated with tartar. Here again, a maximum of two or three years' durability can be expected. In consideration of the density and viscosity of saliva, the substructure should be designed so that the implant head is exposed for easy daily cleaning (Fig. 153). This serves to extend the life span of the implant.

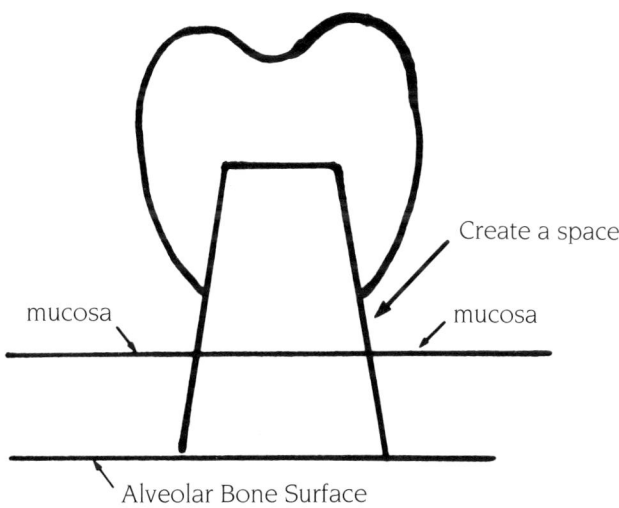

Fig. 153 This part of the implant head should be exposed.

8.2.2.6 The patient and heart disease or anemia

Before performing an implant operation, it is crucial to ascertain whether the patient has suffered from heart disease or anemia. The patient must also be checked for high blood pressure. If the patient has any of these symptoms, the implant operation may need to be avoided.

I was once called for an opinion during a subperiosteal implant operation because the patient had taken a turn for the worse. I asked that the operation be stopped at once and the incised wound be sutured. Arriving at the scene of the operation I found the patient extremely anemic and his pulse irregular. The operator later told me that his patient had suffered from anemia. Had this operation not been stopped when it had, the patient might have died. This medical accident should never have happened.

The subperiosteal implant operation is a serious one. As discussed, it involves removing a relatively wide portion of oral mucosa and bleeding may be extensive. With diabetic patients, bleeding may not be stopped by the normal techniques, and the amount of bleeding is usually much greater.

8.3 PARTS OF THE SUBSTRUCTURE

8.3.1 Abutment
Most of the metal substructure will be covered by the mucosa. Only the abutment remains exposed in the oral cavity. The abutment of the substructure corresponds to the head of the blade. The substructure makes use of the abutment as its base.

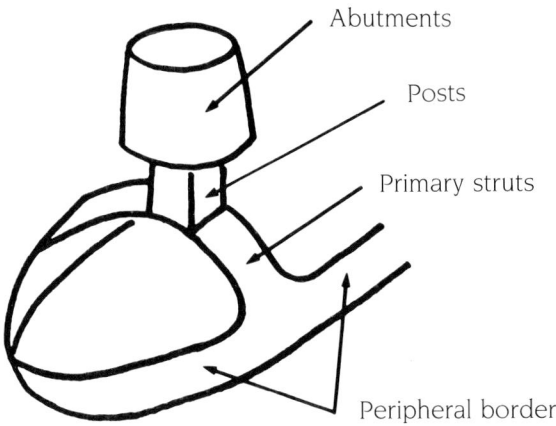

Fig. 154

The abutment should be implanted in the mandibular bone where the condition of the bone is best and is in the best position with respect to bone bite to the opposing tooth. The number of abutments used depends on the design of the substructure and/or the condition of the mandibular bone.

8.3.2 Post
The post is the lower part of the abutment. It is 2 or 3 mm in length, depending on the dimension of the mucosa. Its diameter should generally not exceed 2 mm. The post may be compared to the neck of the blade; it is, however, somewhat different in function. Ideally, the post should be covered and held by the surrounding mucosa. In order to prevent possible exposure of the metal, care must be exercised in suturing the mucosa around the post.

8.3.3 Peripheral border
Most of the occlusal pressure on the substructure is transmitted to the mandible through the peripheral border. The metallic peripheral border is covered with periosteum, with which, ideally, it is completely united, just like a part of the natural mandibular bone. No gap should be left between the peripheral border and the surface of the mandibular bone. Such a gap may occur if the substructure was prepared according to an inaccurate impression.

The peripheral border should be less than 2 mm wide and less than 1 mm thick. If a thicker peripheral border is implanted, the covering mucosa cannot remain flat but will be partly raised where it covers the peripheral border. This in turn makes the oral cavity narrower, spoiling the natural feeling of the tongue and sometimes causing difficulties in pronunciation.

The right side of Figure 155 shows a substructure that is fitted improperly to the bone surface. Periosteum is wedged between the bone surface and the substructure, and the substructure is covered directly by mucosa. This sandwiched periosteum always causes a problem afterward.

The left side of Figure 155 shows a substructure that is perfectly fitted to the bone surface; the substructure is covered tightly first by the periosteum and then by the mucosa.

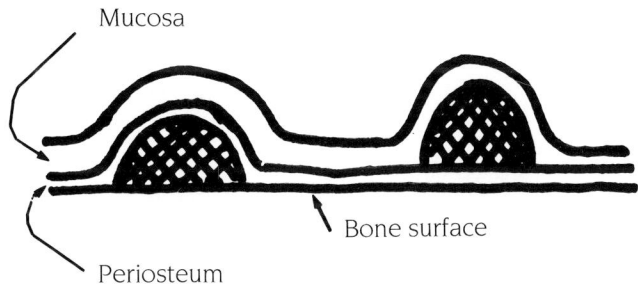

Fig. 155

8.3.4 Primary strut

The primary strut connects the peripheral border to the post. As with the peripheral border, the primary strut must be fitted perfectly to the bone surface. A misfitted primary strut will cause continual pain, so that another operation will be necessary to remove it. Moreover, resorption of the bone is accelerated around the misfitted parts. Thus, if the primary strut is found misfitted during the second stage of the operation, a more precise impression should be taken at this point.

The best results are usually obtained by using fewer pieces of primary strut. Generally speaking, the optimum number of pieces is as follows:

Maxillary bone: 1 piece in the buccal side, 2 pieces in the lingual side.

Mandibular bone: 2 pieces in the buccal side, 1 piece in the lingual side.

Use of more pieces of primary strut will not bring favorable results.

Before proceeding to the next section, I would like to add a word of warning. Although there are principles for designing the substructure, clinical cases may vary significantly. An inexperienced implantologist should therefore obtain the advice of an experienced colleague or simply leave the whole design to the expert.

8.4 MUCOSA STRIPPING

8.4.1 General remarks

The key point of successful subperiosteal implantation is taking an accurate impression. This requires stripping the mucosa and, more precisely, the periosteum in sufficient dimensions.

In order to take an accurate impression on the exposed bone surface after stripping the mucosa, the mucosa usually should be stripped in broader and wider dimensions than an inexperienced implantologist would estimate.

There are two primary principles for taking an implantological impression on the bone surface:

1. No more than 70% of the dimensions of the bone surface where the mucosa and periosteum have been stripped can be used for taking an impression.
2. No more than 70% of the dimensions of the resultant impression is usable for the substructure.

At first sight, the stripped mucosa may appear to have sufficient dimensions. However, frequently the prepared plaster model is found later to be much smaller than expected, and consequently the prepared substructure is also much smaller and therefore ineffective. This is because of the short dimensions of the stripped mucosa, as explained above.

It is important to remember that for a subperiosteal implant operation the mucosa must be stripped as widely as possible. In this regard here is my theory of 70% x 70% = 49%, which I have repeatedly published for ten years in connection with the annual meetings of the AAID. According to this theory, less than one-half the dimensions of the stripped mucosa can be used to design the substructure.

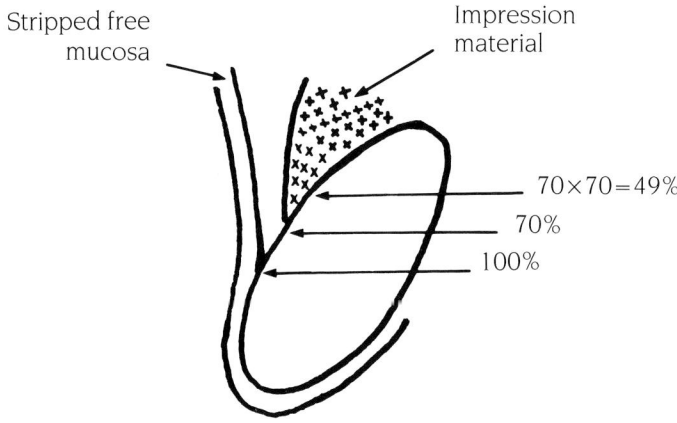

Fig. 156 Usable portion of plaster model prepared from the impression.

My theory is now widely accepted, and many prominent implantologists in the world recognize its merit. It is my regret, however, that only in Japan has my theory not yet been accepted by many self-appointed experts in the field of implantology.

The theory of 70% x 70% = 49% is explained by the following. An impression is made by pressing and pushing impression material on the bone surface after the mucosa has been stripped. Then there are only small spaces left between the bone surface and the stripped-free mucosa. Moreover, due to the force of restitution of the stripped mucosa, impression materials pushed into the deepest regions of the operation site are pushed back again with strength.

Suppose the impression could fortunately be taken into the deepest regions. The impression obtained after hardening of the material is usually found to be very thin in the outermost parts. The plaster model thus might be deformed in the outer regions. Such deformed parts, of course, cannot be used for precise design of the substructure to be implanted.

After the substructure is inserted, it may happen that the metal part of the substructure emerges, breaking the sutured mucosa and becoming exposed in the oral cavity. This is because the dimensions of the stripped mucosa were quite insufficient with respect to the flexibility of the mucosa to containing the substructure after suturing. That is, the sutured mucosa cannot hold the substructure inside.

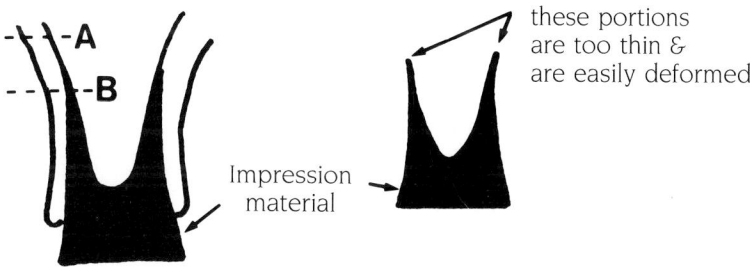

Fig. 157 Stripping is insufficient and thus the impression material is pushed back at the deepest portion.

Exposure of the substructure in the oral cavity is, of course, one of the most dangerous consequences of a subperiosteal implant. Much care must be exercised, therefore, to strip the mucosa wide enough.

Before stripping the mucosa, always keep in mind the following three points:

1. Restitution of the force of the free mucosa: the small space between stripped mucosa and the bone surface.
2. Deformation in the outermost parts due to thinness of the obtained impression.
3. Precaution when exposing substructure metal in the oral cavity.

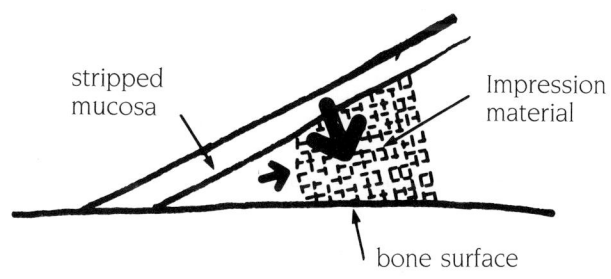

Fig. 158 Impression material inserted in the deepest region is pushed back by restituting reaction of the stripped mucosa.

8.4.2 Preliminary arrangements

The thickness of the mucosa should be measured precisely. This can be done with an injection needle during the time of applying the local anesthetic.

The study model is made in advance, and the location of the abutments should be tentatively determined before performing the operation. By measuring the thickness of the mucosa where the abutments are to be implanted, the length of the substructure post is determined. Measuring on the study model is, however, restricted to rough planning. More accurate measuring is done following anesthesia.

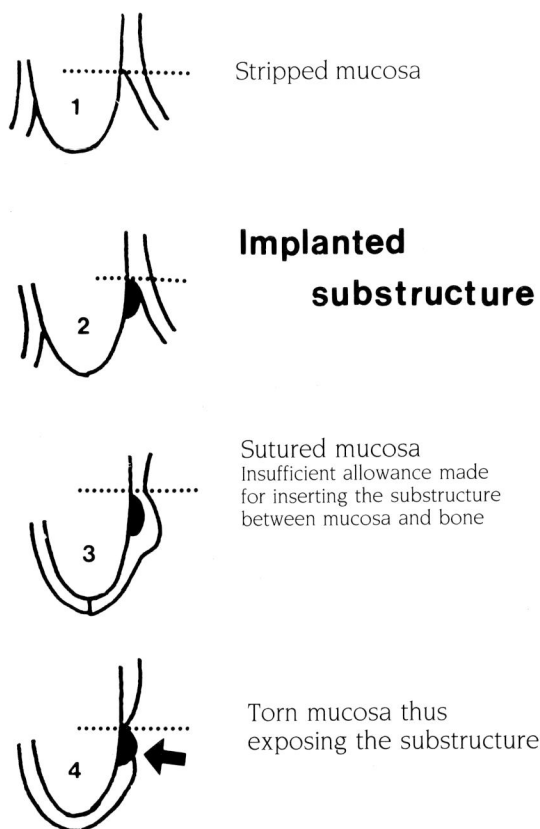

Stripped mucosa

Implanted

substructure

Sutured mucosa
Insufficient allowance made
for inserting the substructure
between mucosa and bone

Torn mucosa thus
exposing the substructure

Fig. 159

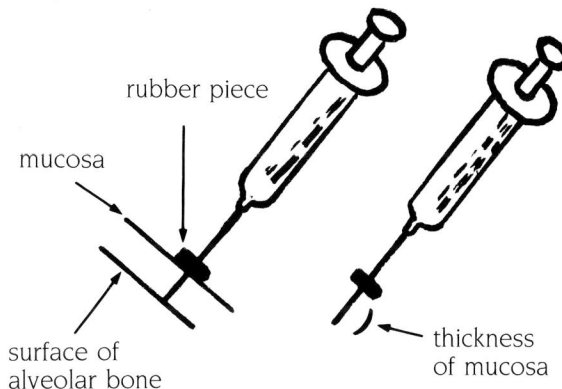

Fig. 160

A cross incision is done along the lip frenulum, whether the operation is performed in the maxillary bone or the mandibular bone (Fig. 161). An incision in another region could mean that part of the primary strut of the peripheral border is exposed in the oral cavity. Thus, a cross incision should never be attempted in the cuspid root or molar root region.

Where the mandible has atrophied, the mandibular canal is sometimes exposed in front of the ramus in the oral cavity. Ordinarily, the mandibu-

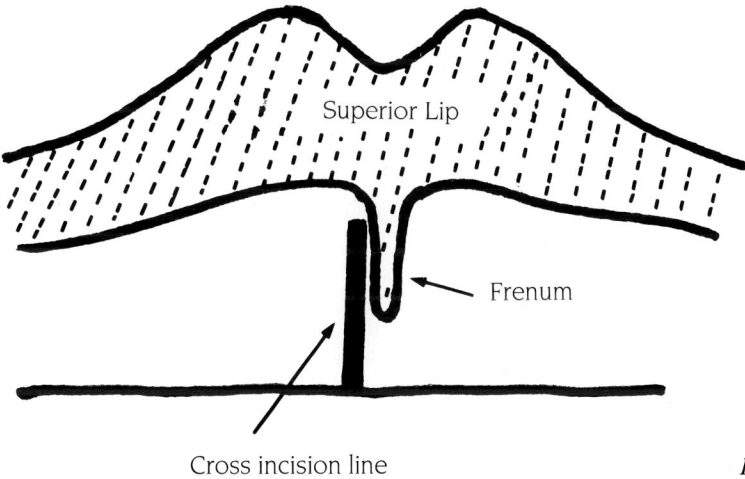

Fig. 161

lar canal is located inside the mandibular bone near the lower end of the mandible. Because atrophy of the bone progresses in this area, however, the canal appears to shift upward.

This shift functions to protect the canal from fracture, which is a more serious possibility, because the mandible has become thinner.

With an atrophied mandible, therefore, the location of the mandibular canal should be carefully confirmed in advance, through x-ray diagnosis. In addition, special precautions should be taken when the incision is made.

For a safer incision, wherever possible, instead of incising the middle portion of the mandibular mucosa, the lingual side should be selected. Never try to incise the buccal side of the mandibular mucosa. As already explained, this is to be avoided because of the difference in size between the mandibular alveolar arch and the maxillary alveolar arch.

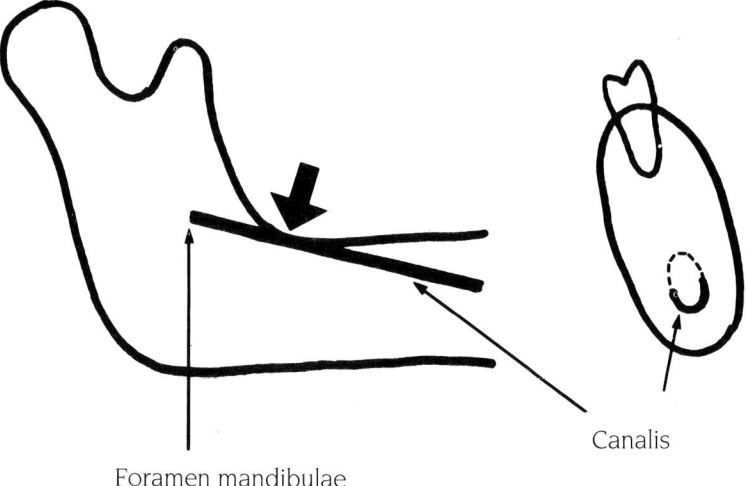

Foramen mandibulae

Canalis

Fig. 162

The posterior abutments of the substructure for the mandible are implanted along the lingual edge. The incision line of this portion is therefore set in the lingual side. This is also helpful to avoid possible damage to the exposed mandibular canal.

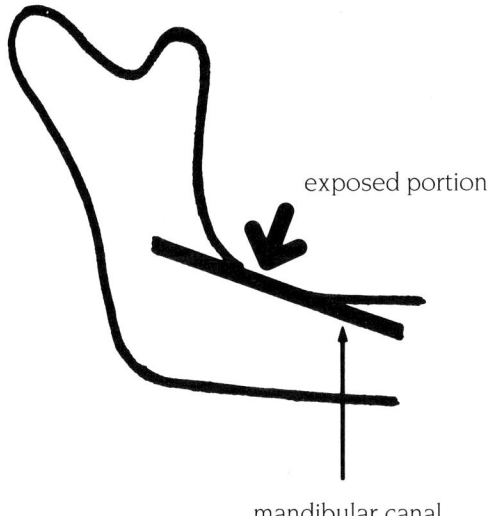

exposed portion

mandibular canal

Fig. 163

8.4.3 Detailed steps

8.4.3.1 Nasal palatine nerve (Foramen incisivum)

In the case of an atrophied maxilla, the foramen incisivum may be located in the median apex of the alveolar bone moved from its original anatomical position (Fig. 164).

Care should be taken not to damage nerve fibers in making the incision, although these fibers are also stripped later when stripping the mucosa. The mucosa is stripped approximately 15 mm from the incisor foramen to the palatine side. This is the optimum dimension of the mucosa to be stripped in this region.

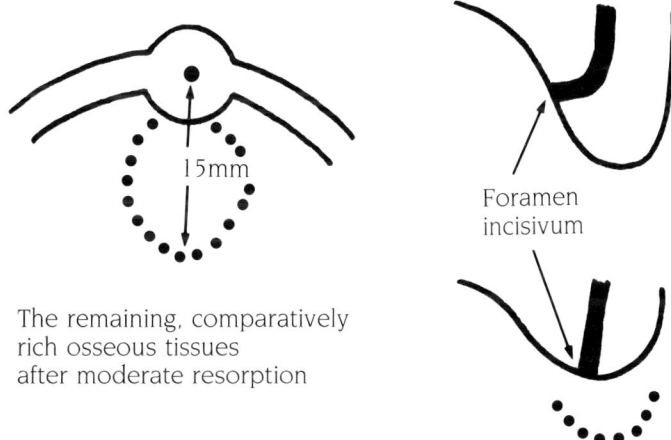

The remaining, comparatively
rich osseous tissues
after moderate resorption

Foramen
incisivum

Fig. 164

Nerve fibers are stuck to the mucosa; peel off the fibers from the mucosa carefully. Never try to cut away fibers with scissors or a scalpel to avoid this rather tedious work.

Because nerve fibers are apt to be elastic, they might spring into the incisive foramen as soon as they are cut. Stray nerve fibers, of course, cannot regenerate after the operation, and thus it is necessary to dissect away nerve fibers neatly and skillfully at this stage of the operation.

At the third meeting of the Japan Academy of Implantology, held in Fukuoka City, I was informed of a case report of maxillary subperiosteal implant. Frankly speaking, the reported procedure of mucosa stripping was quite ridiculous to me. For fear of severing the nasal palatine nerve, according to the operator, he did not strip the mucosa around the incisive foramen and made the impression in a hurry. Such an impression is, of course, very inaccurate and useless. This is simply because the operator had no knowledge or experience of how to strip the mucosa in this region. In the discussion that followed, I questioned him as to why he had not stripped the mucosa in this region and how expert implantologists of the world would feel if they learned this ridiculous method of subperiosteal implantation.

It was, of course, an example of the poor standard of implantology in Japan only ten years ago. Today, as is widely known, no implantologist would hesitate stripping the mucosa in this region.

The remarkable developments that have been achieved in the field of
dental implantology, developments never dreamed of before due to the fact
that Sapphire Implant was successfully introduced, and an energetic cam-
paign sponsored by Kyoto Ceramic and others pushed on and accelerated
Japanese implantology to the level it is now.

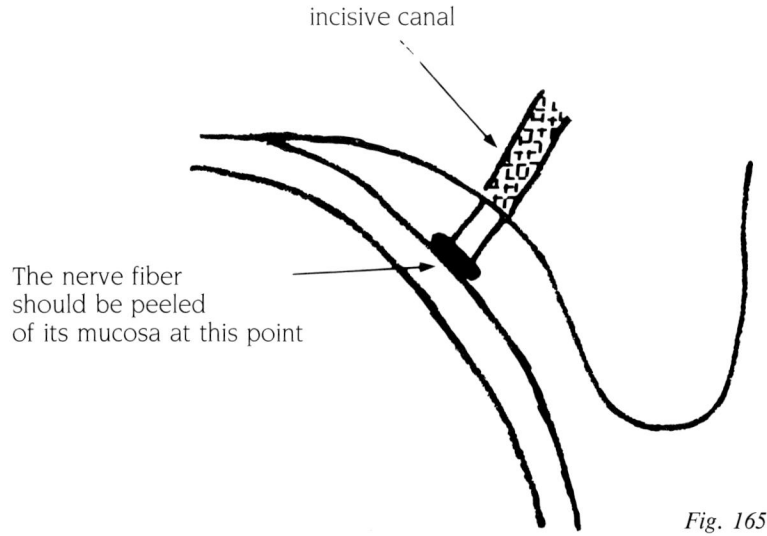

incisive canal

The nerve fiber
should be peeled
of its mucosa at this point

Fig. 165

The dimension of mucosa to be stripped on the palatine side is approximately 10 mm starting from the lower part of the palatine eminence,
that is, from the base of the alveolar crest to the oropharynx (Fig. 166).
Recently, I have been stripping the mucosa much wider, up to 20 mm, almost reaching the center of the palate.

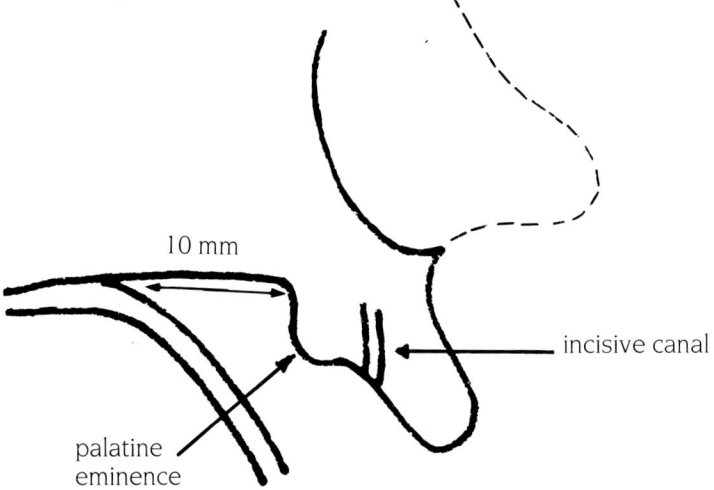

10 mm

incisive canal

palatine
eminence

Fig. 166

8.4.3.2 Spina nasalis

The spina nasalis is the only dependable supporting point for the substructure on the buccal side of the anterior teeth region; this region is accordingly exposed. Performing a maxillary subperiosteal implant without making use of the spina nasalis is of little value.

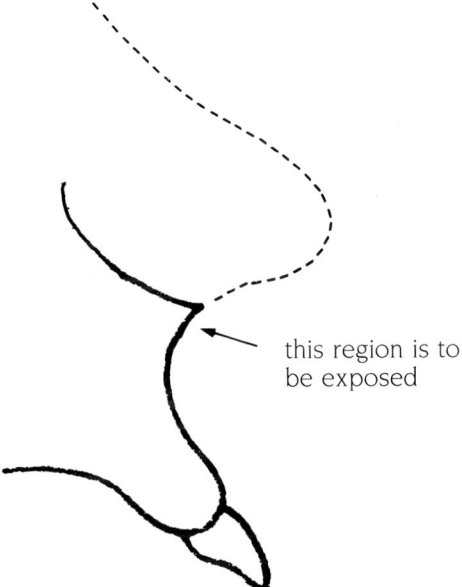

this region is to
be exposed

Fig. 167

8.4.3.3 Maxillary molar palatine side

On the palatine side, the mucosa is stripped approximately 10 mm from the base of the alveolar crest. In practice, the substructure is set on the alveolar crest only; however, by exposing a wider area of this region, the location of both the major and minor palatine foramen is clearly confirmed.

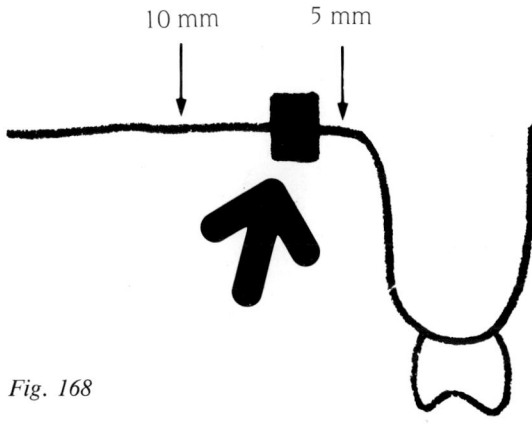

Fig. 168

Implanting the peripheral border at the point indicated by the arrow is dangerous, since the thickness of the bone is insufficient here. Sometimes this part is performed by the sinus.

8.4.3.4 *Maxillary molar buccal side*

In the maxillary molar buccal side, strip the mucosa up to the alveolar crest; then continue stripping to buccal side as for as reaching the zygomatic arch.

The bone of this region is very thin; care must be exercised, therefore, not to perforate into maxillary sinus during stripping operation. The maxillary bone here is a kind of cortical bone and its surface is very smooth; osseous tissue is, however, very thin. When the surface of bone is tapped lightly by the tip of forceps and the like, a light tone is heard in response, indicating the location of the maxillary sinus. The light tone is suggesting small quantity of osseous tissue. Continue stripping further, approximately 15 mm from the base of the alveolar crest; as far as reaching just below eyeball, or below the ourter canthus. The depth corresponds to the distance to the center of the nasal cavity.

Continuing to strip the mucosa from this region, the parallel plane to palate is reached. This plane is located just in front of the spot where maxillary bone and zygomatic arch are firmly sutured together.

In order to confirm the plane without fail, here is a helpful tip phrase: "Parallel to palate", please note. Do not fail to find out this parallel plane while stripping mucosa; this is no treasure hunting and the operator can surely find the plane.

The substructure is to be designed so that it fits the surface of this plane perfectly; it is, therefore, necessary to strip the mucosa to a considerably deep area; the operator who has limited knowledge of anatomy and little surgical experience may hesitate to perform this wider and deeper mucosa stripping - it is a pity.

Before reaching this plane, the exposed surface of the bone appears, a typical feature of the cortical bone. This part of bone is, however only to enclose maxillary sinus; therefore, it is very thin.

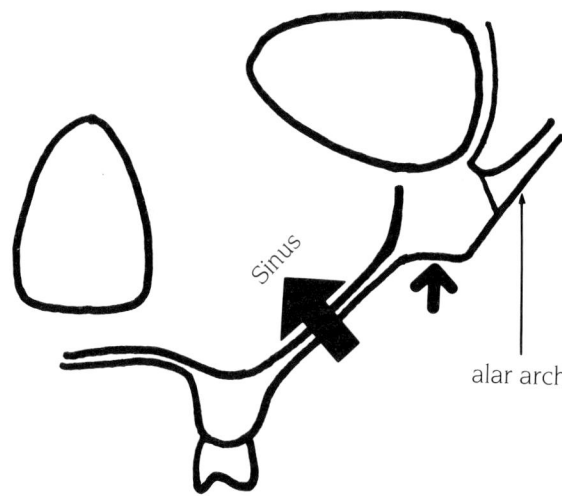

Fig. 169

Designing a substructure in this part should be avoided; otherwise, dangerous perforation to maxillary sinus may happen as a very unfavorable side effect.

Start stripping the mucosa from the molar region; stripping the mucosa starting from the molar region may hurt facial nerve fibre extended from the inferior orbital foramen. Hurting nerve fibre would cause troublesome facial paralysis.

As explained above in detail, this is one of the most difficult kind of mucosa stripping.

8.4.3.5 Surroundings of the mental foramen

By stripping the mucosa close to the mental foramen, do not try to strip the mucosa from the occlusal plane with the help of the elevator. Stripping the mucosa from upside would take downward force;
consequently, there is the possible danger of hurting or cutting off nerval fibre. Do not strip the mucosa from upside, please!

Instead the mucosa should ge stripped carefully parallel to the occlusal plane. By the way, the mental nerve is easily sought.

Mucosa stripping from this region has possible chance of injuring mental nerve

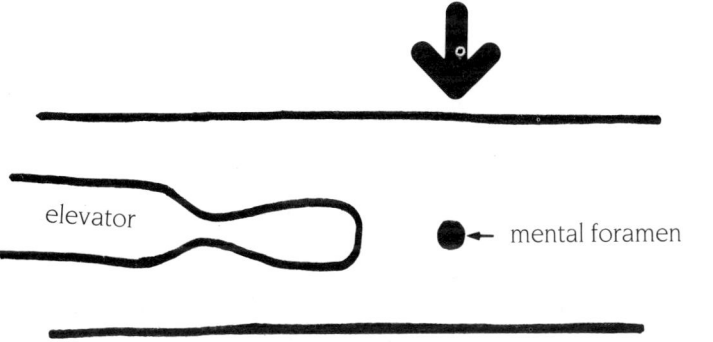

Fig. 170

In the surroundings of the mental foramen, particularly along the lower edge of the mandibular bone, the mucosa should be stripped approximately 10 mm, without cutting off the mental nerve, of course.

Mental nerve fibre may become as long as 5 to 10 mm when it is expanded; it is seldom broken by expansion.

After confirming the location of the mental foramen, continue to strip the mucosa in the way explained above, parallel to the occlusal plane; stripping the mucosa around the mental foramen is thus achieved successfully and it is much easier than expected.

In case of atrophied mandible, the mental foramen is frequently found in the alveolar crest. Care must be taken in confirming the accurate location of the mental foramen in advantage by analyzing a pantoma x-ray film.

If necessary, take again a pantoma x-ray film until the accurate location is confirmed. Usually it is not easy to find out the mental foramen when located on the alveolar crest. Besides, the mental foramen is sometimes found in the lingual side. In this case particular care must be taken, of course, when incising the mucosa.

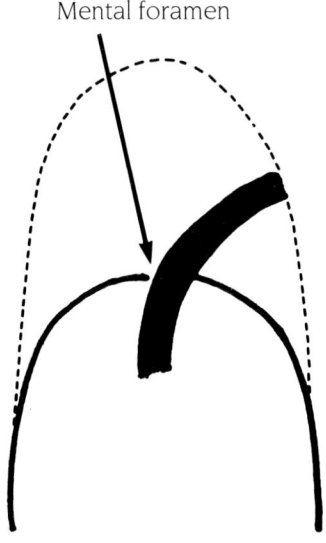

Atrophied mandible   *Fig. 171*

8.4.3.6 *Protuberance of the mental tubercle*

The mental protuberance or protuberance of the mental tubercle is the apex part of the mandible. This part of the mental tubercle has no nerve fiber; strip the mucosa to the inferior edge of the mandibular bone to expose the bone surface completely. To prevent vibration of the substructure and disperse the palatine pressure, this part is the most dependable supporting place.

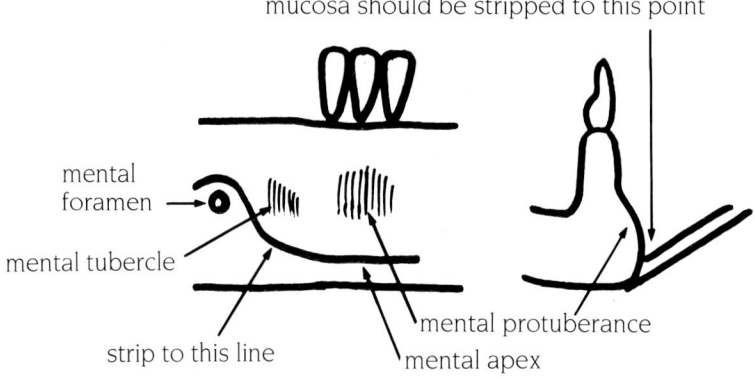

Fig. 172

Dr. Robert Todd of Illinois, USA, as well as Dr. Chercheve of France, design the substructures of mandibular subperiosteal implants so that best use is made of this part, as well as the surroundings of the mental foramen. When complete resorption of osseous tissue has occurred, and the alveolar crest is lost (the lingual side is connected directly to the buccal side), it is then necessary to perform a preliminary operation prior to the main one. This entails preparing an artificial substitute for the alveolar crest.

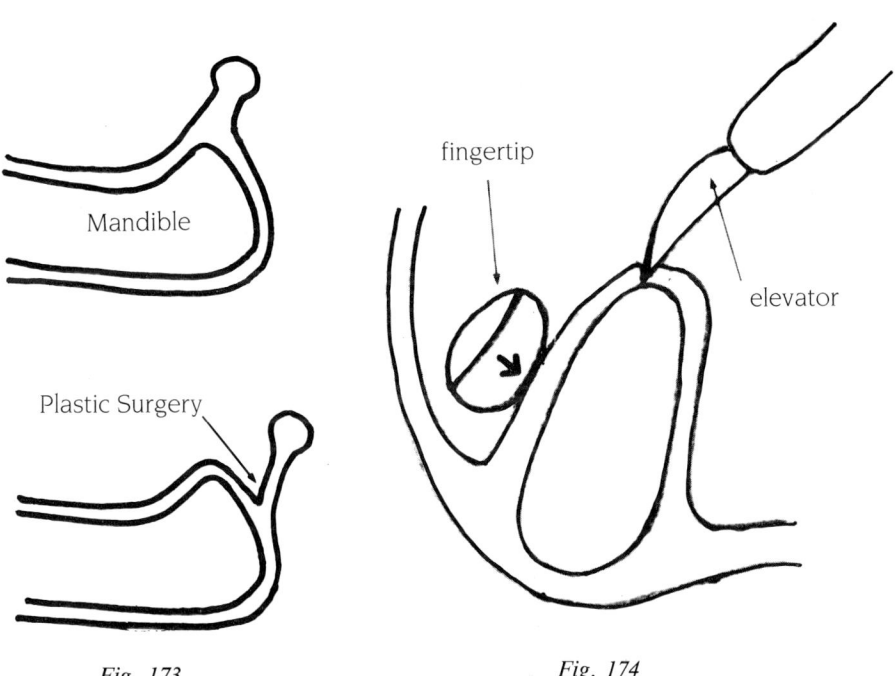

Fig. 173   Fig. 174

Without this preliminary work, the stitching thread can be broken by the strong pressure of the muscle shortly after suturing. The surface of the mandibular bone is exposed following the day of the operation, causing considerable pain. The patient is thus unable to eat.

8.4.4 Cautions to be exercised when stripping the mucosa

Stripping the mucosa for the subperiosteal implant operation does not require too much force by the operator. Too much force might cause stripping too broad a dimension of the mucosa than is really necessary, perforating the mucosa by the tip of the elevator, or even perforating the skin over the mucosa.

Always strip the mucosa carefully and skillfully. To do this, either in the mandible or maxilla, either on the buccal or lingual side, strip the mucosa with the help of an elevator and holding the mucosa firmly by pressing it with the fingertips.

The metal substructure may become exposed in the oral cavity after the operation, as mentioned in the preceding chapter; this is due to insufficient room beyond the flexibility of the mucosa, which is in turn caused by too narrow a dimension of stripped mucosa. Again, the first step of a successful subperiosteal implant is stripping the mucosa wide enough.

8.4.5 Dealing with free mucosa

By stripping the mucosa on the buccal side, some space results between the mucosa and the bone surface, however widely and broadly the mucosa is stripped. This is because of the strong facial muscles affecting the mucosa.

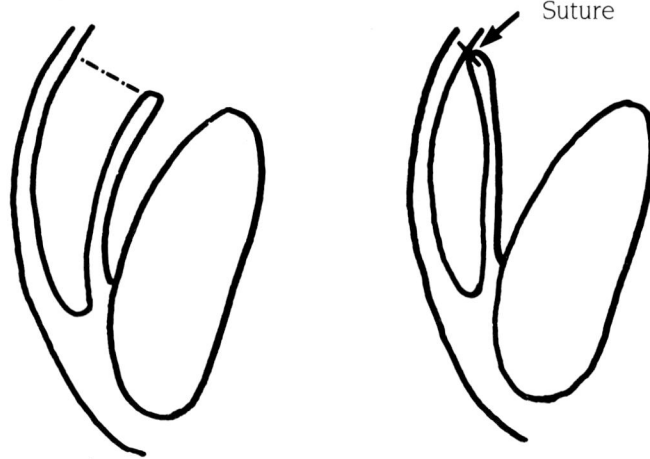

Fig. 175

Also, the free or isolated mucosa often found in this region hinders taking an accurate impression. In order to take an impression smoothly into the deeper parts, it is advised to fix the burdensome free mucosa by a temporary suture to the buccal mucosa in the molar region, or onto the lip mucosa in the anterior teeth region.

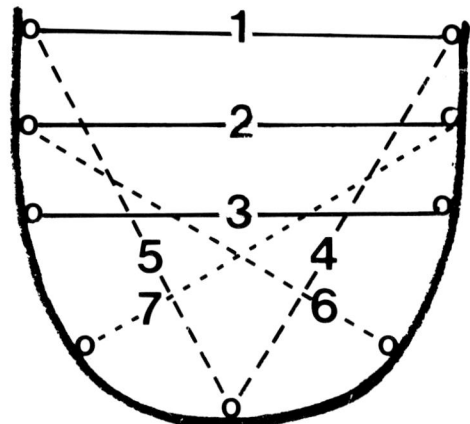

Fig. 176

The palatine mucosa is comparatively thick, and is provided with a natural power of restoration. In order to prevent moving of the stripped mucosa, it is better to fix it temporarily from right to left, from the front to the rear, so that the restoration power may interfere as little as possible.

Figure 177 shows the directions and steps for suturing the free mucosa.

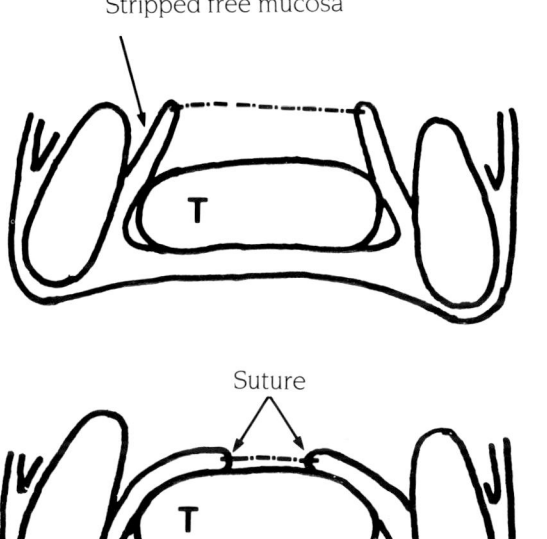

Fig. 177

Free mucosa on the mandibular lingual side is thin naturally; the mucosa is apt to roll up. If the impression should be taken upon the rolled-up free mucosa, a precise impression cannot be obtained. Free mucosa in this region is to be fixed temporarily by suturing it from right to left, then from left to right, so that the tongue is enclosed.

8.4.6 Taking a bone impression

Both the material and method for taking an impression have changed in accordance with developments in oral implantology. When subperiosteal implantation was introduced, the impression was taken in the normal course of dental treatment, that is, taken on the mucosa. From the obtained model, a tray was made and the model of the bone impression thus proceeded.

Bone impression was also taken in the same way with algenic acid.

Later it was found that, after stripping the mucosa, the prepared tray made from the impression taken on the mucosa was too large or fitted too poorly for effective use. Next came the period during which taking a direct plaster impression without preparing a tray was common practice. Difficulties ensued, caused by heat generated when the plaster hardened, broken pieces of plaster, portions of plaster getting into the undercut, and so on. Furthermore, the impression could be removed only after having been divided into several sections.

Between 1970 and 1980, silicon took the place of plaster, mainly input of Vicon or Coltex and the like; but they also were easy to deform and a precise impression was difficult. Moreover, if the leftover impression material of silicon lingered in the deep part of the operative site, it was very difficult to remove all of the material. Also, bleeding in the site, for instance, further hindered cleaning the area.

An implantologist of my study group used a special material for primary impression-taking, made of silicon mixed with 12% iodoform powder. Immediately after taking a bone impression with this material, a pantoma x-ray film was taken to find leftover silicon in the operation site. This is a practical application of the x ray transmissive nature of iodoform. This helpful idea is to be credited to Dr. Akira Phuchi of Koriyama City, Fukushima. Dr. Charles M. Weiss, one of the leading implantologists of the world, also is using silicon material for taking bone impressions.

8.4.7 Otobe method of taking an impression

My own method of taking a precise bone impression includes the following steps:

1. Immediately after the mucosa is stripped, clean the surface of the bone with physiological saline solution and inspect carefully to determine whether the bone surface is completely exposed. I have used the term «stripping the mucosa,» but this means literally stripping not only the mucosa, but also the periosteum. It would, of course, be impossible to perform a successful subperiosteal implant with an unstripped periosteum.
2. Stabilize the separated free mucosa to the buccal side of the mucosa by temporary sutures. This step, as explained previously, is helpful for taking an accurate impression up to the buccal side of the bone surface.

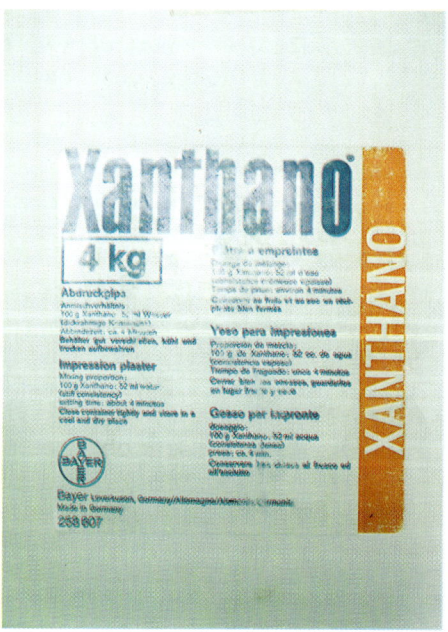

Fig. 178

3. Take an impression of the bone surface with heavy-bodied silicon. The impression is taken two times, the first impression for the purpose of making a tray, the second for the purpose of the bone bite.
4. Pour in plaster of Xanthano.
5. Usually Xanthano completely hardens in three minutes or so. Pouring plaster slower and hesitantly may result in inconsistent harden-

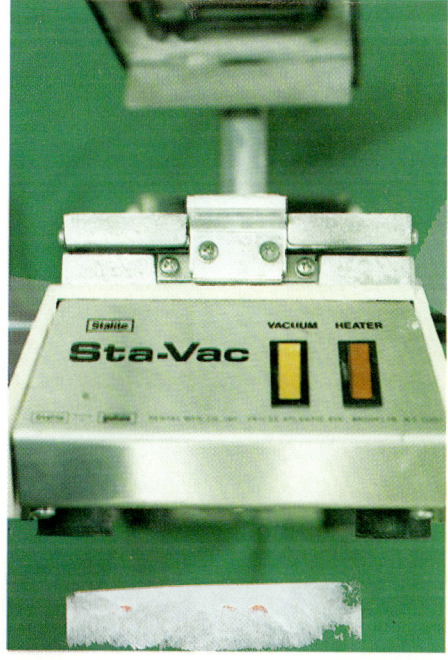

Fig. 179

ing. It is, therefore, helpful to carry out a test in advance to know how many minutes are required for optimum hardening of the plaster.
6. Make a tray of the model with a STA-VAC. Begin heating the STA-VAC while pouring in the plaster; in this way the tray and plaster model are obtained together.
7. Cut off the tray and adapt it to the surface. I use clear, transparent material so that unfitted points can easily be found. Scrape the unfitted points accordingly. The tray may be deformed by heat; dip the tray in alcohol for a minute to cool and sterilize it. The tray should be finished within 15 minutes after taking the impression, for during this time the anesthetic effect is decreasing. Additional anesthesia applied to the stripped mucosa is ineffective.

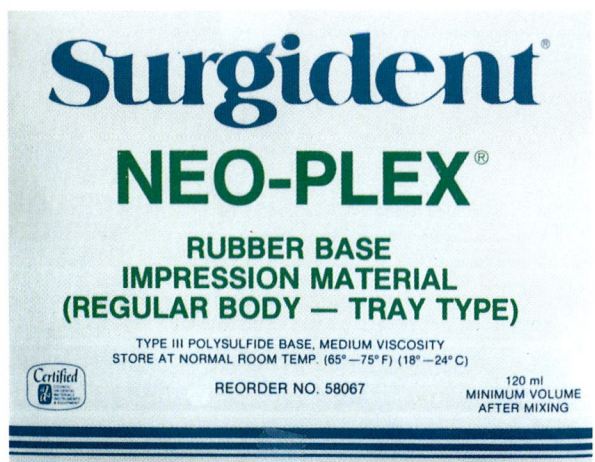

Fig. 180

8. Now is the time for taking the second and major impression. The material used is Surgident Neo-Plex of Lactona. After kneading the material for the tray, the impression is taken. Do not remove the tray before the material is hardened completely. Wait with perseverance, for the operator must be patient at this stage of the operation.

If the impression obtained is found to be unsatisfactory, return at once to step 4 and continue as before. A precise impression is the second key point of a successful implant operation (stripping the mucosa properly, as I mentioned before, is the first). Check carefully for possible leftover impression material in the unsatisfactory impression. Leftover impression material can cause suppuration in the operative site, causing the operator troublesome aftercare and the patient considerable pain.

8.5 BASIC DESIGN OF THE SUBSTRUCTURE

8.5.1 General

The peripheral border, the primary strut, and the other metallic parts to be covered by the periosteum should not exceed 2 mm in width and 1 mm in thickness. A subperiosteal implant can succeed only if the substructure is enclosed tightly in the periosteum. If it is covered only by the oral mucosa instead of the periosteum, the operation cannot succeed. If the peripheral border is designed in a double trapezoid form, a window of 2 mm in diameter should be made in the vent; otherwise, the periosteum will not easily adhere to the vent.

The shape of the post and other parts should be determined as discussed in the preceding section. The neck should be designed with a smaller diameter, so that it will easily be covered and enveloped by mucosa.

The problem of fixing the substructure to the mandibular bone with a screw has already been discussed. Occlusal pressure exerted on the substructure may cause the screw to vibrate and shake, which may in turn accelerate resorption of osseous tissue in the area around the screw.

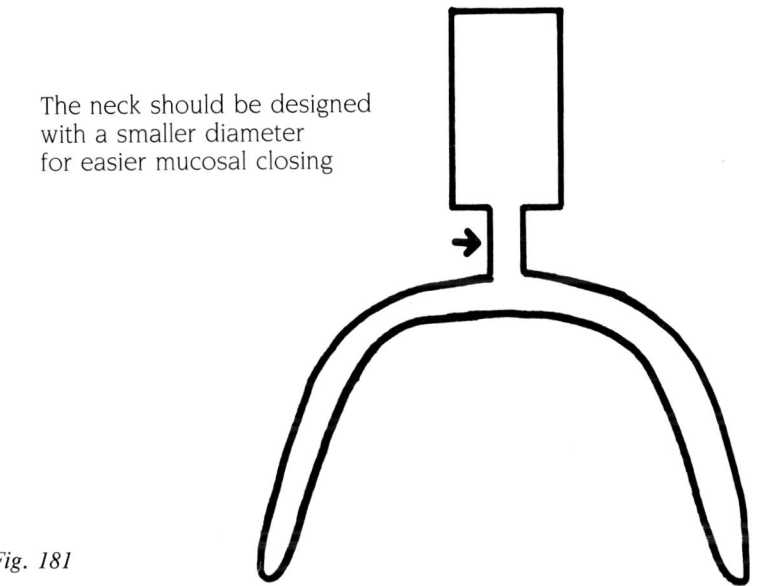

The neck should be designed
with a smaller diameter
for easier mucosal closing

Fig. 181

Today, with the accuracy of impression-taking having greatly increased, no untoward consequences, including resorption of osseous tissue, should ensue if the substructure is fixed to the jawbone with a screw. It is, however, far more preferable to remove the screw once the substructure is firmly enclosed in, and held by, the periosteum.

8.5.2 *Mental foramen*

The design line of the substructure should be set 2 mm apart from the mental foramen. This is particularly important in the upper part of the foramen, where resorption is apt to occur. Should the substructure sink down, pressing against the nerve fiber, a destructive lesion would result.

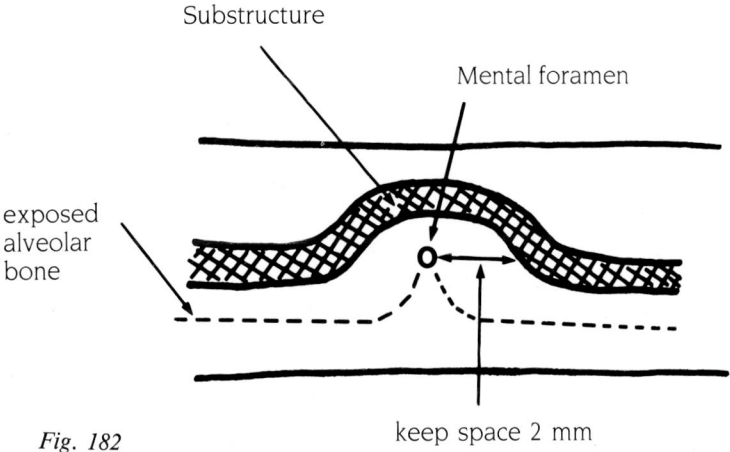

Substructure

Mental foramen

exposed
alveolar
bone

keep space 2 mm

Fig. 182

Around the foramen, muscles are much stronger than in other regions, perhaps in order to protect the nerve fibers. Thus, the substructure should be designed as large as possible. As the foramen should be completely exposed, the substructure should be implanted near the lower edge of the mandibular bone, if possible.

The foramen area is the corner of the substructure, where the substructure metal is particular apt to deform and bend. Bending the substructure metal could have a number of negative consequences. Thus, this part must be carefully designed to withstand strong external pressure.

8.5.3 Mandibular molar region

Do not try to extend the design line of the substructure to the lower part of the undercut in the molar lingual region. The undercut is helpful in stabilizing the substructure during the first stage of the operation.

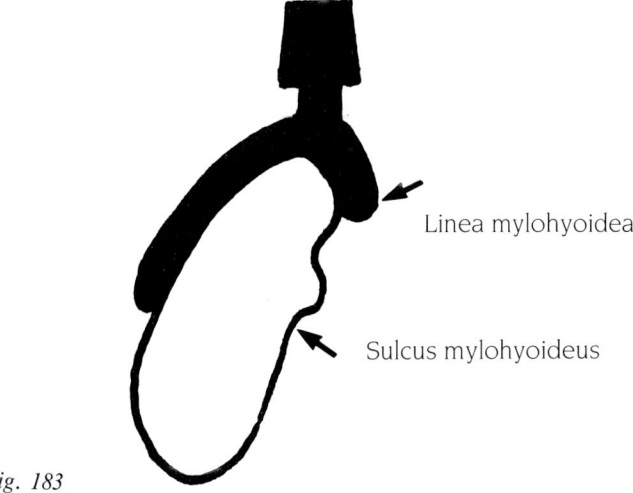

Linea mylohyoidea

Sulcus mylohyoideus

Fig. 183

The substructure is firmly held at first; however, resorption of osseous tissue starts in the linea mylohyoidea region immediately after the insertion of the substructure. The tissue then turns to granulation tissue, causing pain to the patient and sometimes suppuration in the operative site.

Never try to set the design line under the crest of the linea mylohyoidea. Resorption is particularly pronounced under the abutment.

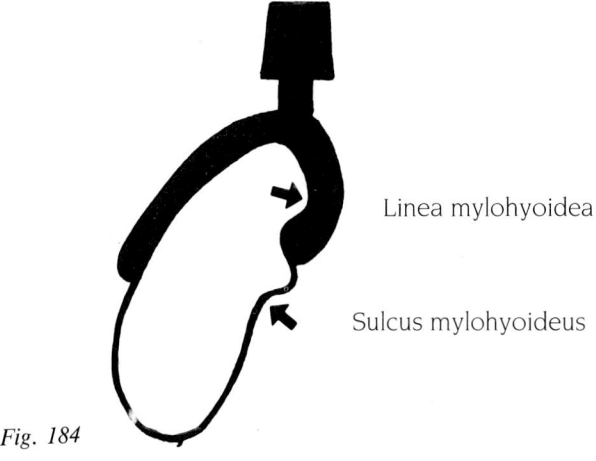

Linea mylohyoidea

Sulcus mylohyoideus

Fig. 184

On the buccal side, this is precisely the region where the masticatory muscle is inserted. The metallic part of the substructure could rub against the muscle and possibly cause an abrasion. Such an abrasion is very troublesome; it is characterized by both significant pain and edematous swelling.

Attempts often are made to cure a hard swelling beneath the mucosa in the operative site through reincision to stop suppuration. Such attempts fail because no pus is found. Hard swelling is no more than accumulated exudate following abrasion or scratching of the muscle by the substructure.

8.5.4 Maxillary molar region

The design line of the substructure should be set so that the buccal palatine alveolar crest is clasped. If this line is set even slightly lower, it will go against the maxillary antrum wall.

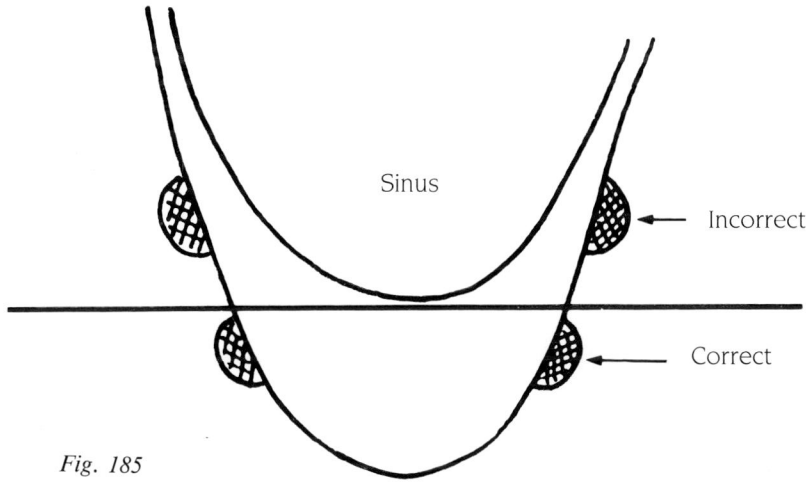

Sinus

Incorrect

Correct

Fig. 185

On the buccal side, in particular, the bone surface is smooth and appears very hard, just like the cortical bone. At first sight, the bone appears strong enough to hold the substructure firmly against the high pressure of occlusion. Actually, there is some danger of perforation of the maxillary sinus because the bone is comparatively thin.

Thus, the design line of the substructure should never be set here. If the substructure perforates the maxillary sinus, it will also penetrate into the oral cavity.

Therefore, after stripping the mucosa, by percussion, two tests should be carried out. The thickness of the bone should be examined, and the question of whether the point is on the maxillary sinus wall or on the alveolar crest should be resolved by tapping. The latter examination is particularly important.

In the palatine region, however, the substructure does not easily perforate the oral cavity even if it has perforated the maxillary sinus. This is because the palatine mucosa is thicker than the buccal mucosa, and contains sufficient fat. If the substructure perforates the sinus, the mucosa encloses it, preventing the exposure of the substructure in the oral cavity.

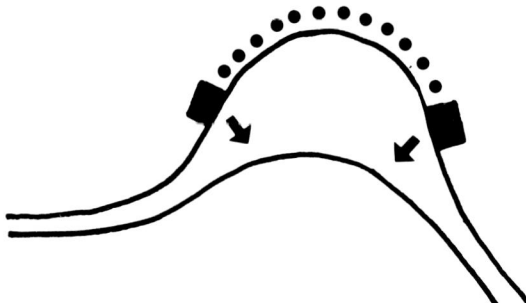

Fig. 186

In my clinical experience, with the maxillary molar bone, resorption of osseous tissue is faster on the buccal side than on the palatine side. The mucosa, of course, moves in accordance with resorption. Consequently, part of the substructure may become exposed. For this reason there is a trend away from designing substructure on the buccal side of this region.

A substructure implanted in the palatine side may perforate the maxillary sinus in a comparatively short time after the operation, and is usually faster than a substructure implanted on the buccal side because the palatine bone of this region is very thin. The perforation is not, however, easily noticed, because the substructure is covered with thick palatine mucosa.

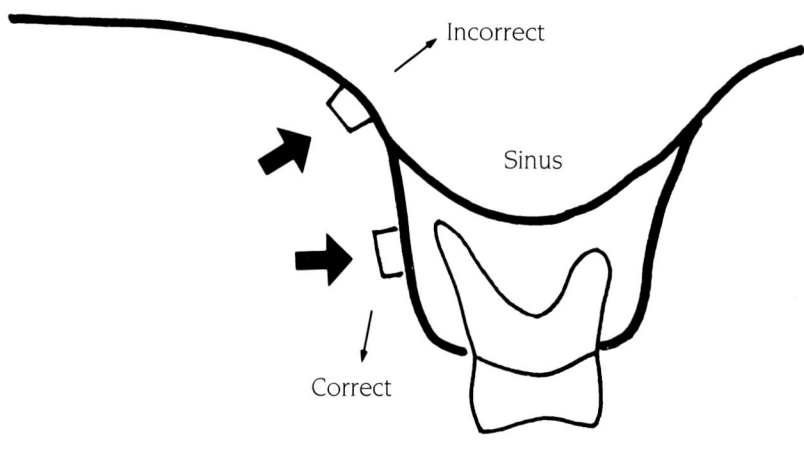

Fig. 187

In short, it is better to design the substructure in this region so that it will clasp the maxillary alveolar crest. The faster resorption on the buccal side is due to the greater occlusal pressure exerted. I would like to mention in passing that, although the problem of occlusion is now receiving more attention in Japan, authors often overlook the most important point. That is, they neglect the significant function of the jawbone in occlusion. Discussion of occlusion that fails to consider the jawbone function has little meaning in implantology.

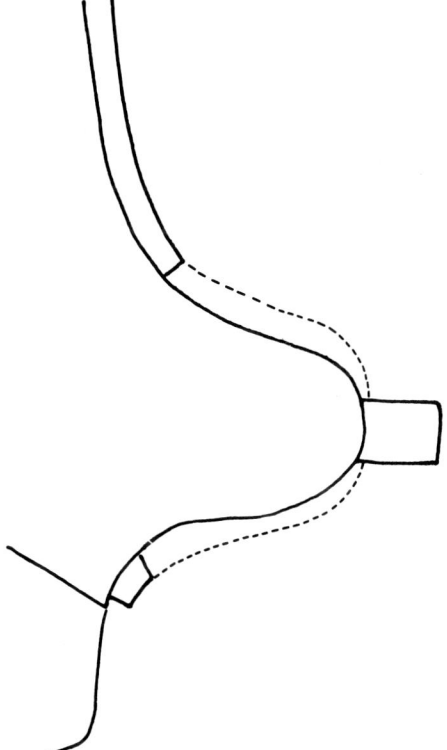

Fig. 188

In stripping the mucosa further in the molar region, a triangle-shaped high crest is encountered. This triangle should not be used. It is part of the maxillary sinus wall connected to the zygomatic arch.

Approximately 5 mm in front of the suture of the zygomatic arch and the maxillary bone, the surface of the bone is found parallel to the palate. This is regarded as the border of the triangle. There is a flat surface, about 5 mm in width, 12-15 mm from the eye socket. This is a spot where the substructure can be effectively supported against the high pressure of occlusion. It is, however, located comparatively deep. Thus, both stripping the mucosa and taking an impression are extremely difficult, requiring much skill and experience on the part of the operator.

Effective utilization of this region makes it possible to eliminate over 65% of the problems associated with subperiosteal implantation. At the same time this is, as already indicated, a very difficult region on which to operate successfully. The operator must be experienced.

8.5.5 *Nasal spine*

Use of a nasal spine is a well-known technique in maxillary subperiosteal implants. The metal should be made thinner when designing the substructure to be used in this region. Otherwise, rubbing of the metal against the skin can cause a painful abrasion. This can happen readily, as it is a human habit to draw in lips and to stretch out skin under the nose.

8.5.6 Nasal wings

This region corresponds to the crest of the cuspid root. At first glance, it appears suitable for an implant substructure. However, it is also a human habit to shake the head from left to right or vice versa. This may cause scratching of the substructure, followed by lasting swelling and pain if the substructure is implanted in the nasal wing region. Hence, this region should not be used for installing the substructure.

8.5.7 Opening of the incisive canal and surrounding area

Some authors say that the substructure for this region should be designed in the shape of a large net fitted on the palate. A wide substructure would diminish the sensitiveness of the tongue and cause pronunciation difficulties after the operation. Also, applying a substructure that covers almost the entire region of the incisive canal opening decreases the capacity of the oral cavity.

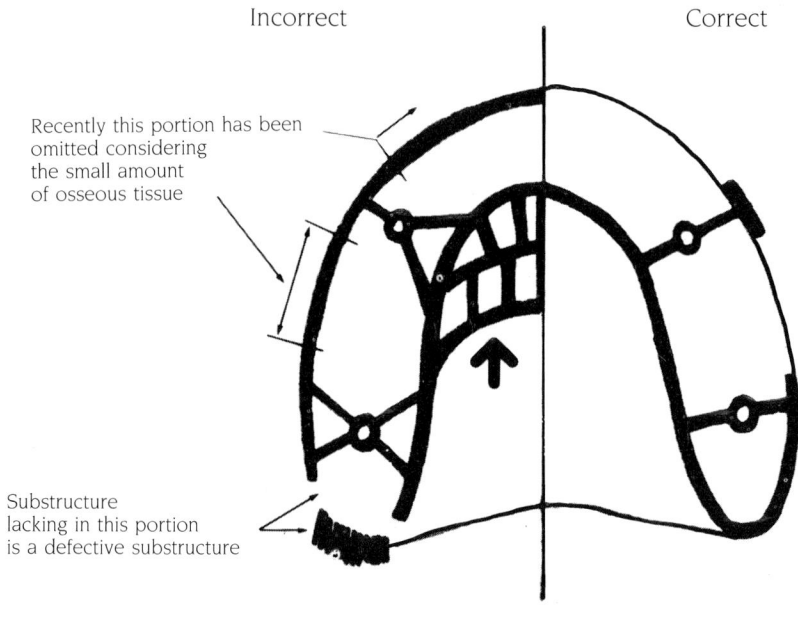

Incorrect   Correct

Recently this portion has been
omitted considering
the small amount
of osseous tissue

Substructure
lacking in this portion
is a defective substructure

Fig. 189

It has also been said that one peripheral border is quite sufficient. In the rapidly advancing field of implantology, and particularly of subperiosteal implant, no established theory can be found. Some have said that in order to prevent possible forward movement of the substructure caused by occlusion, the peripheral border should be made somewhat wider. In my clinical experience, substructures implanted in this region do cause somewhat decreased sensitivity of the tongue and temporary difficulties in pronunciation; the recovered function of biting can be evaluated. However, I feel that, generally speaking, the merits outweigh the demerits. Because this region is connected to the palatine bone, the nasal septum and the cranial base, it is able to hold the substructure firmly against strong occlusal pressure. It is therefore a region that can be used.

8.5.8 Pterygoid extension
Detailed comments on the pterygoid extension are given later.

8.5.9 MUSTs and MUST NOTs
There are three MUSTs in subperiosteal implants:
1. The mucosa MUST be stripped wide enough.
2. The impression of the bone surface MUST be carefully taken and be precise.
3. The substructure design MUST take into account implantological occlusal pressure.

The following is a MUST NOT in subperiosteal implantology:
The frame MUST NOT be placed on the alveolar apex.

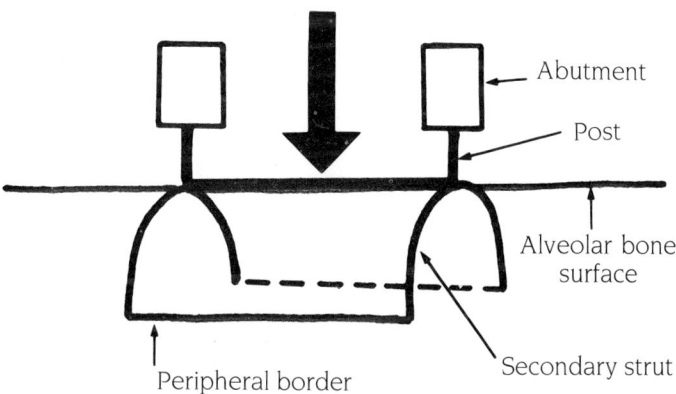

Fig. 190

As resorption starts from the apex, the result would be exposed in the oral cavity. Moreover, the alveolar apex overlaps the incision line. When the metal is left on this line in suturing, the mucosa cannot easily enclose it, and so causes exposure of the metal after the operation. Exposure of metal is, of course, to be minimized.

8.6 CLASSIFICATION OF SUBPERIOSTEAL IMPLANT: OTOBE THEORY

Subperiosteal implant cases vary in grades according to the condition of the remaining natural teeth. The dimension of the mucosa to be stripped and design of the substructure also vary in accordance to the grade. In 1978, at the annual meeting of the AAID, I presented my lecture on the four classes of subperiosteal implant as follows:

Class 1. Lost anterior teeth
Class 2. Lost molars - free end molar
Class 3. Lost molars in one side only
Class 4. Fully edentulous

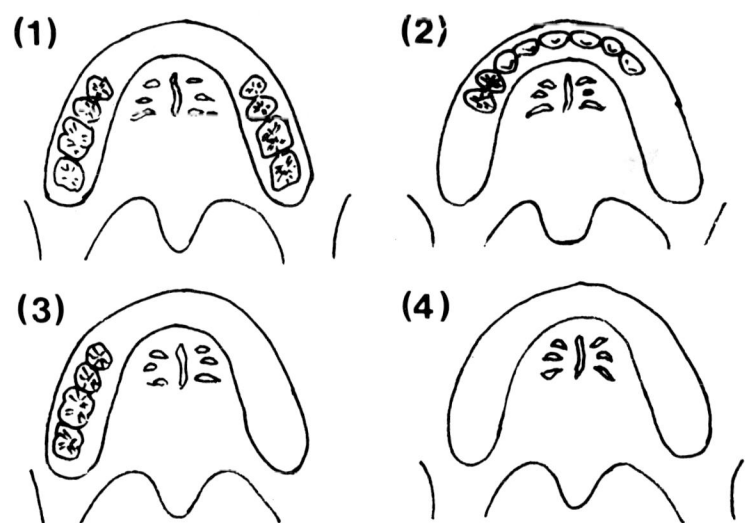

Fig. 191

Figure 191 shows the dimension of mucosa to be stripped.

Figure 192 shows the basic design of the substructure. Letter X indicates the point of the spina nasalis. Letter P indicates the post of the substructure. Letter Z indicates the point of the incisive canal.

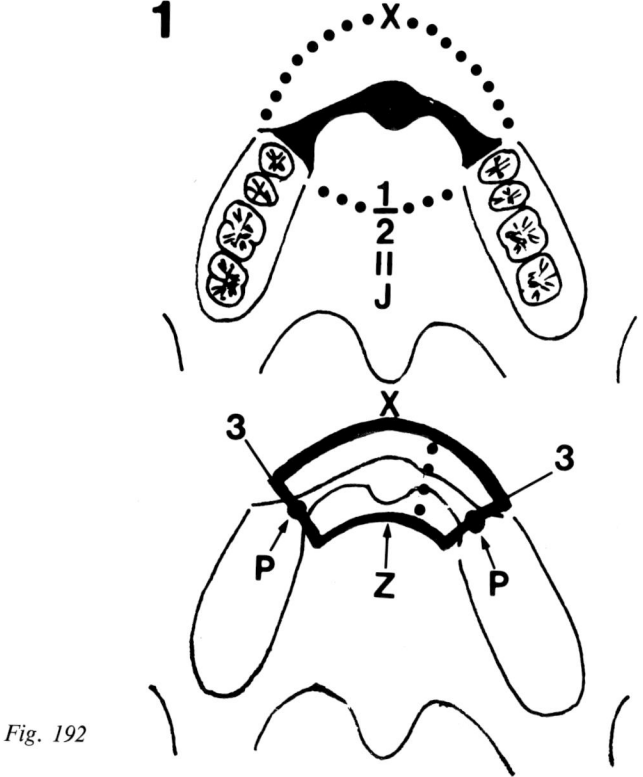

Fig. 192

8.6.1 Class 1

In Figure 192 the dimensions of the mucosa to be stripped are shown with a dotted circle. In particular, the nasal spine must be exposed accurately. On the palatine side, in general, approximately one-half of the mucosa of the determined dimensions is stripped; the opening of the nasal palatine nerve is, in particular, fully stripped. Stripping this half of the palatine mucosa to perfectly expose the surface of the palatine bone is by no means an easy operation; much skill of the operator is required, as well as a very long operation time.

In this region the substructure base and bone surface should be fitted precisely; otherwise, later there may occur a pushing forward of the substructure by occlusal pressure, causing considerable pain to the patient.

If the implanted substructure should begin vibrating in the mucosa, the mucosa begins to grow fat and thick. Occlusal pressure applied to the substructure is broken down and absorbed on the bone surface; vibrating substructure hinders the proper function of bone and, as a substitute of bone, the mucosa becomes as thick as 5 mm or more in order to disperse the pressure of occlusion. This is a kind of instinctive defense mechanism of the tissues.

In the conventional dental clinic, such a symptom is infrequently observed. The thickened mucosa is very difficult to incise because of its increased hardness; it is very difficult to stitch as well. Stripping and turning up such mucosa is, of course, also very hard and troublesome. After a long operation, the unfitted substructure is finally removed--a typical case of failed subperiosteal implantation.

The thickened mucosa of this region naturally causes many other problems, including difficult and imperfect pronunciation.

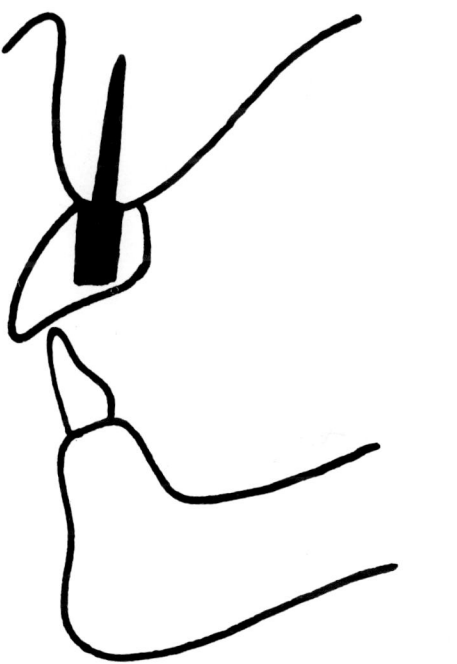

Fig. 193

As for the subperiosteal implant in the region of the nasal spine and the incisive canal opening, I have considered this topic previously.

Before going into the substructure design, the relationship between the mandibular arch and the maxillary arch should be considered. The abutment of the anterior teeth region is implanted in the alveolar ridge when the condition of the osseous tissue is found to be most suitable. This is, however, from the occlusal point of view, the worst place.

The substructure is designed with an extremely prognathous shape to be fitted on the buccal side instead of on the alveolar crest. If the substructure is designed with an extremely prognathous shape, however, care must be taken so that the substructure does not strike against the mandibular front teeth. If the patient agrees, from the viewpoint of the longer life span of the implant, the substructure is better designed in the shape of a reverse occlusion. The implantologist should always aim at the longest life span of the implant.

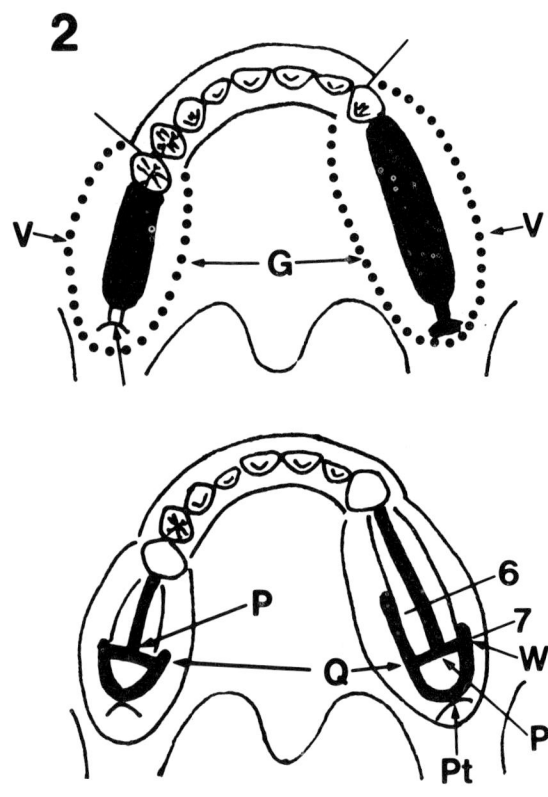

Pterygoid Extention (PT)

Fig. 194

8.6.2 Class 2

For the pterygoid extension implant, the symphysis to the rear maxillary bone and hamulus pterygoideus is used for implanting the substructure. Number 7 in Figure 194 means 7/7; the abutment is implanted here. Never try to implant the abutment behind 7/7.

The mucosa behind 7/7 is a kind of movable, layered, flat epithelium resembling the mucosa of the pharynx rather than oral mucosa. In the mucosa of this region it is, therefore, difficult to enclose an implanted post, which can frequently cause pericolonitis.

The letters Q and W in Figure 194 refer to section (4) of Basic Design in the preceding chapter. The letters Pt indicate the pterygoid region. This is located comparatively posteriorly, almost bordering the pharynx. The extension bur should never be touched by mucosa, and preferably should be separated from it by 2 mm or more.

This is the overall design of the pterygoid extension implant.

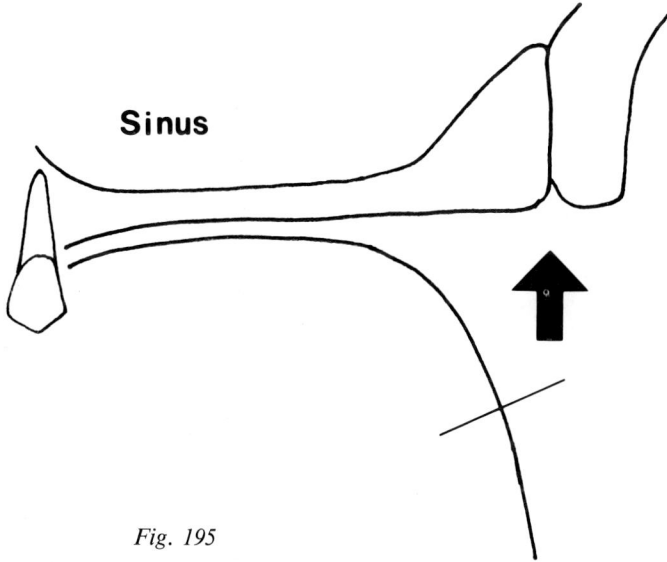

Sinus

Fig. 195

The arrow in the above figure indicates a suture section approximately 10 mm long. This region can bear the strong pressure of occlusion, and resorption of osseous tissue is infrequently observed. It is, however, located in a far posterior position, bordering the pharynx region.

The line under the arrow in the pharynx region shows the starting point of the incision for stripping the mucosa wide enough to completely expose the bone surface of the pterygoid. Confirming the exposed pterygoid tendon of the tensor palatine muscle located here is very helpful.

In Classes 3 and 4 (mentioned later), this region can be used effectively for the bed of the substructure.

The problems of the pterygoid extension implant operation are the following:

1. An accurate impression of the bone surface is very difficult to take.
2. The substructure base is accordingly difficult to fit on the bone surface.
3. Stray muscle may get between the substructure and the bone surface.
4. Infection may frequently occur.

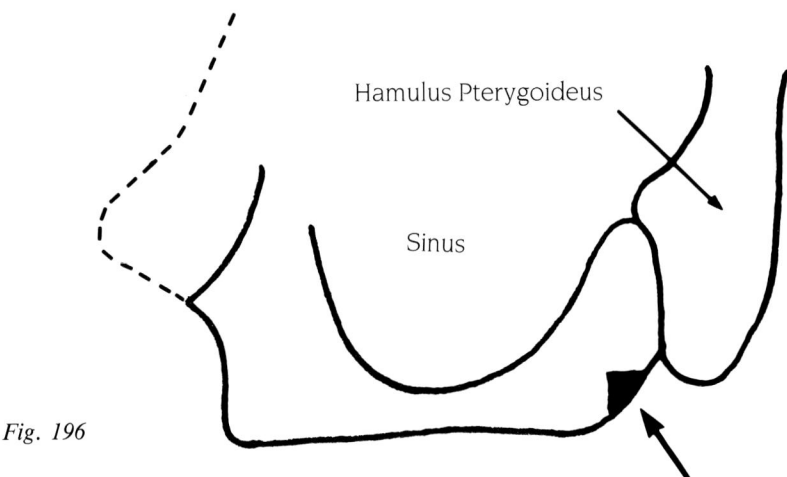

Fig. 196

From the occlusal point of view, the pterygoid extension is a suitable region for implanting the substructure; it is, however, very difficult to make effective use of this region due to the problems listed above. In this regard, instead of inserting metal in the pterygoid and causing the in-

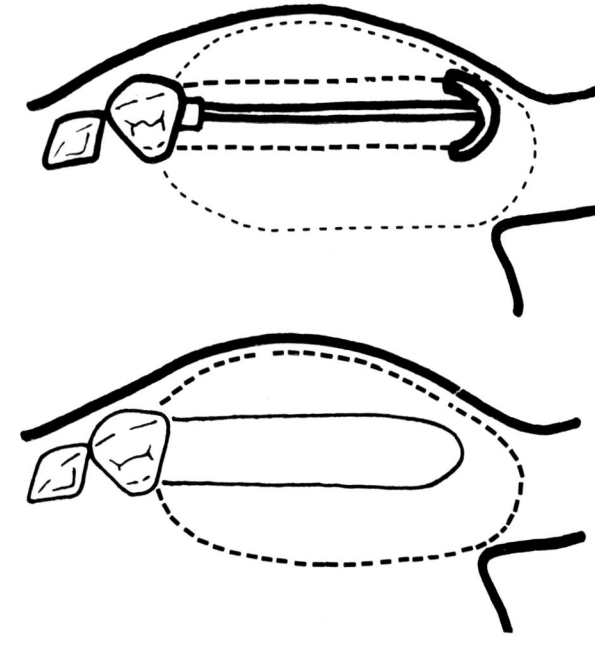

Fig. 197

creased capacity of this region, I prefer to set a channel on a part of the maxillary posterior wall as a substitute for the pterygoid. This has been shown to be better clinically.

Previously, cases belonging to Class 2 of my classification were treated with pterygoid extension implantation; after 1989, however, when Dr. Linkow developed the tuber blade, more than 80% of cases of Class 2 can be treated with tuber blade implant instead of pterygoid extension implant.

Figure 197 illustrates an earlier type of pterygoid extension implant. The extension bur was extended from the hindmost part as seen. A design of this type is not presently used, mainly due to hygienic reasons. In order to connect dentures to the remaining natural teeth, however, this earlier type of pterygoid extension implant has proved helpful.

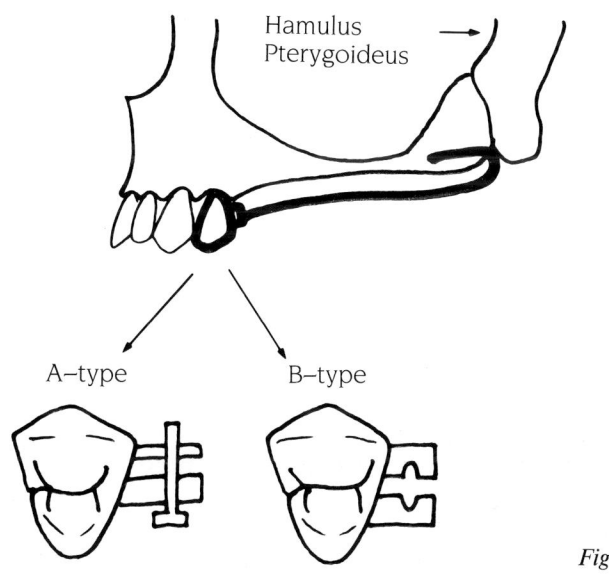

Fig. 198

8.6.3 Class 3

Class 3 is a complex of Classes 1 and 2. The dimension of the mucosa to be stripped and the design of the substructure are also decided considering the combined factors observed in each case.

On the anterior buccal side, the nasal spine should be used; on the palatine side, the incisive canal opening. On the molar buccal side, do not design the substructure in the surrounding area of the first molar because the bone is too thin.

The problem of a subperiosteal implant for this class of patients is that high pressure is exerted to the substructure in the direction of the cuspid buccal side according to the design of the substructure. As a consequence, the substructure is apt to be pushed diagonally. This happens mainly in the cuspidate region, as well as in the posterior pterygoid region.

The possible migration of the cuspidate region in the diagonally forward direction is characteristic, particularly in those cases belonging to Class 3; the substructure implanted in the molar region is pushed upward.

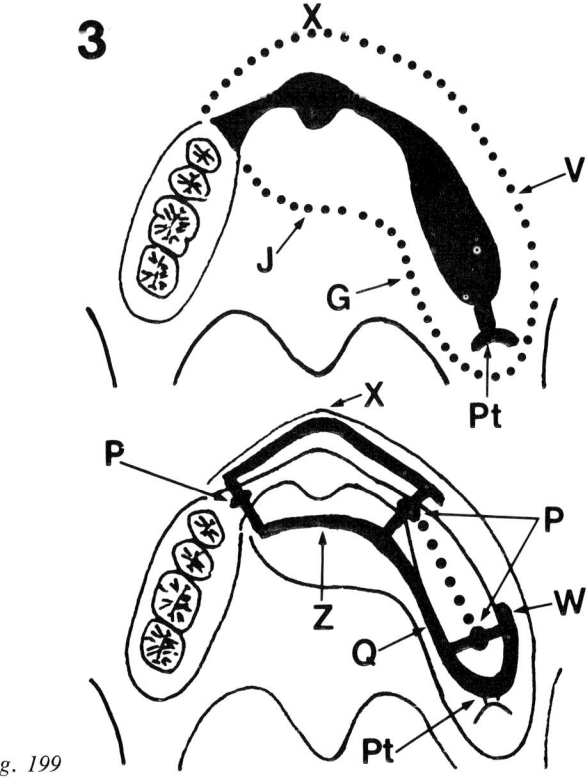

Fig. 199

Consequently, soft tissue may stray in between the substructure and the bone surface, causing pain to the patient.

At the stage of designing the substructure, the operator should attempt to devise a means of preventing the diagonally forward movement. The same may be said of the design of the superstructure as well.

8.6.4 Class 4

Class 4 is that of the so-called fully edentulous jaw. In Japan, patients belonging to this class are the majority. For them, a subperiosteal implant is to be applied without exception. Until now, they had to be content with rather imperfect dentures.

This is the most difficult case of subperiosteal implantation. First of all, a wide and large area of mucosa must be stripped. Second, a precise impression must be taken, which, as mentioned previously, requires much skill.

Recently, I have used the region just in front of the suture of the maxillary bone with the buccal arch in order to stabilize the structure and to break down occlusal pressure. The difficulty associated with the mucosal stripping and impression taking are beyond description. At the second stage of the operation a bucket is successfully inserted.

The final stage is designing the superstructure; as I explained, I concentrate all my attention on how to eliminate or minimize the extraordinarily high pressure of occlusion occurring as a result of the maxillary

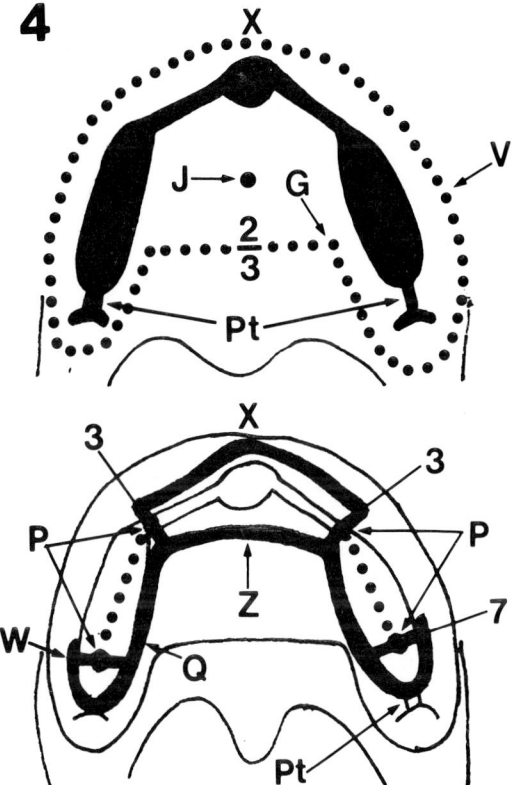

Fig. 200

arch. Basically, I take a serious look at the occlusal pressure rather than an overview of the superstructure.

Generally speaking, the expected life span of a denture-type super-structure is 15 years and that of a bridge-type is 10 years, according to Dr. Linkow. In view of the ease of cleaning, the denture type is much better. Most Japanese patients, however, psychologically prefer the bridge-type, saying it's none the better for the change having dentures again after a painful operation.

In order to extend the life span of the implant, a mouthpiece of soft type originally designed for boxers is helpful to prevent the hard bite possibly taking place during sleep. The mouthpiece is easily prepared to fit the patient individually with a STA-VAC.

According to the balance of power, a design line is set in a triangular form from A to D and A to E. This line is actually not a straight one, but via K and K' as illustrated in Figure 202.

The substructure is twisted when the pressure is given to K and K'; this twist is turned to the extraordinary pressure.

The peripheral border is not set in so deep a position of the cuspidale bone crest. If it is set too deep, movement of the nasal wing may cause abrasion.

Figure 202 also shows the situation for the mandibular bone; it is the same for the maxillary bone as well. Care should be taken not to use too

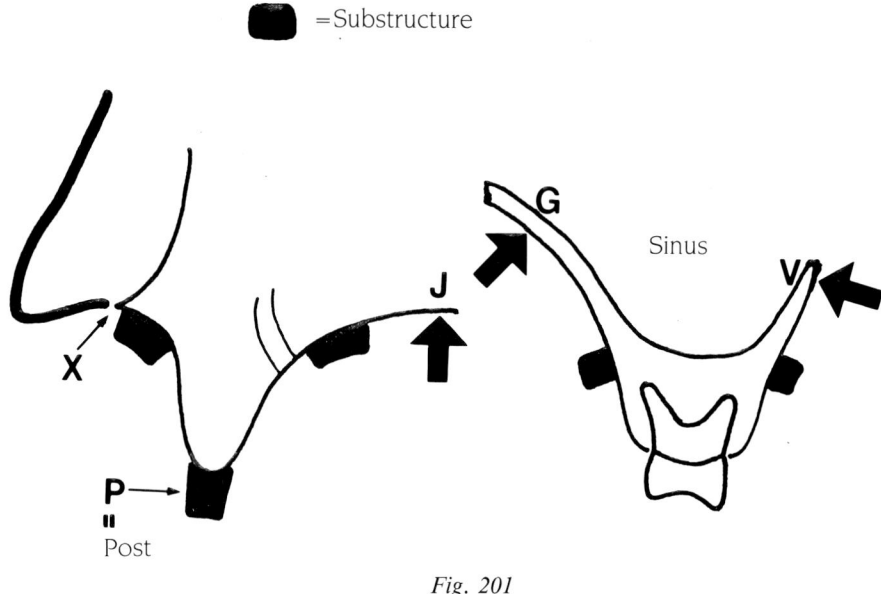

Fig. 201

much strength when moving the jaw horizontally. Inordinate pressure may be frequently given to the implant by occlusion; I once observed a case in which the implant bridge was broken in two. An ordinary bridge is seldom broken by occlusal pressure; hovever, an implant bridge is, given, as it is sometimes, to much stronger pressure by occlusion. This is because the implant bridge has no reflex action of innervated muscle.

In testing the occlusal pressure, natural teeth always score higher as a numerical value than artificial teeth, including an implant. I believe that one of the reasons is that the human brain orders and controls the target organ to bear the high pressure of occlusion after being informed the test is to be given.

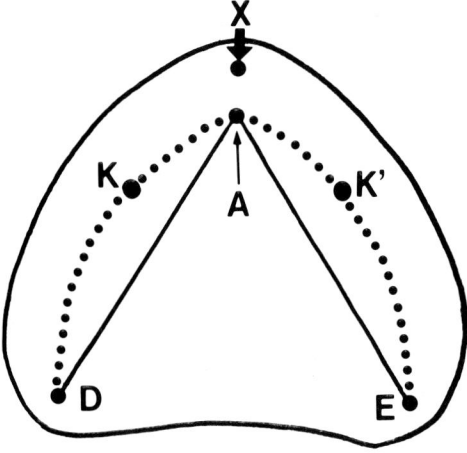

Fig. 202

As for the superstructure of Class 4, it must be realized that the maxillary alveolar arch is smaller than the mandibular alveolar arch, and that the mandibular bone is somewhat prognathous in the anterior teeth region. I have insisted on the above two points repeatedly, for they have a very important relationship to the implants of Class 4.

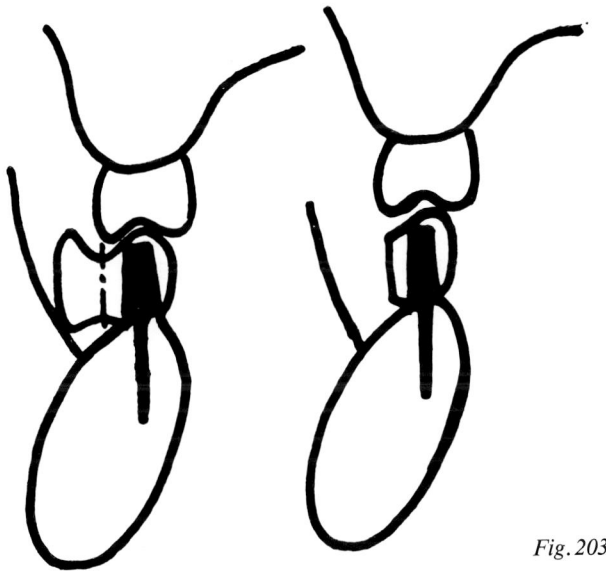

Fig. 203

If the superstructure is prepared in the normal way of denture design, the substructure is pushed forward in the anterior teeth region and raised upward in the molar region at the same time. Both the forward and upward movement are the most unfavorable ones in respect to maintaining the life of the implant. The substructure should be designed so that the given pressure of occlusion is effectively decreased and movement of the substructure is halted.

The anterior part is better designed according to the arrangement of reverse occlusion.

SUMMARY

1. Strip the mucosa completely to the nasal spine.
2. Strip the palatine mucosa to the prescribed position.
3. Strip the mucosa completely on the molar buccal side and pterygoid region.

After stripping the mucosa to the prescribed position completely and neatly, a precise impression can be obtained.

The steps for a successful implant operation are as follows:

A. The diagnosis and treatment plan.
B. The surgical technique.
C. The design of the substructure.
D. Occlusion and rehabilitation by prosthetic equipment.
E. Oral hygiene and aftercare.

Let me repeat the most important tips leading to a successful implantation:

1. Strip the mucosa widely enough.
2. Take an accurate impression of the bone surface.
3. Design the substructure considering the occlusal pressure.

S-Case 1 (a)

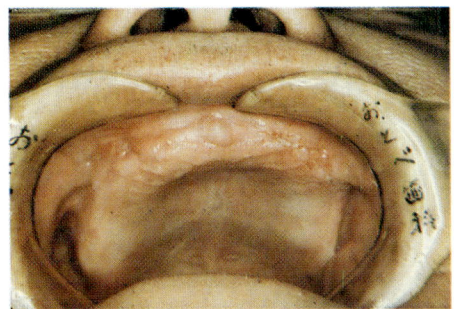

1.

Edentulous case (before operation).

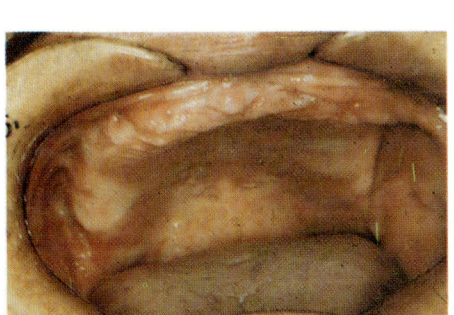

2.

Preoperative photo.

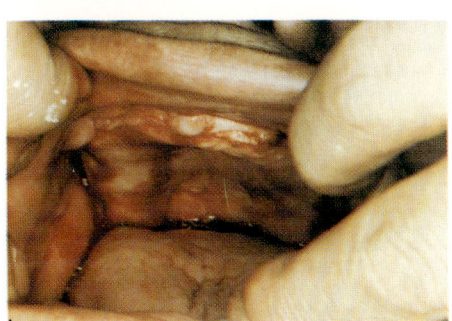

3.

Incision of mucosa.

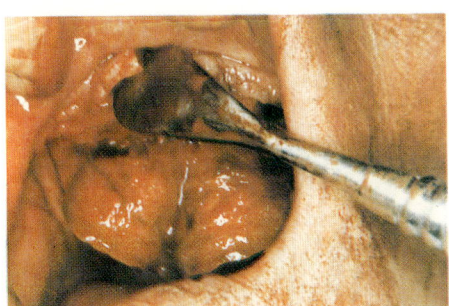

4.

Reflection of mucosa.

S-Case 1 (b)

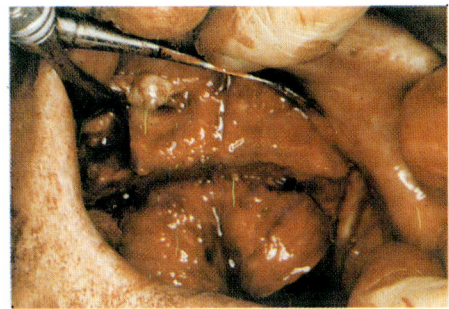

1.

Bone is exposed, the center being the anterior nasal spine.

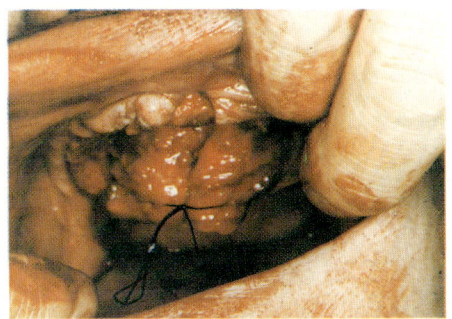

2.

Reflected mucosa is sutured.

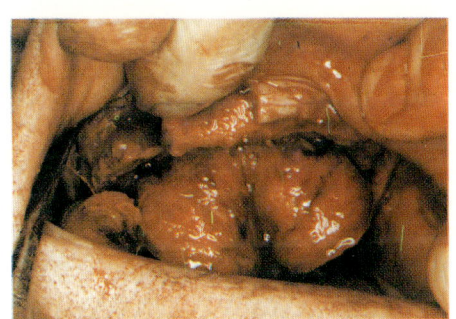

3.

The cavity caused by cuspid extraction two months prior to the operation. Soft tissue in the cavity is removed to expose the bone.

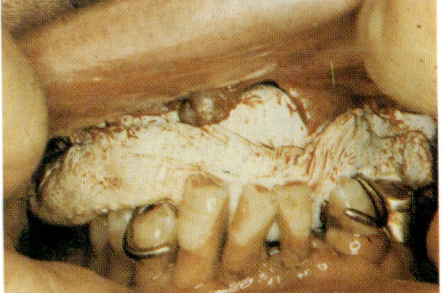

4.

Bone impression and bone bite.

S-Case 1 (c)

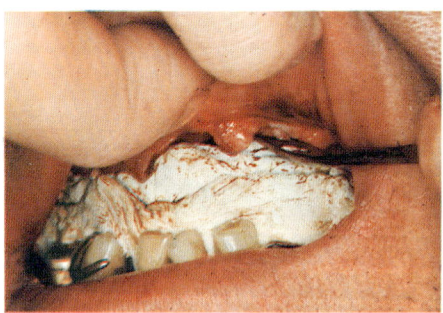

1.

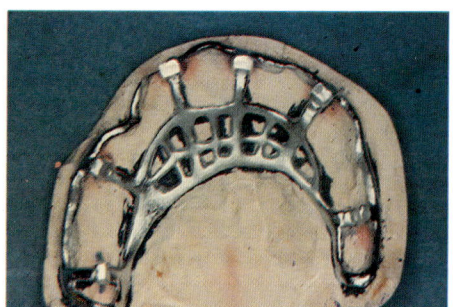

3.

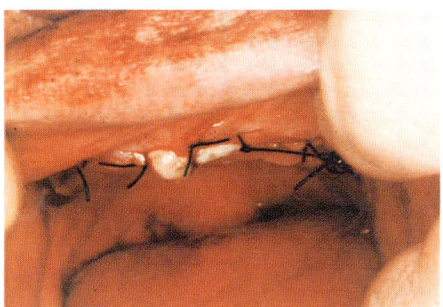

2.

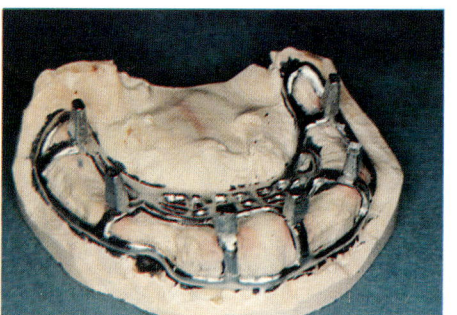

4.

1. Bone impression material. Until about 17 years ago, a bone impression was taken only once. Now it is taken twice to ensure a more precise model.
2. Suture.
3. Substructure: palatal side view.
4. Substructure: front view.

S-Case 1 (d)

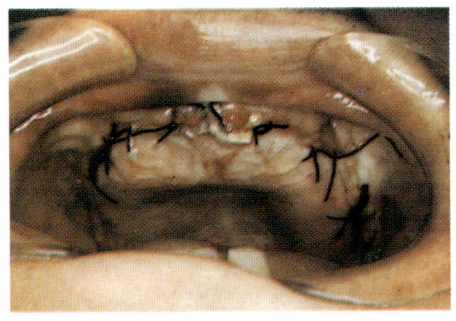

1.

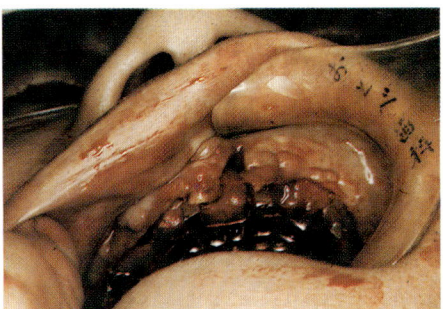

3.

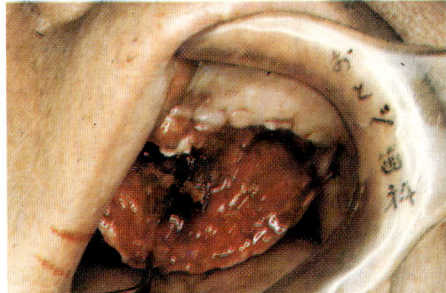

2.

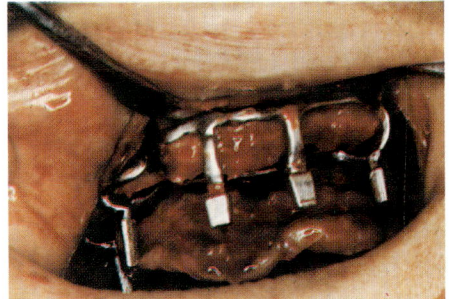

4.

1. One week after the initial operation and prior to the second stage.
2. Mucosa is reflected again. Cyanosis is seen in the center of mucosa.
3. The superstructure is fitted to the bone.
4. The superstructure is inserted. The tightness of the fit is examined and confirmed.

S-Case 1 (e)

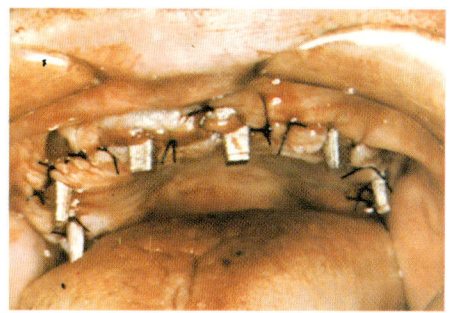
1.

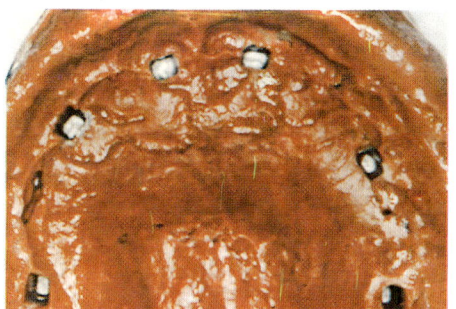
3.

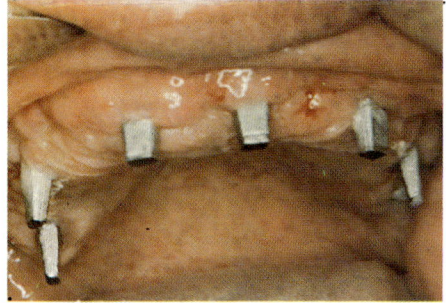
2.

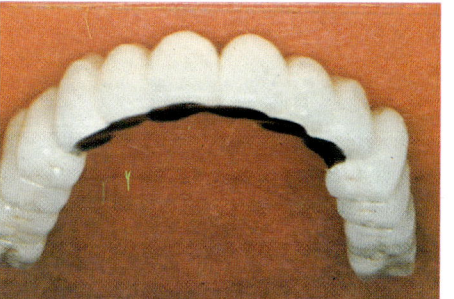
4.

1. Mucosa is sutured.
2. Ten days after the operation the mucosa is completely healed.
3. Final impression with agar.
4. Superstructure.

S-Case 1 (f)

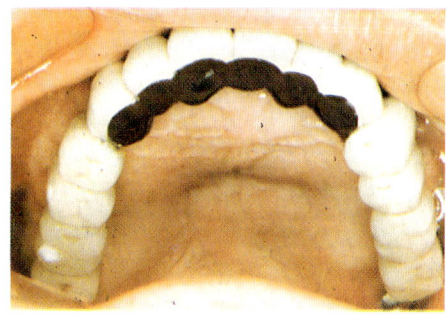
1.

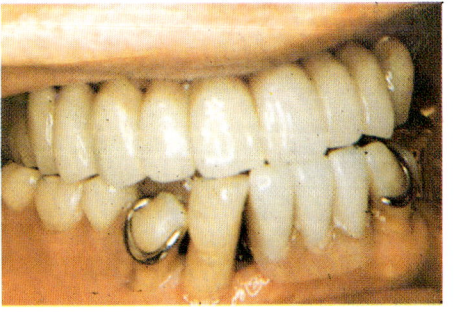
2.

1. Superstructure is set in the mouth.
2. Postoperative photo.

S-Case 2 (a)

S-Case 2 (b)

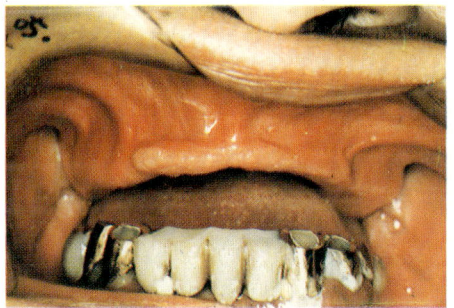

1.

Preoperative photo:edentulous case.

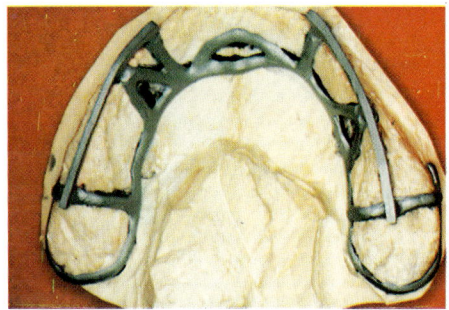

1.

Substructure: palatal-side view.

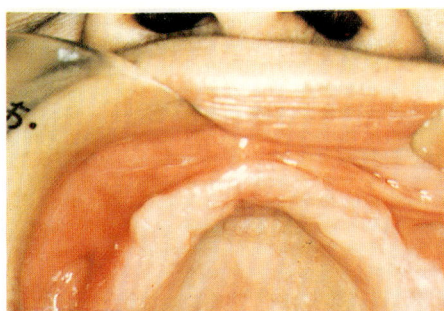

2.

Preoperative photo

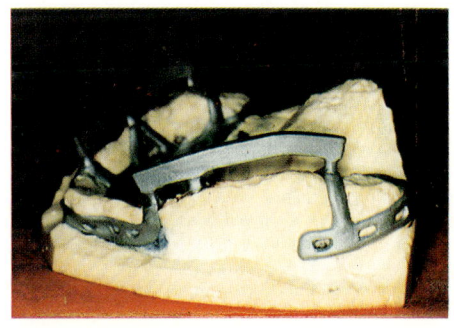

2.

Substructure: buccal-side view.

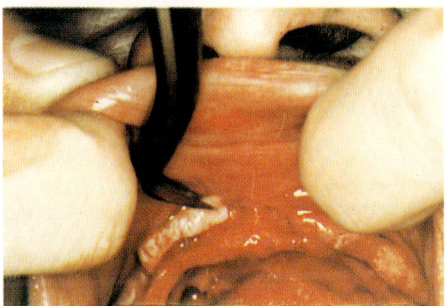

3.

Bone is exposed: anterior nasal spine must be exposed.

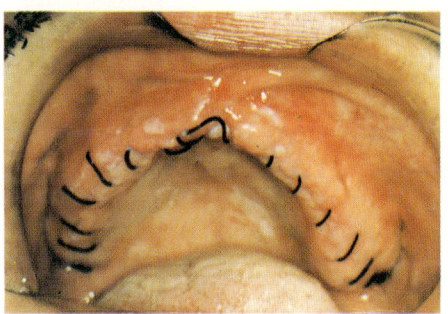

3.

One week after 1st stage operation.

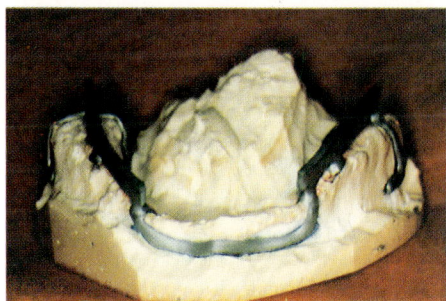

4.

Resorption of bone is more severe in the front than the molar part.

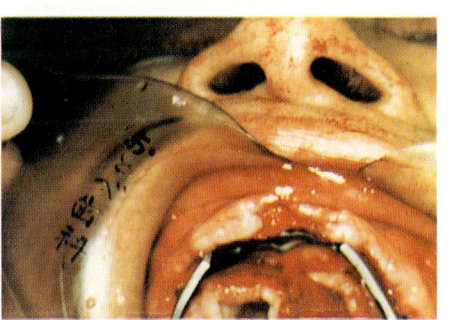

4.

Photo of 2nd stage operation. The mucosa is reflected again and the substructure is fitted.

S-Case 2 (c)   **S-Case 2 (d)**

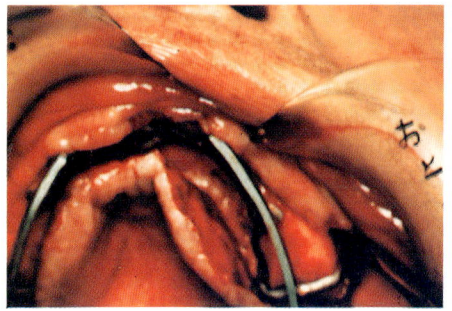

1.

Photo of 2nd stage operation.
The accuracy of the fit is noted.

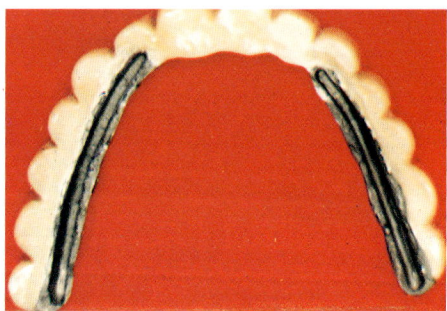

1.

Superstructure.

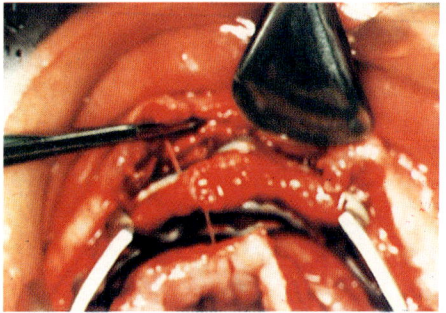

2.

Photo of 2nd stage operation. Fitting is
wonderful.

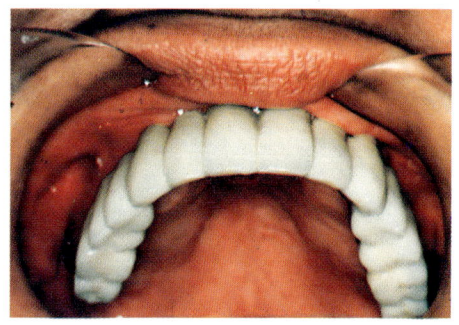

2.

Cementing superstructure.

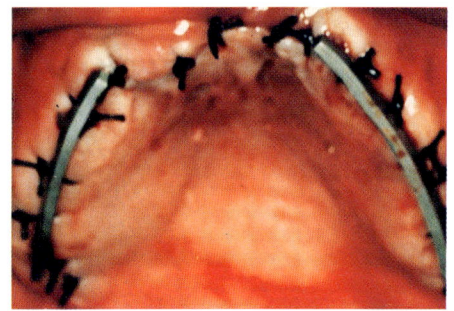

3.

Sutured.

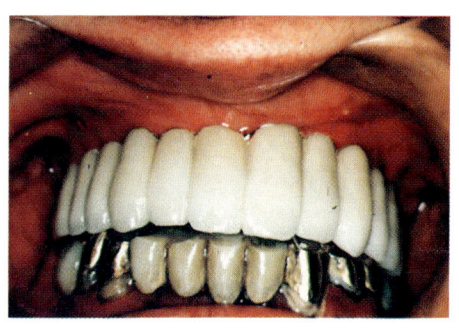

3.

Superstructure.

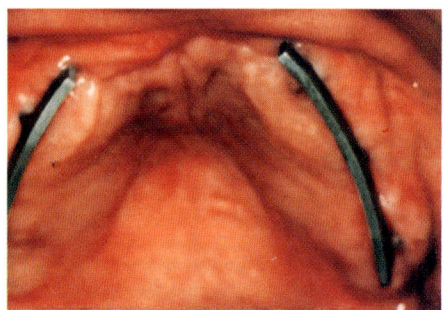

4.

Ten days after operation. Beautiful oral
cavity.

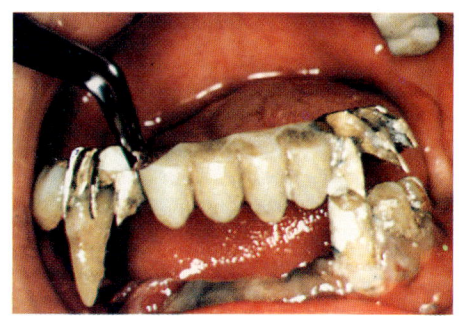

4.

Removed old bridge.

S-Case 2 (e)

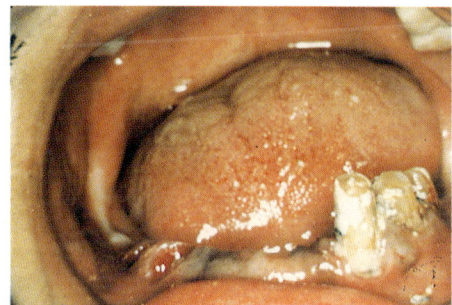

1.

Pre operative oral cavity.

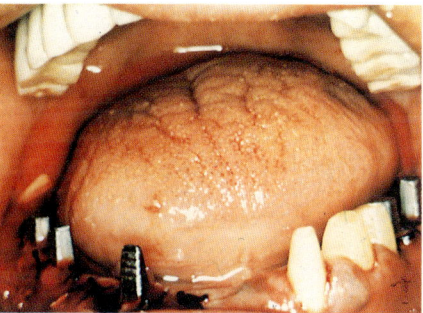

2.

Inserting blade.

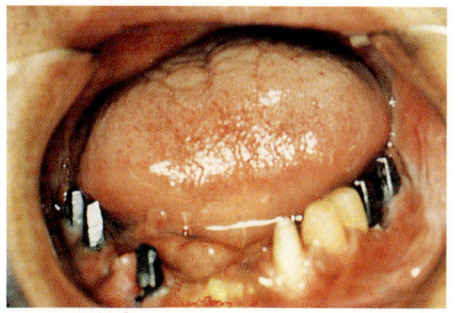

3.

After 1 week.

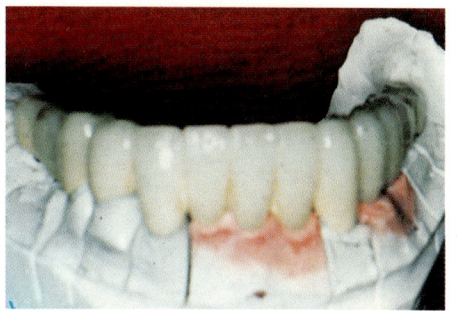

4.

Superstructure.

S-Case (f)

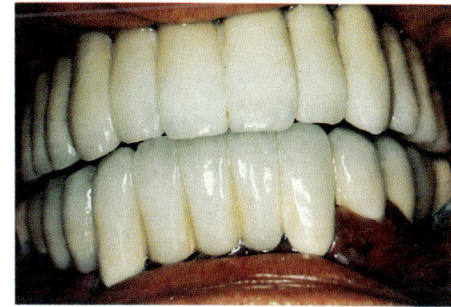

1.

Cementing superstructure.

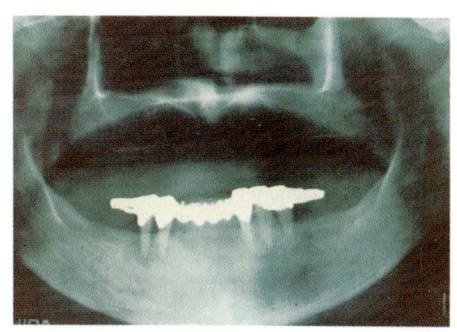

2.

Before operation.

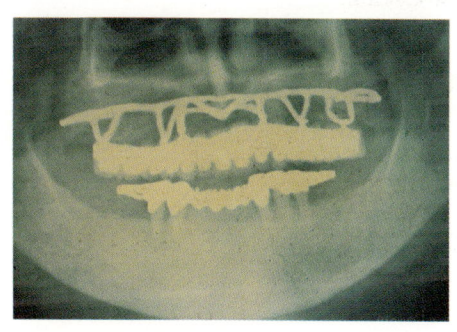

3.

After subperiosteal implant.

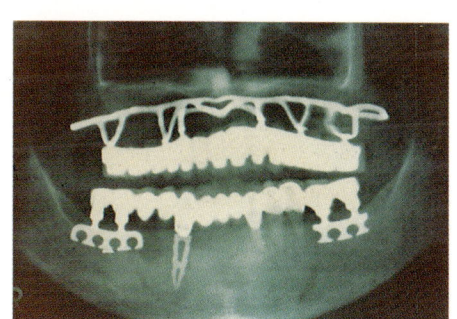

4.

Inserting the lower blade.

S-Case 3 (a)   **S-Case 3 (b)**

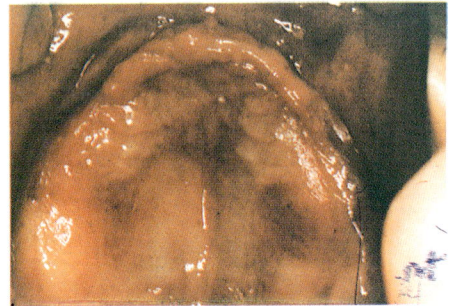

1.

Preoperative photo. Edentulous case.

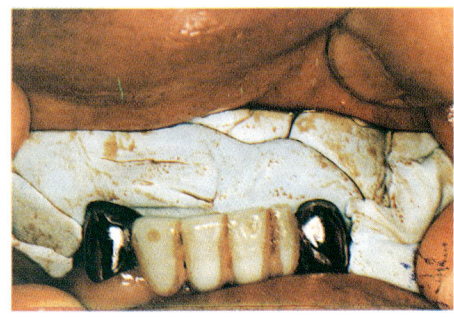

1.

Bone impression and bone bite are taken.

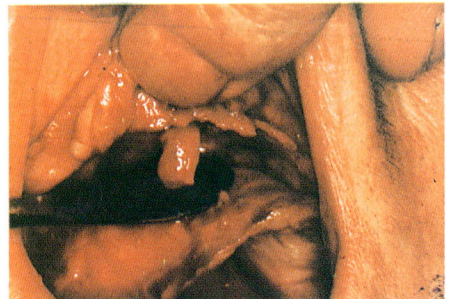

2.

Mucosa is reflected. It is important not to cut along the sphenopalatine at the level of incisive foramen.

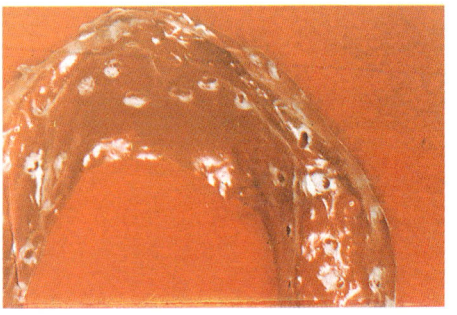

2.

Plastic impression tray. It must be made within 15 minutes.

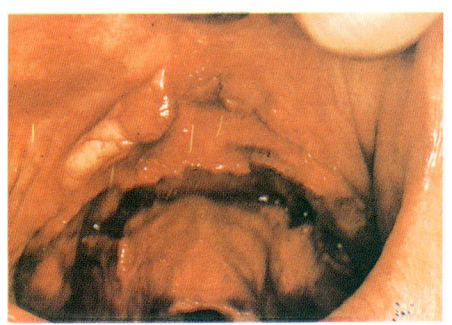

3.

Bone is exposed.

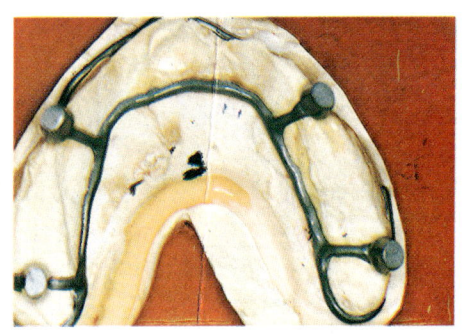

3.

Substructure.

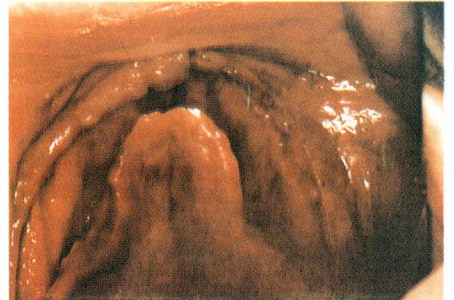

4.

Bone is exposed (maxilla).

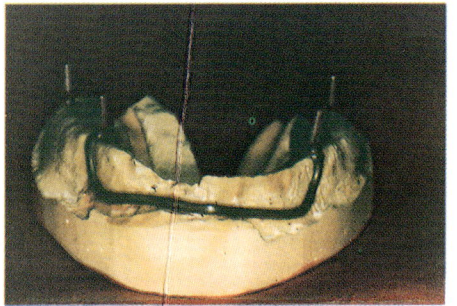

4.

Substructure: front view.

S-Case 3 (c)

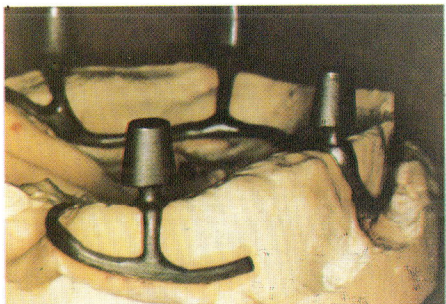

1.

Substructure: buccal-side view.

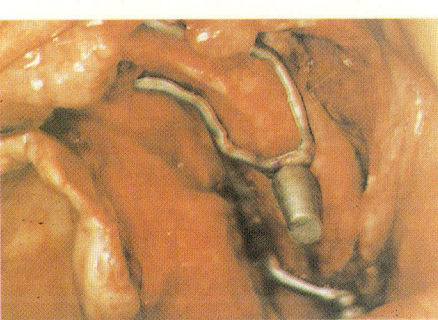

2.

1 week after the 1st stage operation.

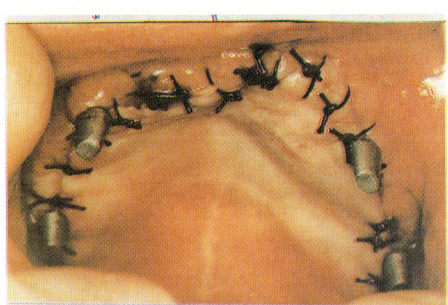

3.

Second stage operation. Tight fitting is confirmed.

4.

Suture. Soft tissues are repositioned and sutured.

S-Case 3 (d)

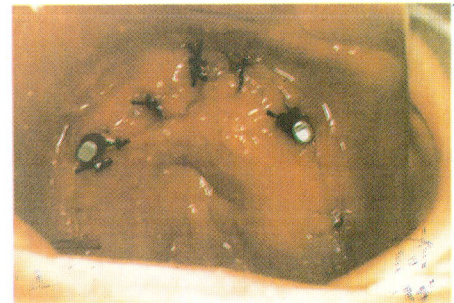

1.

10 days after the 2nd stage operation.

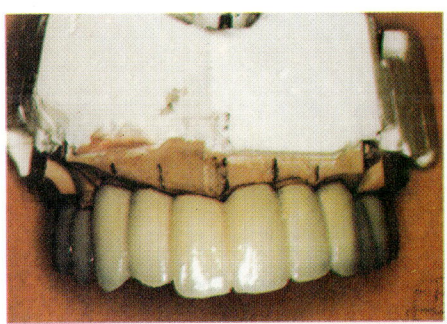

2.

Superstructure.

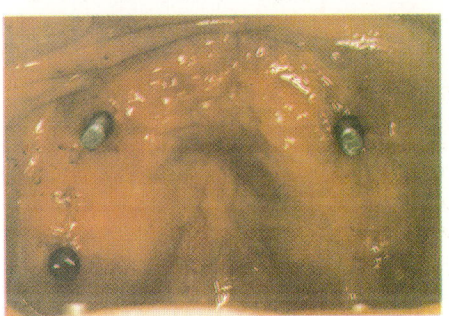

3.

2 weeks after the 2nd stage operation. Mucosa is very normal.

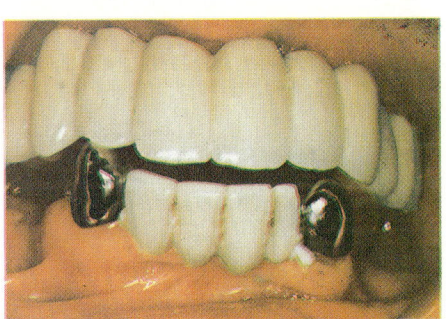

4.

Superstructure is cemented.

S-Case 3 (e)   **S-Case 3 (f)**

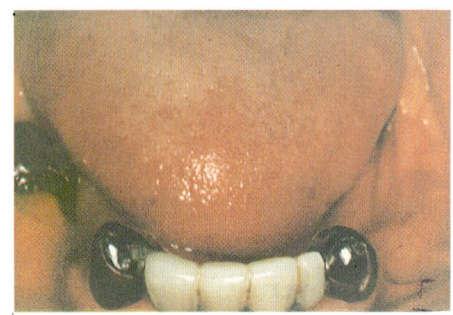

1. Preoperative photo.

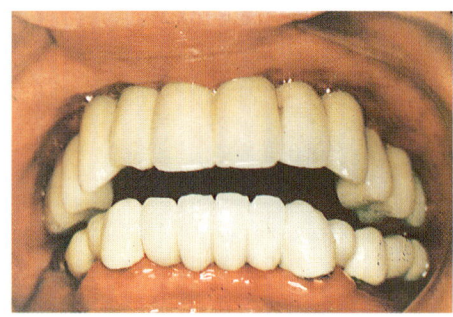

1. Postoperative photo.

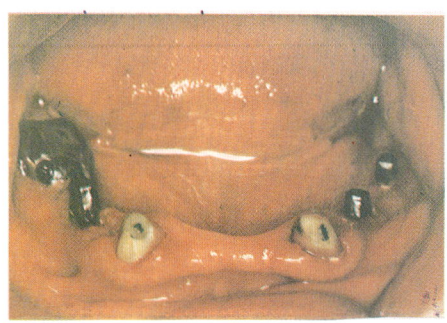

2. Bridge is removed and implants are inserted on both sides at the same time.

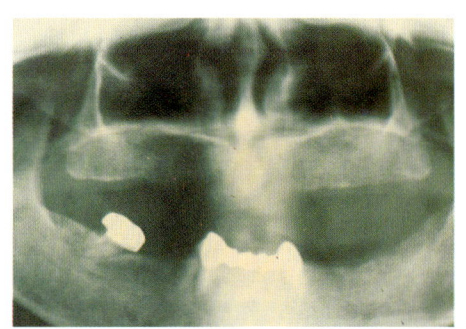

2.

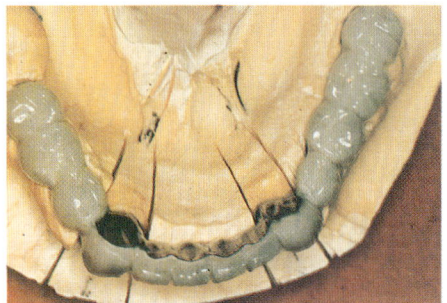

3. Superstructure.

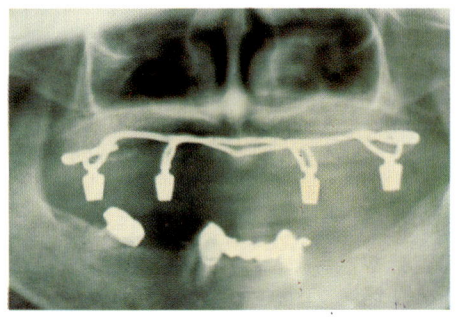

3.

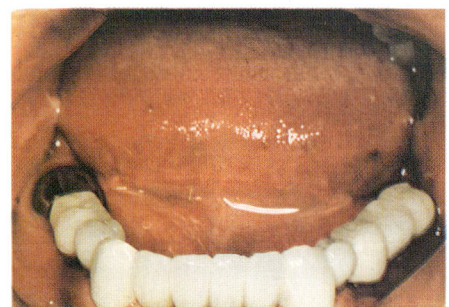

4. Superstructure is cemented. Front view.

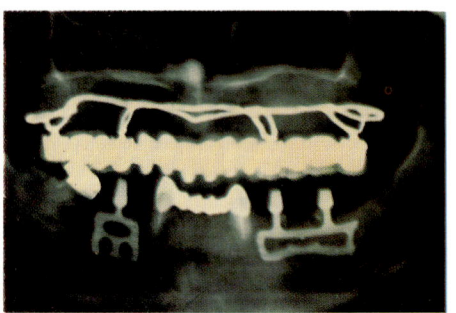

4. Postoperative panoramic X-ray.

S-Case 4 (a)   **S-Case 4 (b)**

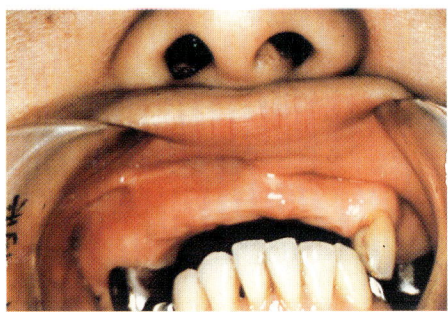

1.

Preoperative photo. Frontal view.

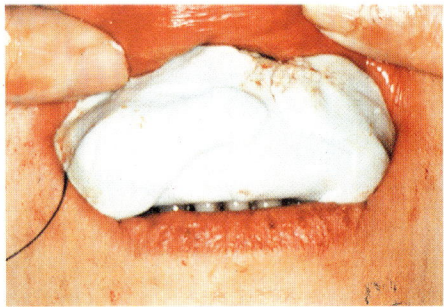

1.

Photo of bone impression.

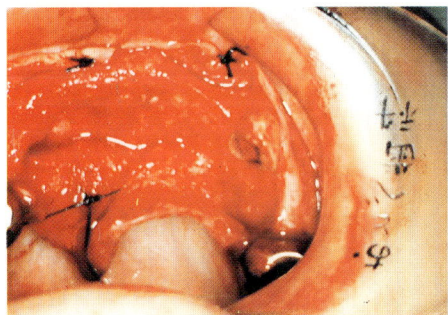

2.

Mucosa is reflected as widely as possible.

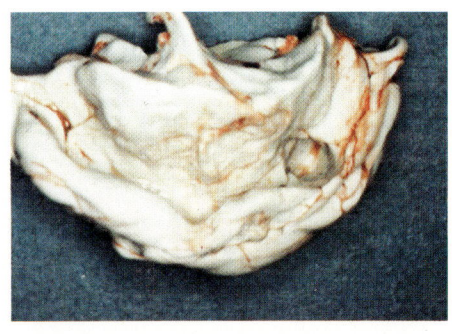

2.

Substructure: lingual-side view.

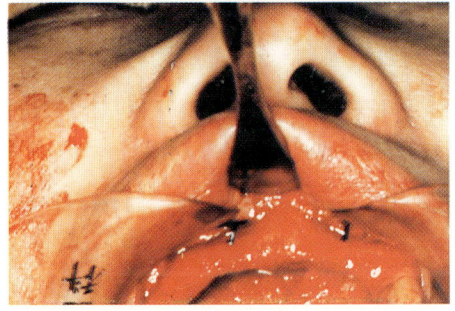

3.

Anterior nasal spine is exposed.

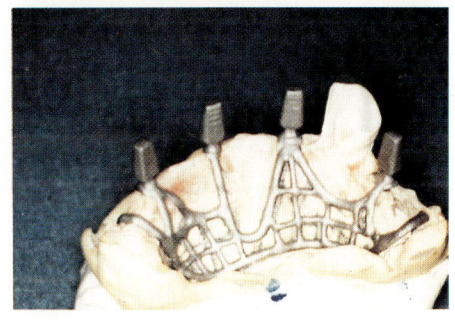

3.

Substructure: buccal-side view.

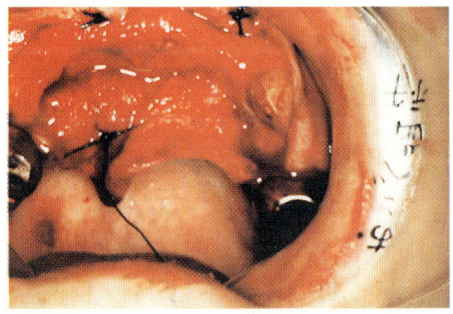

4.

Mucosa is reflected.

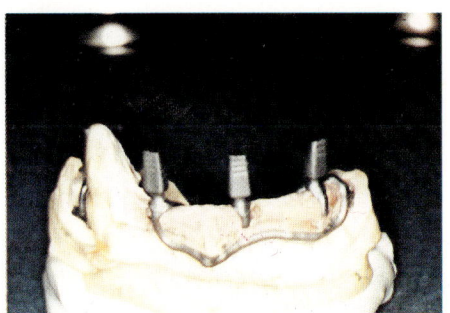

4.

Bone impression and bone bite are taken.

S-Case 4 (c)   **S-Case 4 (d)**

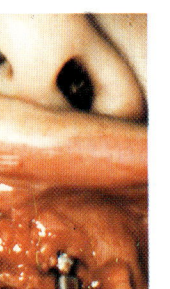

1.

The substructure is fitted to bone.

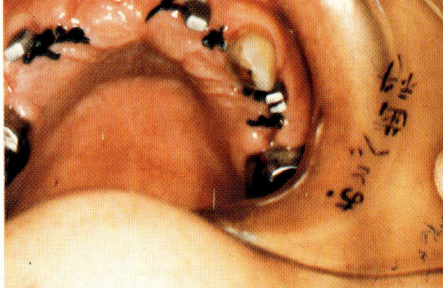

1.

1st days after the 1st stage operation.

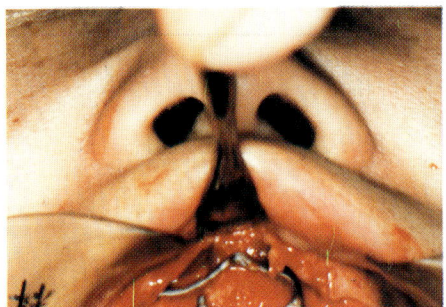

2.

Substructure is fit correctly on the anterior nasal spine.

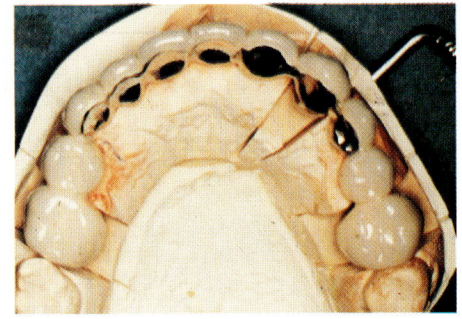

2.

Superstructure.

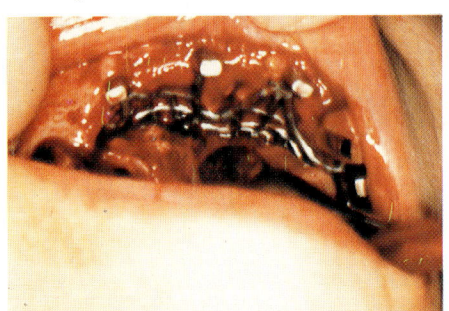

3.

Substructure is inserted. Fitting is examined and accuracy is confirmed.

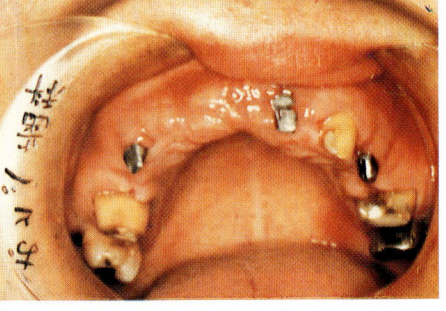

3.

Mucosa is completely healed and normal.

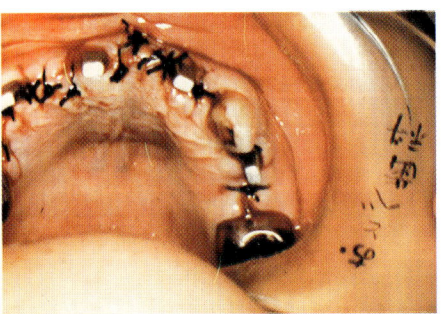

4.

Mucosa is sutured.

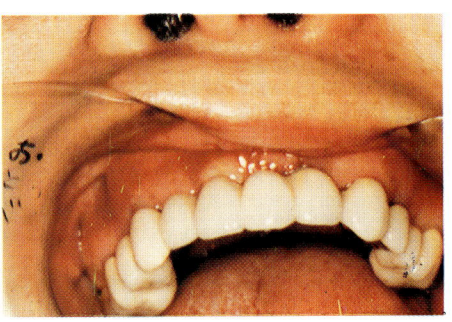

4.

Superstructure is cemented.

S-Case 4 (e)

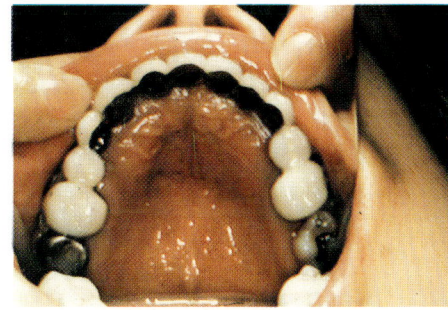

1.

Superstructure. Palatal-side view.

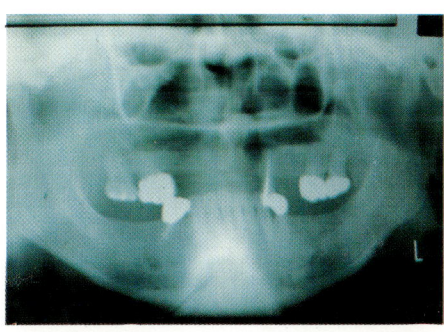

2.

Panoramic X-ray taken right after the 2nd stage operation.

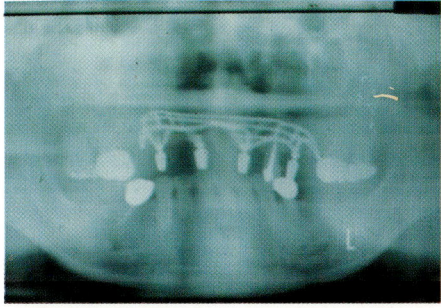

3.

Preoperative panoramic X-ray.

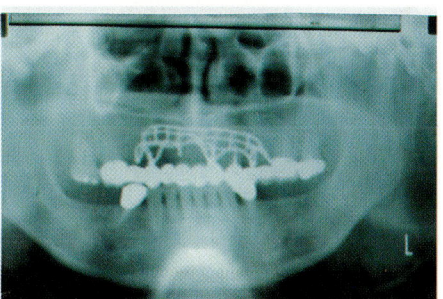

4.

Postoperative panoramic X-ray.

S-Case 5 (a)   **S-Case 5 (b)**

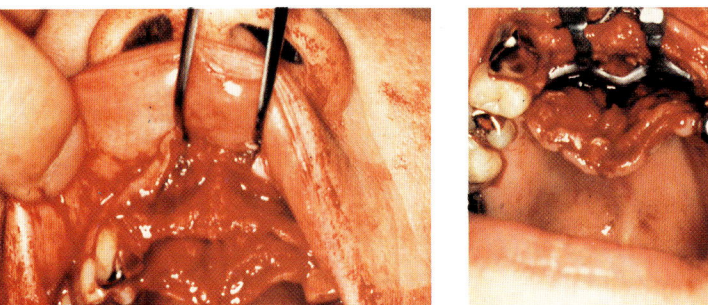

1.

Preoperative photo.   Substructure: front view.   1.

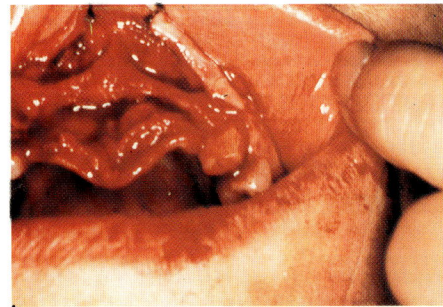   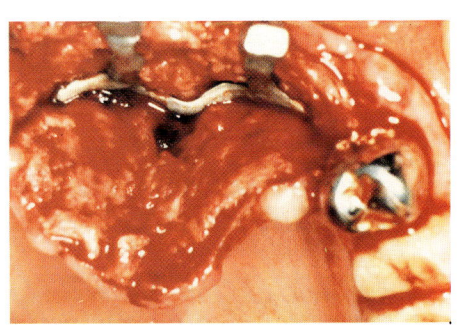

2.

Incision.   Substructure: palatal-side view.   2.

3.

Mucosa is reflected.   Substructure is fit.   3.

4.

The nasal spine is very important to ident-   Substructure. A tight fit is observed.   4.
ify in the anterior exposure.

S-Case 5 (c)

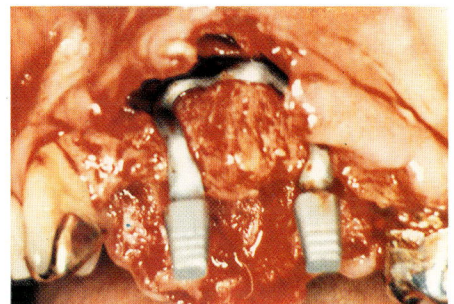

1.

The substructure is set on the anterior nasal spine correctly.

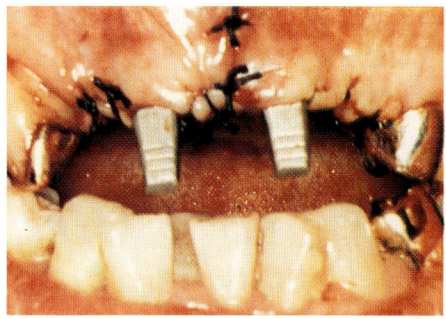

2.

Suture.

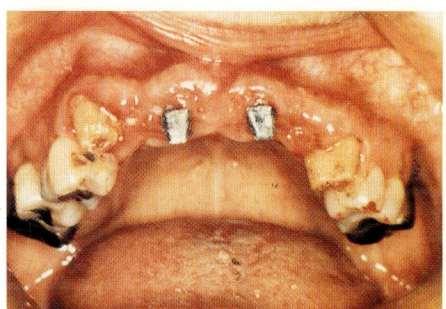

3.

2 weeks after the 2nd stage operation.

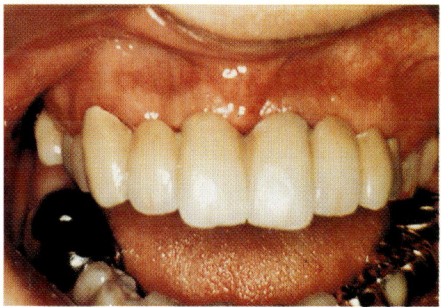

4.

Superstructure.

S-Case 6 (a)   **S-Case 6 (b)**

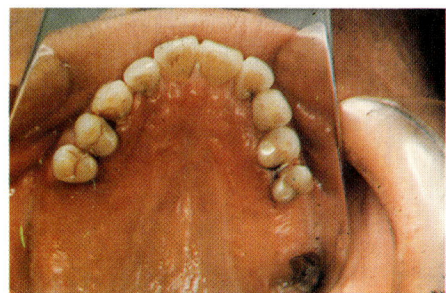

1.

Preoperative photo.

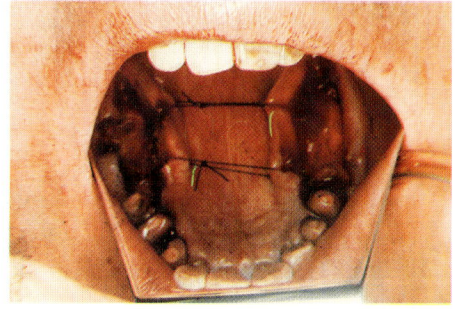

1.

Photo of 1st stage operation. Mucosa is reflected on both sides and pterygoid extension are exposed.

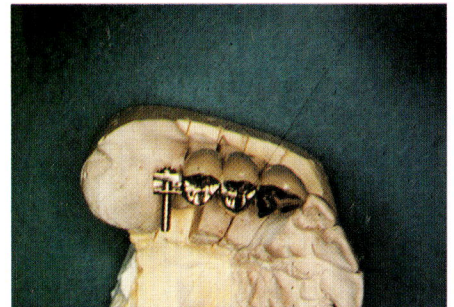

2.

Crowns with a key anchor at their ends are tried.

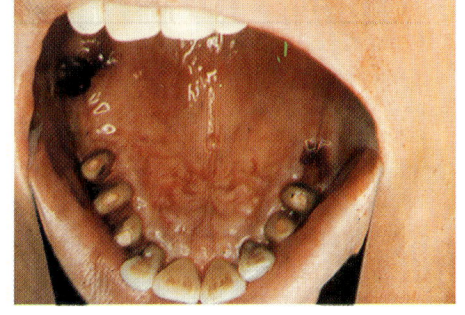

2.

Crowns are tried in the mouth cavity.

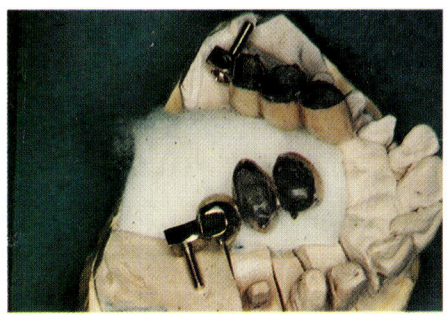

3.

Crowns with screw coupling at ends are made for molars.

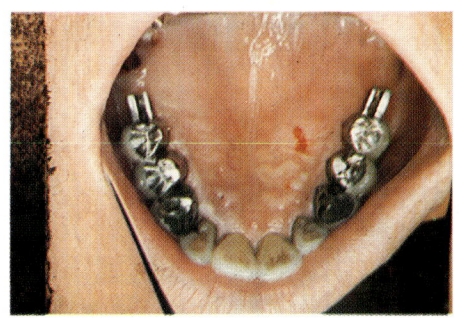

3.

Preoperative photo.

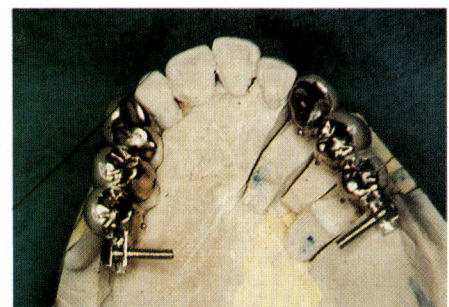

4.

Same as above.

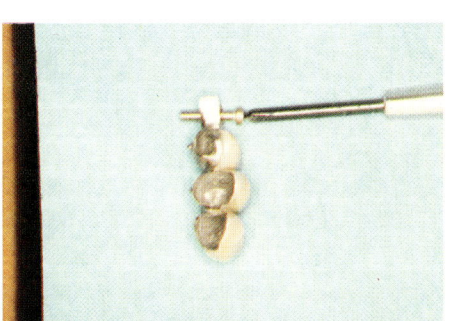

4.

Screw coupling

S-Case 6 (c)

S-Case 6 (d)

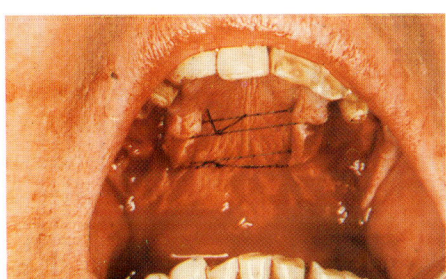

1.

Reflected mucosa is sutured to operate easily.

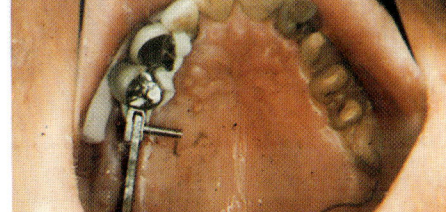

1.

Crowns are cemented in the mouth. The extension bar is fitted to the bone. Crowns and extension bar are connected.

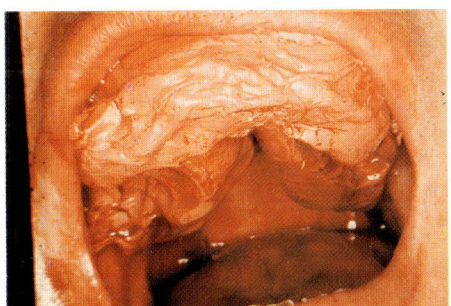

2.

Bone impression is taken.

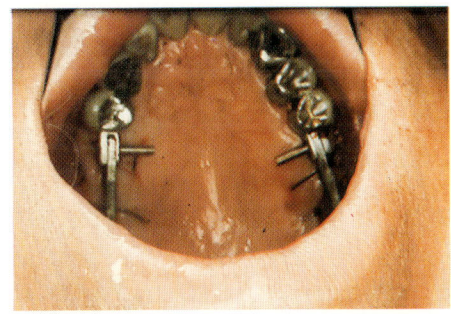

2.

After suturing, the unnecessary parts of the screws are cut off.

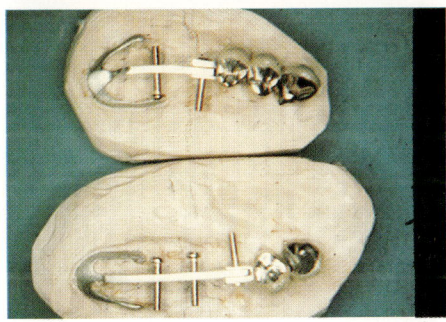

3.

Substructure and extension are connected.

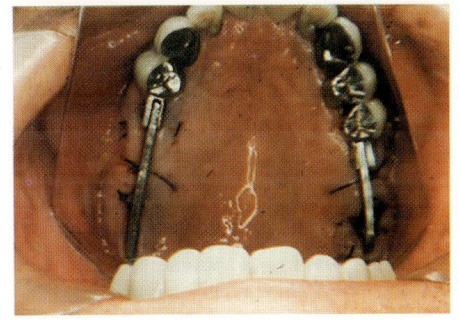

3.

Suture.

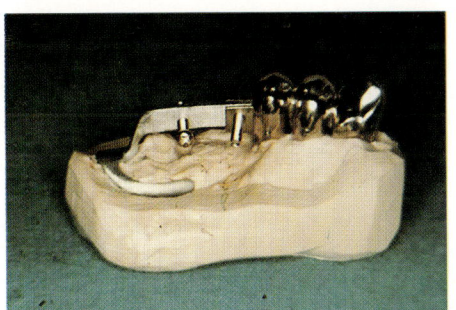

4.

Substructure and extension, lingual side view.

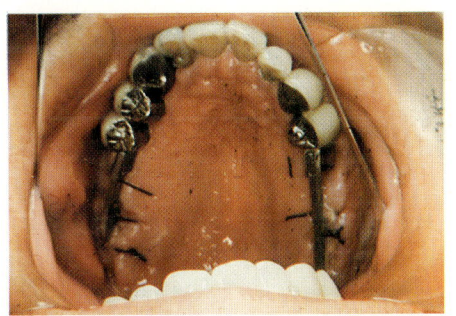

4.

Ten days after the 2nd stage operation mucosa is beautiful.

S-Case 6 (e)   **S-Case 6 (f) THIS CASE IS PTERYGOID EXTENSION**

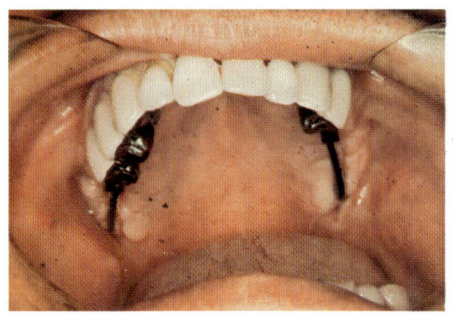

1.

Superstructure is tried in.

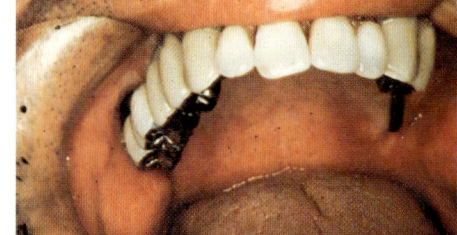

1.

Superstructure is tried in.

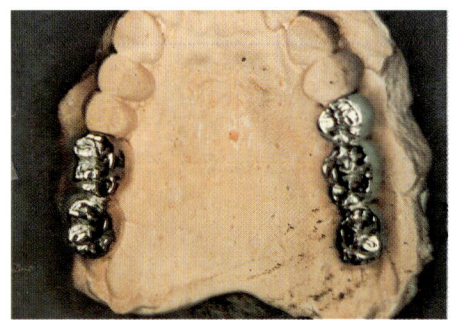

2.

Superstructure.

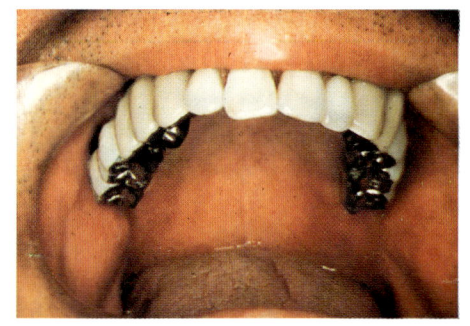

2.

Superstructure is cemented.

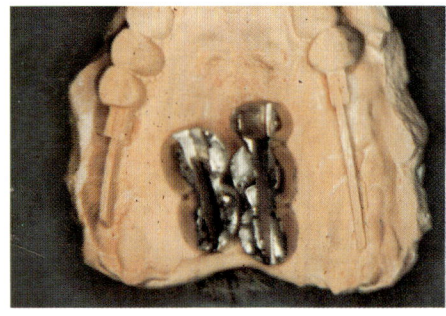

3.

Superstructure.

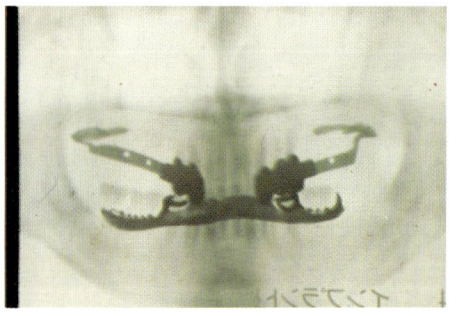

3.

Postoperative panorama X-ray.

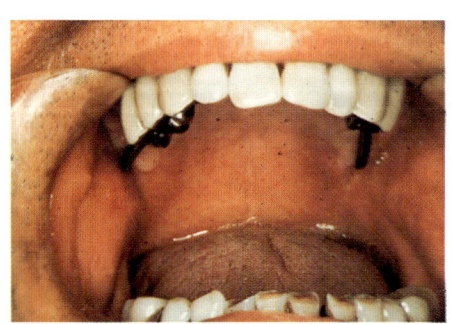

4.

S-Case 7 (a)

S-Case 7 (b)

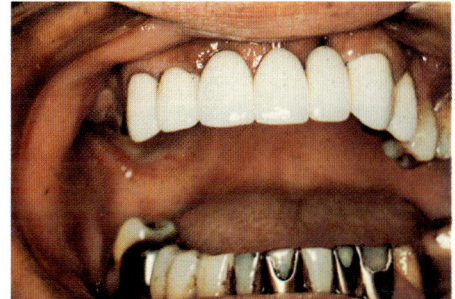

1.

Preoperative photo.

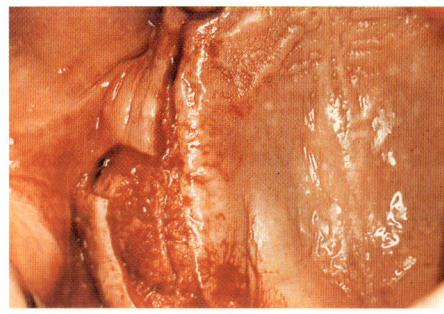

1.

Reflection of soft tissues.

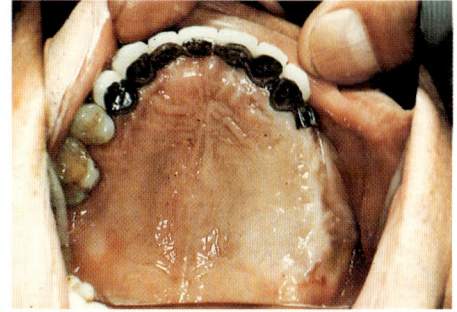

2.

Preoperative photo (palatal-side view).

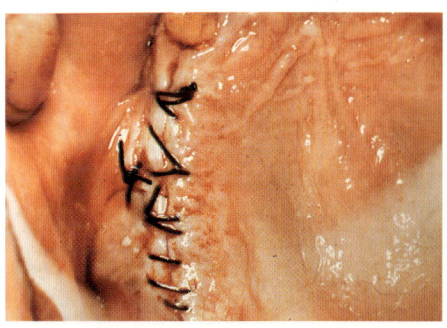

2.

Suture after bone impression taking.

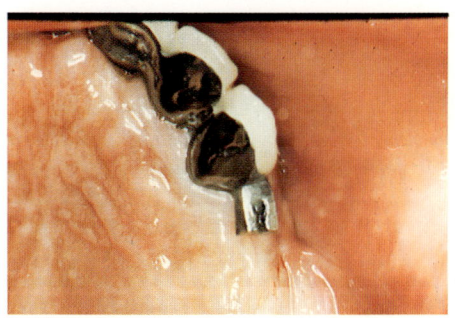

3.

Crown with a key anchor at its end is tried.

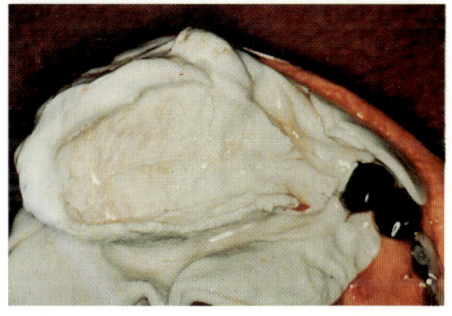

3.

Bone impression - mucosa-side view.

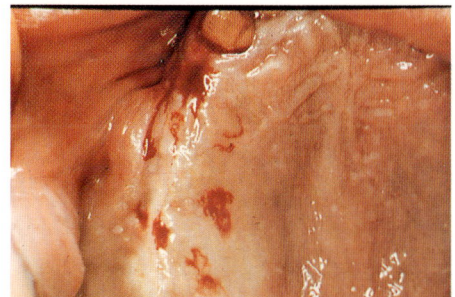

4.

Incision.

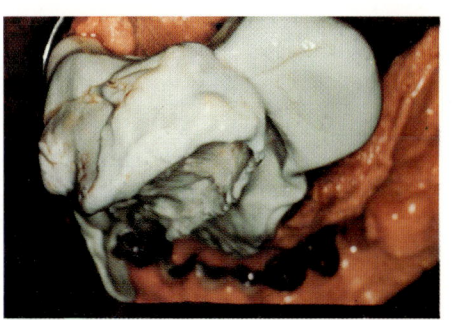

4.

Bone impression - buccal-side view.

S-Case 7 (c)   **S-Case 7 (d)**

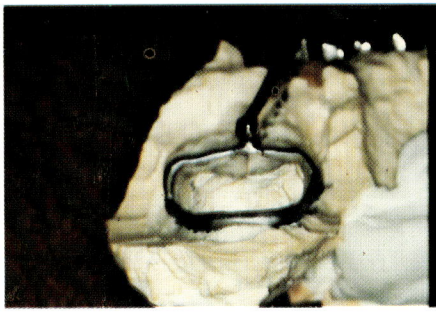

1.

Substructure - Pterygoid extension is utilized.

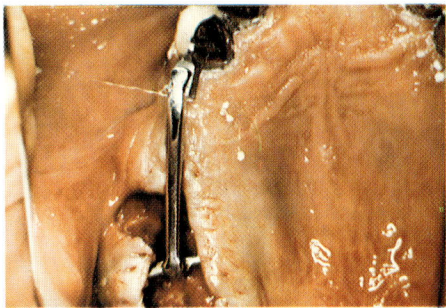

1.

Pterygoid is exposed and substructure is implanted.

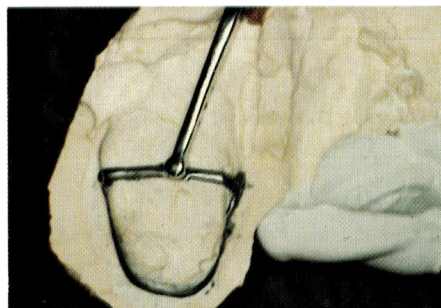

2.

Substructure.

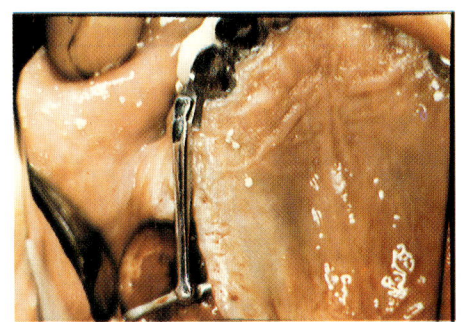

2.

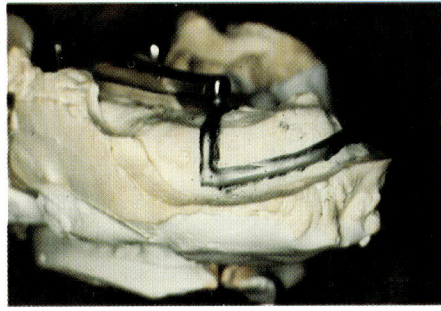

3.

Substructure.

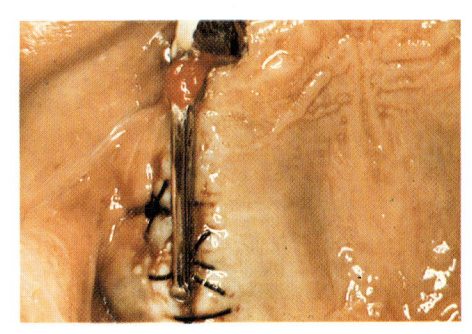

3.

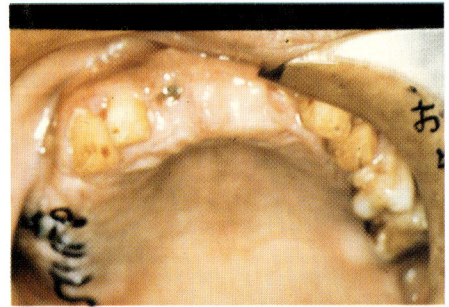

4.

Ten days after the 1st stage operation.

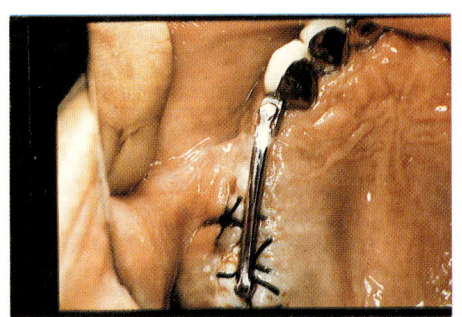

4.

4. Suture.

S-Case 8 (a)

S-Case 8 (b)

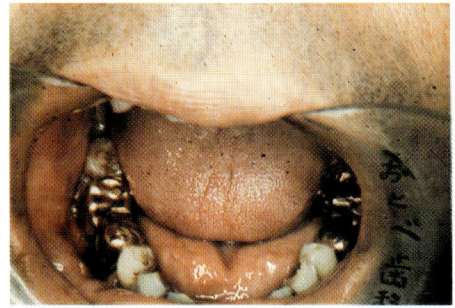

1.

Preoperative photo.

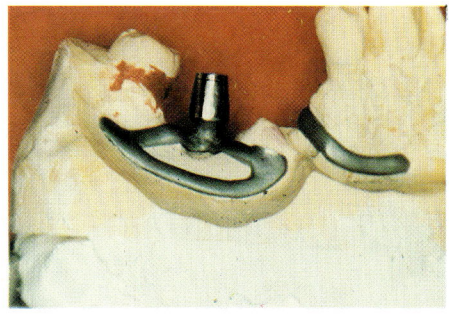

1.

Substructure: buccal side view.

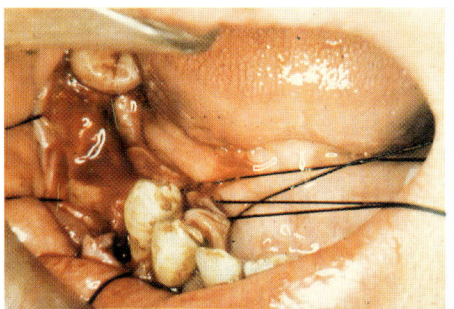

2.

Mucosa is reflected in exposing bone.

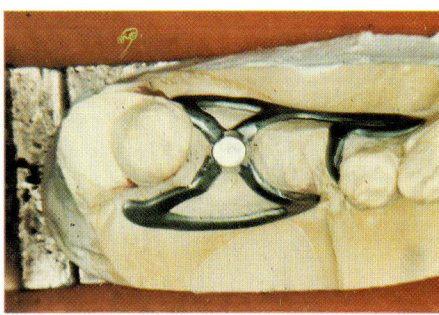

2.

The part on the right side of the line was unnecessary.

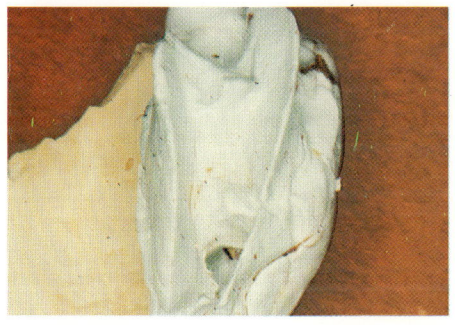

3.

Bone impression.

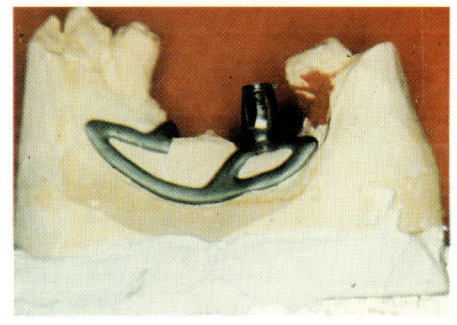

3.

Substructure: lingual side view.

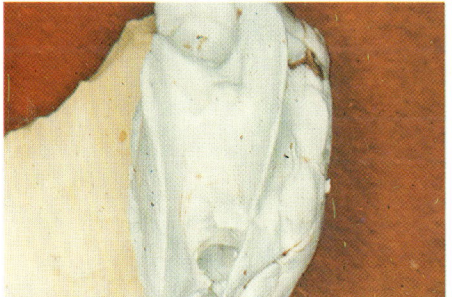

4.

Bone impression.

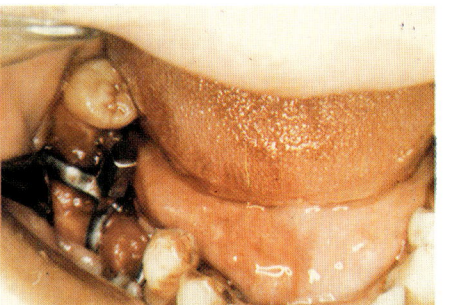

4.

Second stage operation. Implant is inserted.

S-Case 8 (c)   **S-Case 8 (d)**

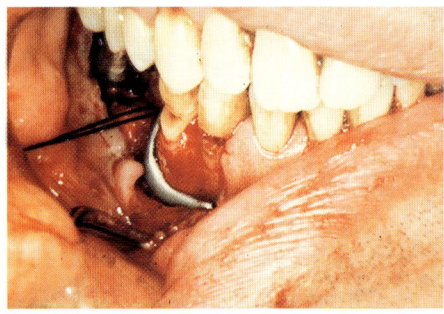

1.

Second stage operation.

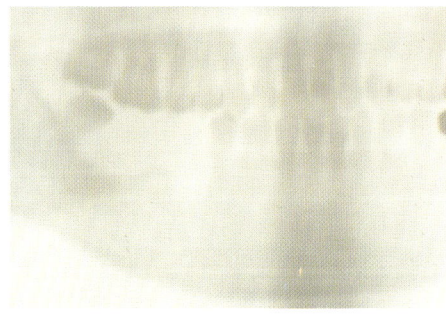

1.

Preoperative panorama X-ray.

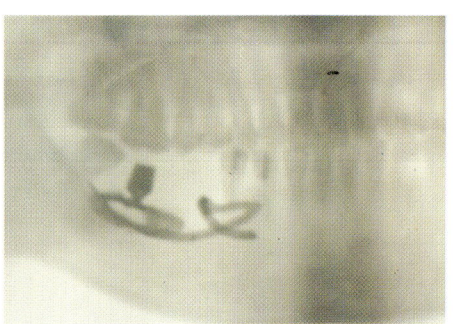

2.

Second stage operation. Tissues are sutured.

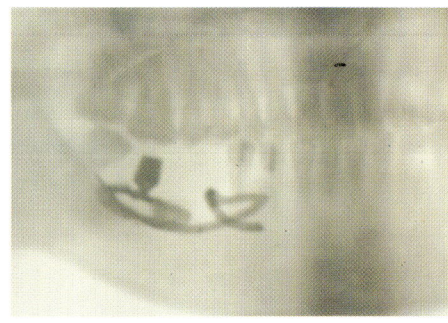

2.

Panoramic X-ray after second stage operation.

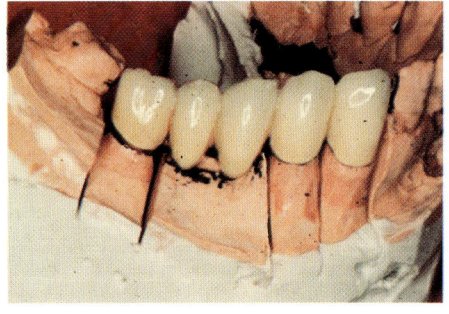

3.

Substructure is attached to model.

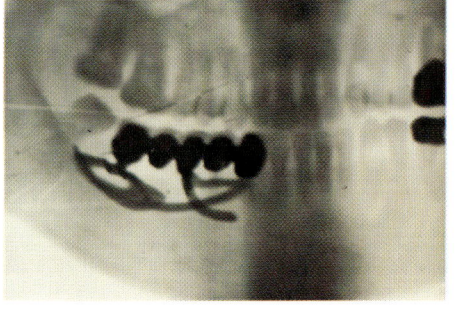

3.

Postoperative panorama X-ray.

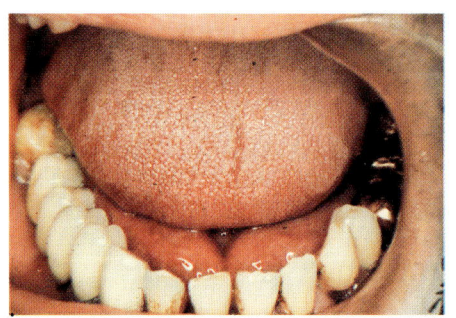

4.

Superstructure is set in the mouth.

LOWER UNILATERAL

S-Case 9 (a)

S-Case 9 (b)

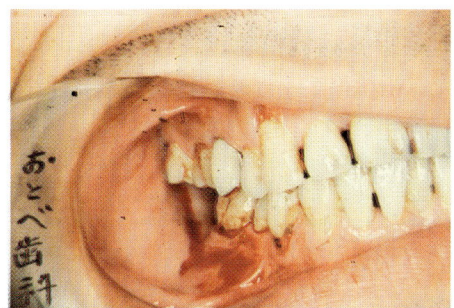

1.

Preoperative photo.

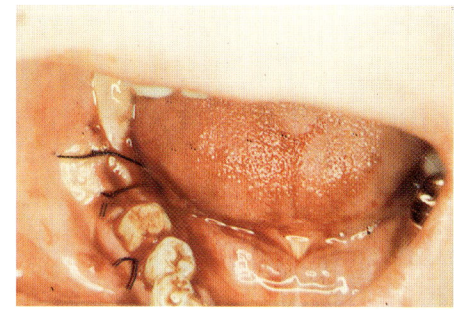

1.

Suture.

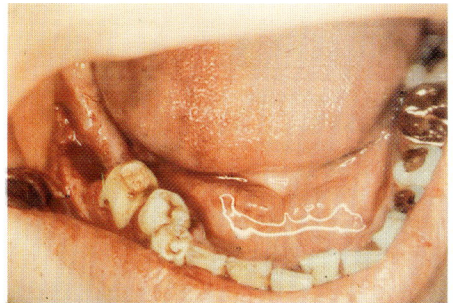

2.

Reflection of soft tissues.

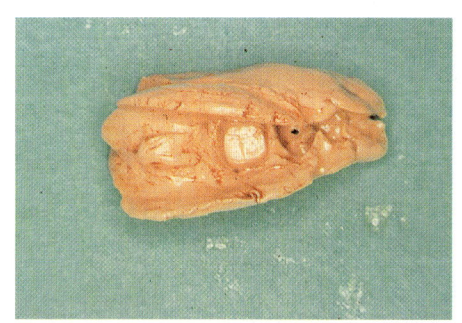

2.

Bone impression.

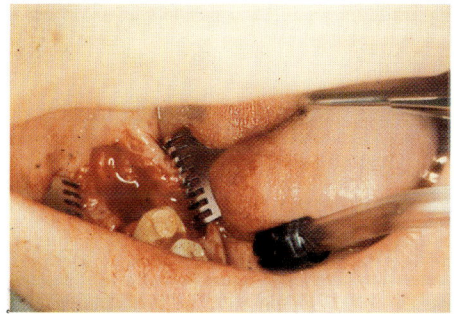

3.

Bone is exposed.

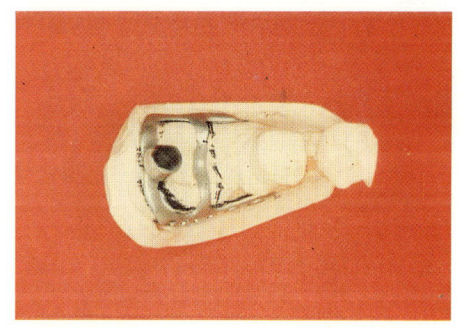

3.

Substructure.

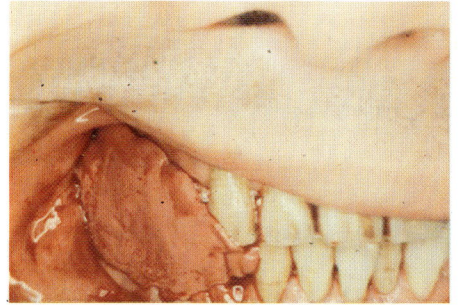

4.

Bone impression and bone bite are taken.

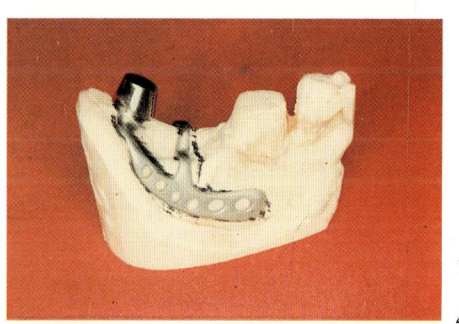

4.

Substructure: buccal-side view.

S-Case 10 (a)   **S-Case 10 (b)**

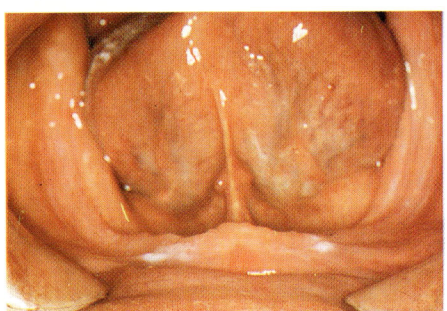

1.

Preoperative photo.

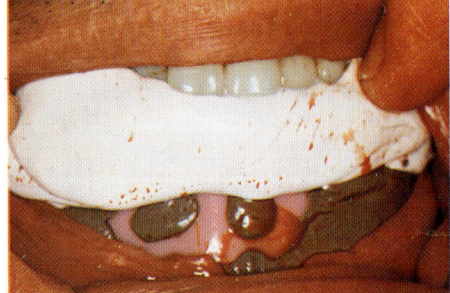

1.

Bone impression and bone bite are taken.

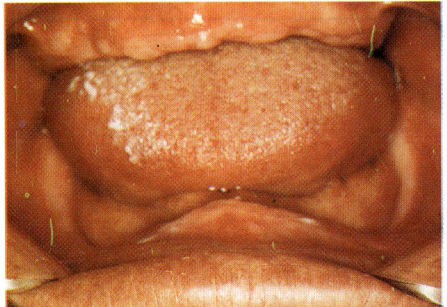

2.

Preoperative photo.

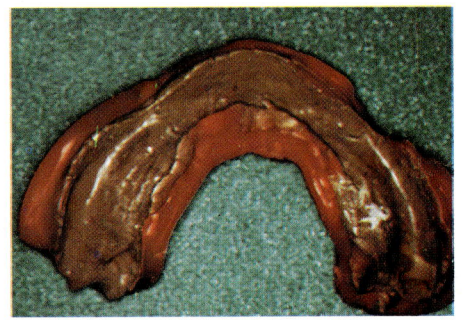

2.

Bone impression (mucosa-side view).

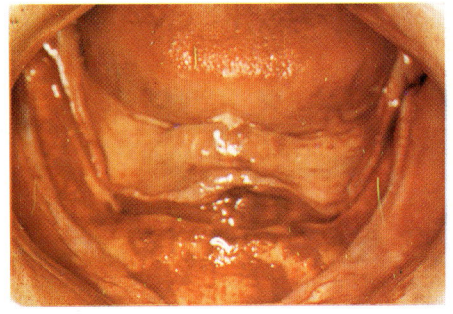

3.

Photo of 1st stage operation. Bone is exposed.

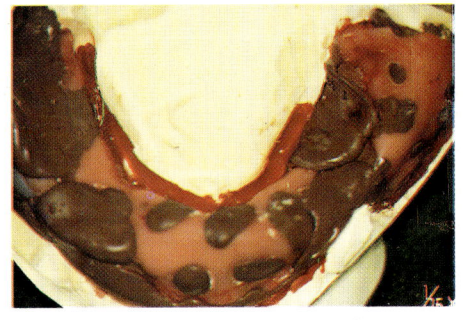

3.

Plaster is poured into the impression.

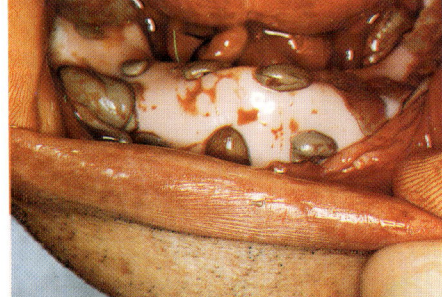

4.

Bone impression.

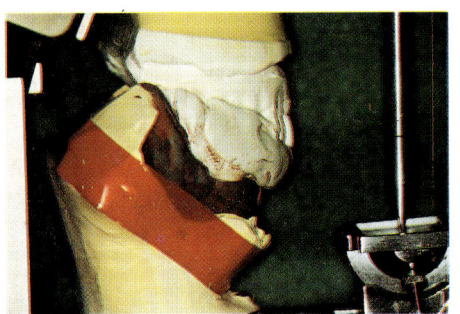

4.

Model attached to the articulator.

S-Case 10 (c)

S-Case 10 (d)

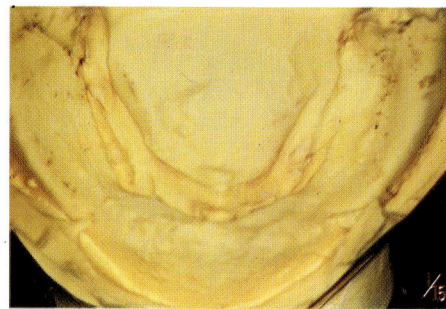

1.

Model.

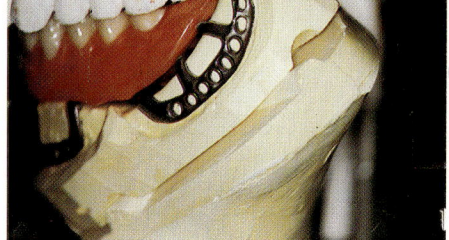

1.

Substructure and superstructure on model.

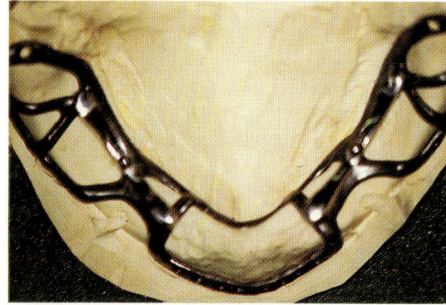

2.

Substructure.

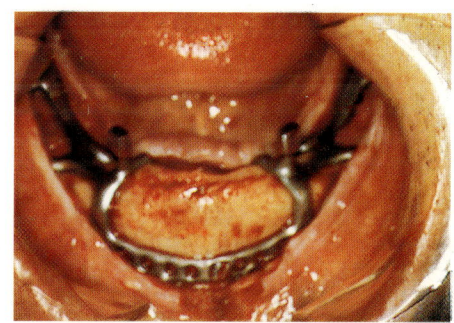

2.

Photo of 2nd stage operation. Superstructure is fitted to the bone beautifully.

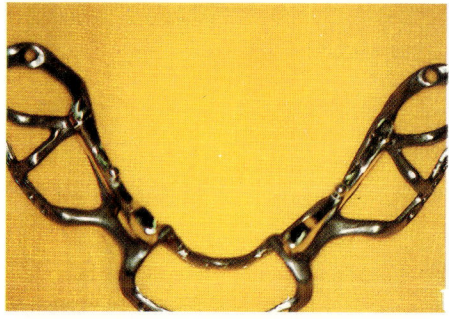

3.

Substructure.

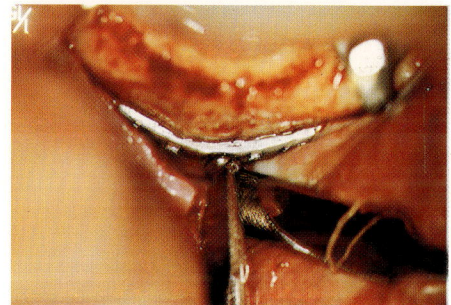

3.

Photo of 2nd stage operation. Tight fitting is observed.

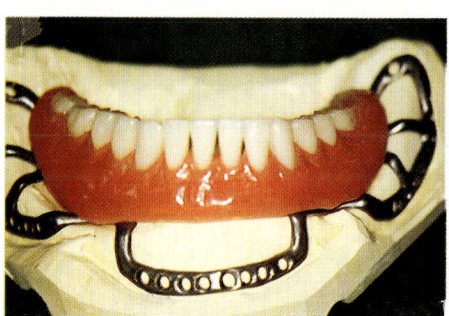

4.

Substructure and superstructure.

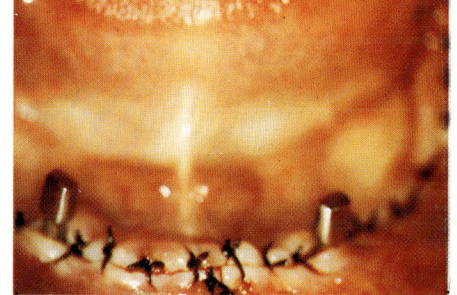

4.

Suture.

S-Case 11 (a)

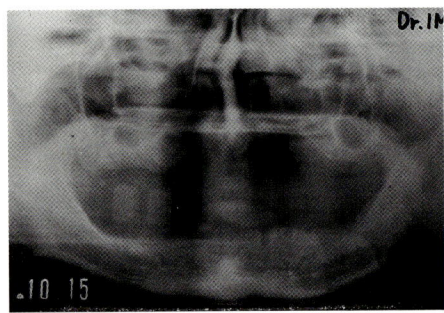

1.

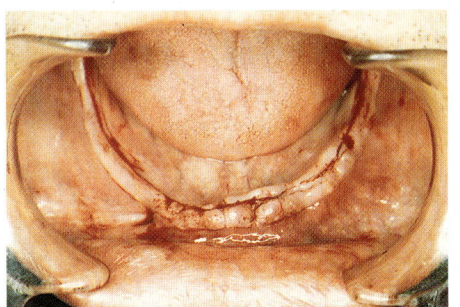

3.

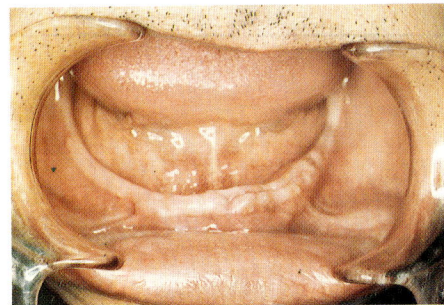

2.

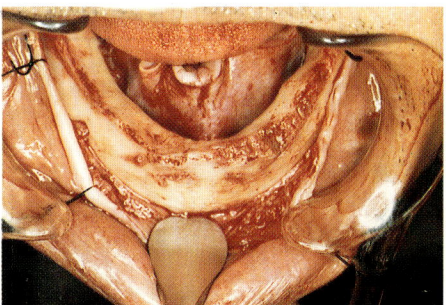

4.

1. The radiograph demostrates moderate atrophy of the mandible, with a minimal amount of residual alveolar ridge in the region of the molar teeth, and no odontogenic tumours and no dental anomalies.
2. The patient was unable to function with his lower denture because of the excess gum tissue and the severe atrophy of the mandible.
3. Care was taken to create a definite atraumatic incision line completely through the attached gingiva and periosteum.
4. The tissues were reflected carefully to expose all the landmarks.

S-Case 11 (b)

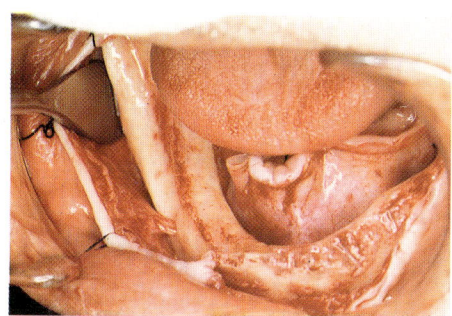

1.

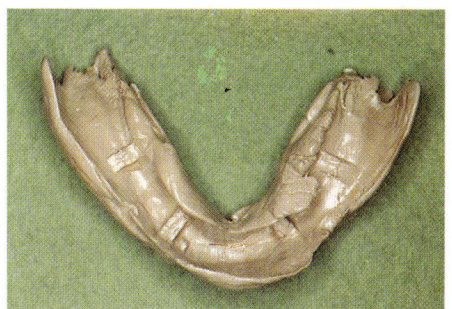

3.

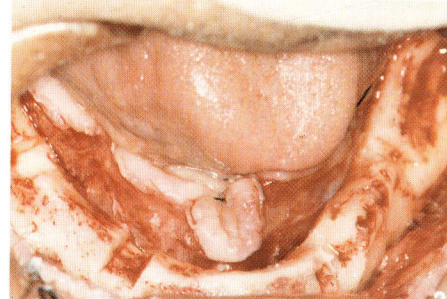

2.

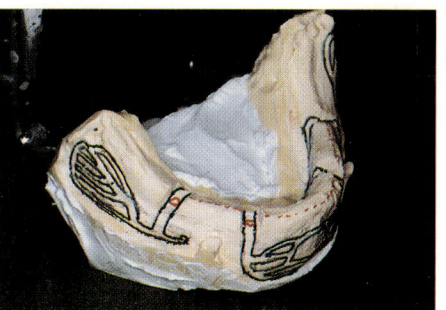

4.

1. Extreme care was taken in the mental foramen areas to avoid any disruption of the neurovascular seaths.
2. The groove of the residual alveolar bone in the region of the connecting struts of the substructure was prepared so that the connecting struts could be prevented from exposure.
3. The impression was checked thoroughly for the presence of voids and the registering of all anatomical landmarks.
4. The cast was mounted utilizing the surgical bites obtained and the framework was designed on the cast.

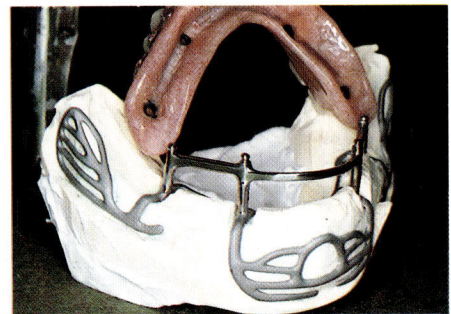

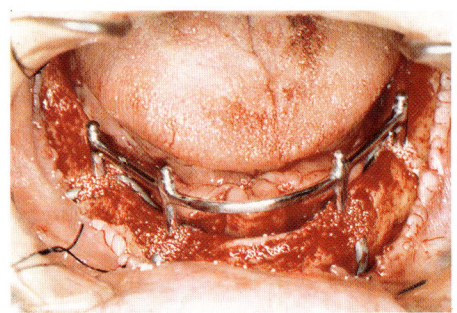

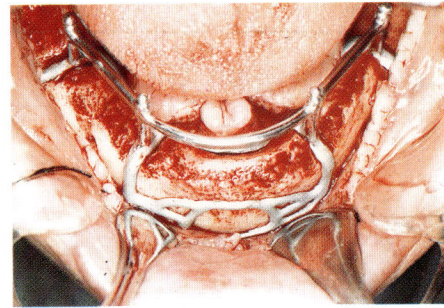

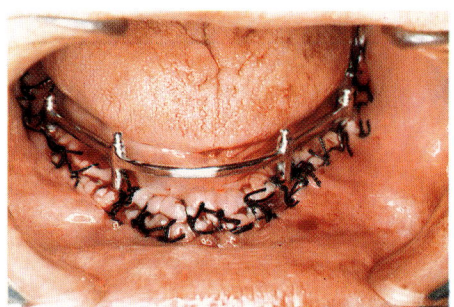

1. Upon return, the frame-work was evaluated, approved and sterilized in an autoclave for surgery. The lower denture with O-ring attachment was completed.
2. The completed implant was inserted. A close evaluation was made to see if a tight fit existed.
3. The hydroxylapatite particles were packed in the bone groove so that new bone might deposit on the surface of hydroxylapatite forming a strong attachment and facilitating the repair of bony defects.
4. Purse-string sutures were placed closely around each protruding neck, making sure that the tissue closely adapts to the necks. Interrupted surgical ties were placed between the posts and the necks. Any tissue that seemed to resist closing was augmented with a mattress suture.

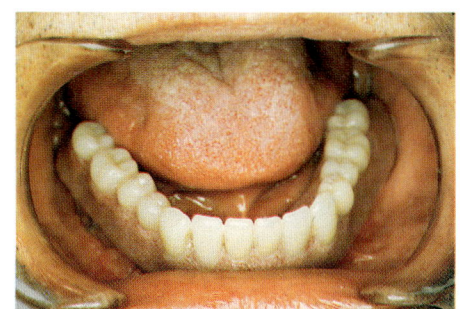

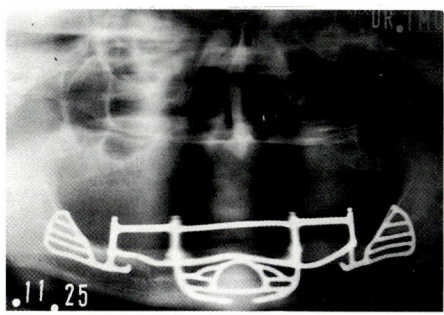

1. The lower denture with O-ring attachment was placed into sub-periosteal posts and the patient was reminded to eat soft foods. No mobility, infection and discomfort were present.

2. Panoramic x-ray.

NEXT 21 CASES ARE EXHIBITED AS SAMPLES OF SUBSTRUCTURE DESIGN

Upper full edentulous

Case 1   **Case 2**

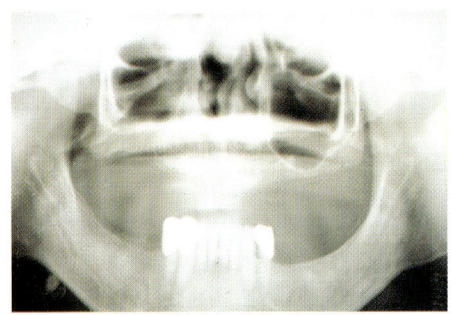

1.

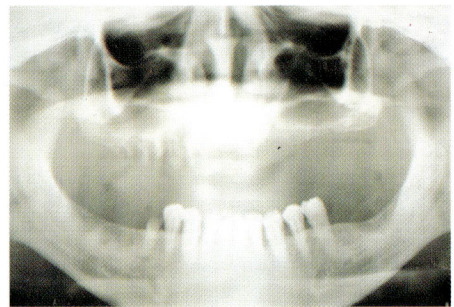

1.

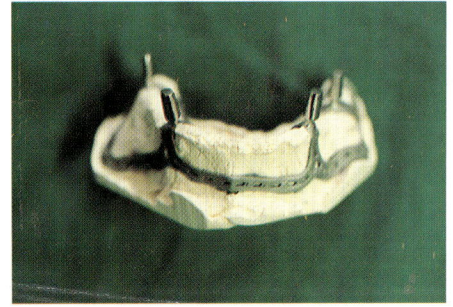

2.

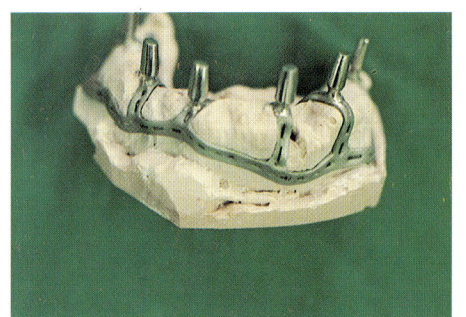

2.

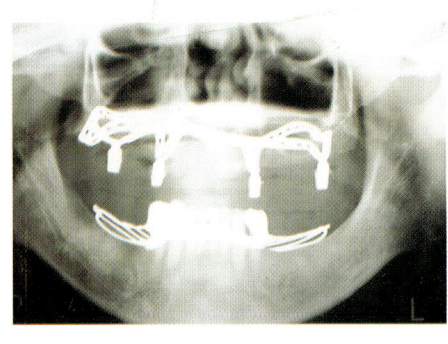

3.

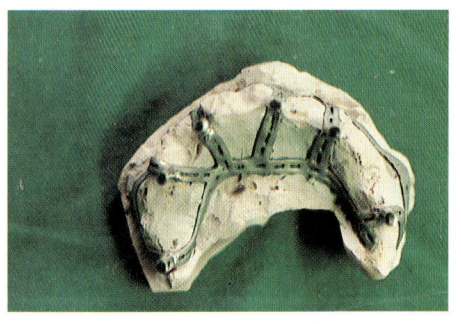

3.

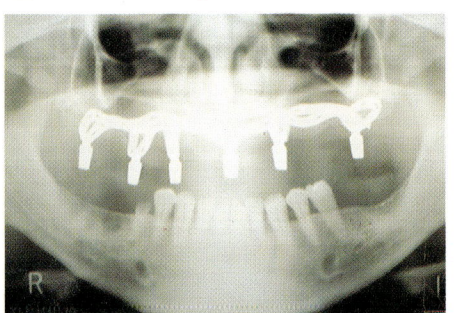

4.

4.

**Fully edentulous
Case 3**

**Fully edentulous
Case 4**

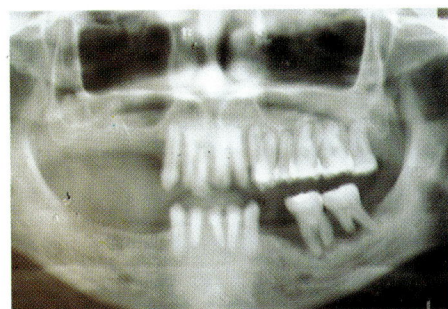

1.

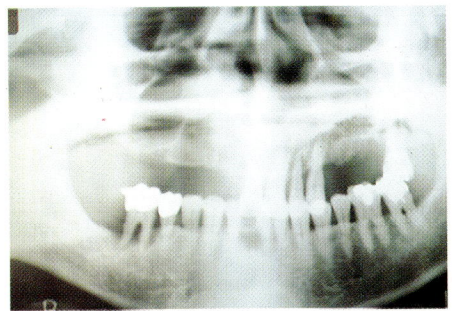

1.

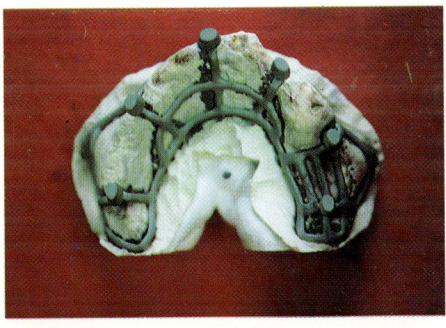

2.

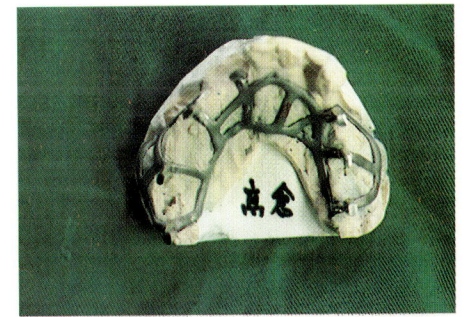

2.

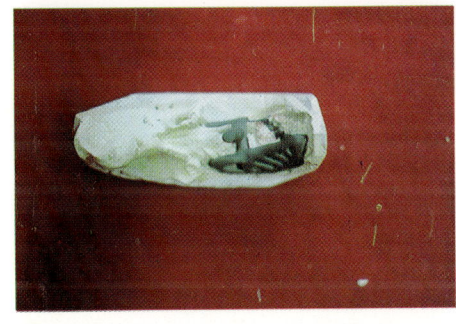

3.

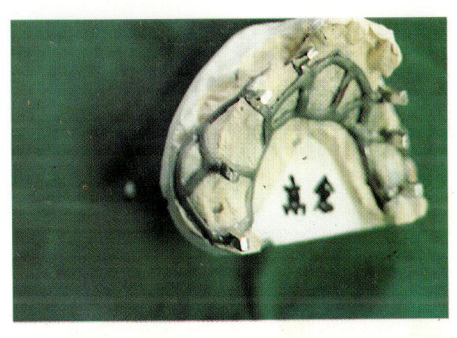

3.

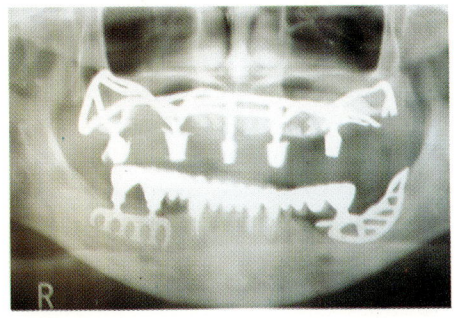

4.

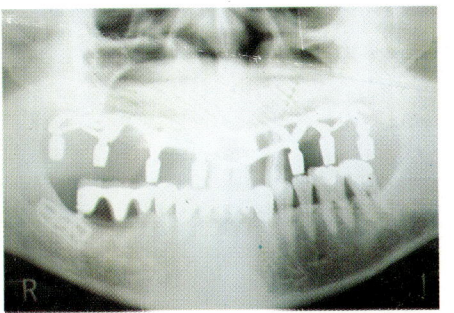

4.

**Full substructure
Case 5**

**Full substructure
Case 6**

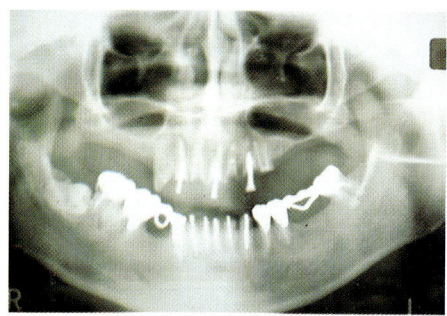

1.

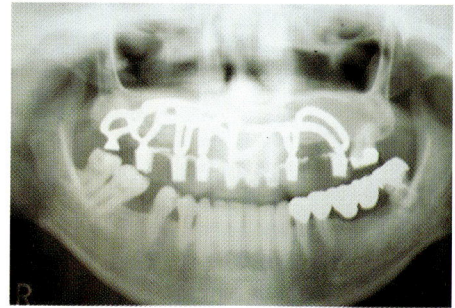

1.

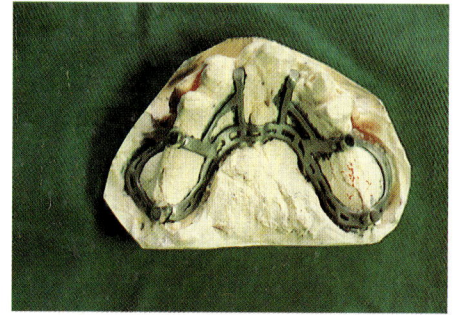

2.

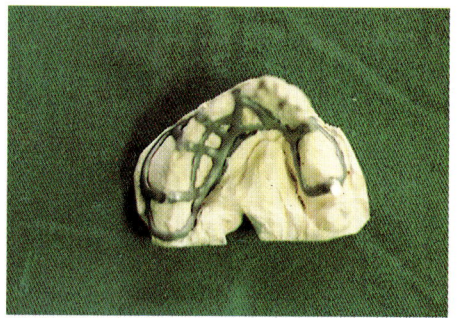

2.

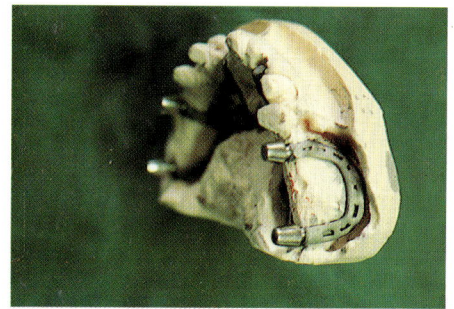

3.

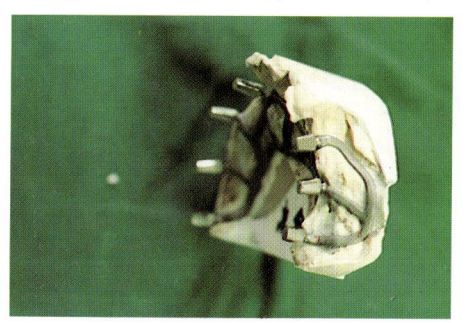

3.

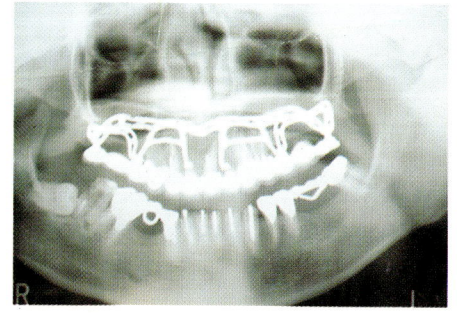

4.

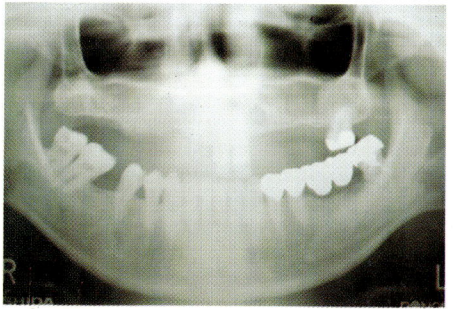

4.

**Full substructure
Case 7**

**Full substructure
Case 8**

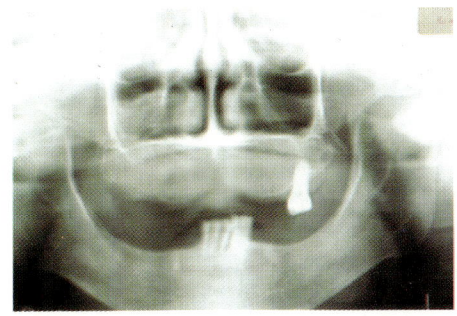

1.

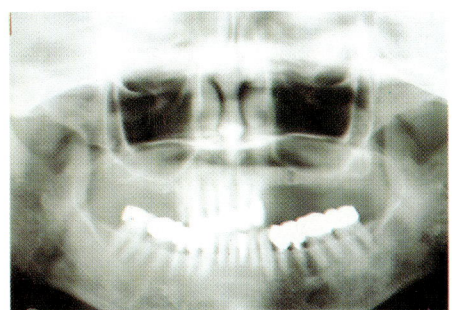

1.

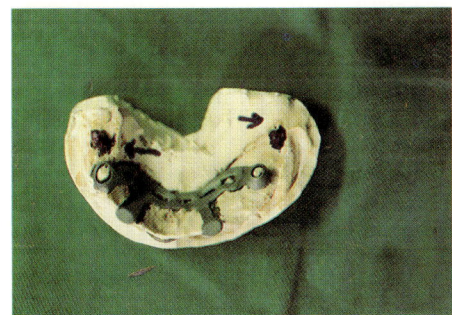

2.

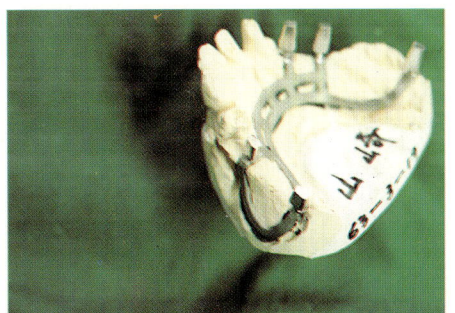

2.

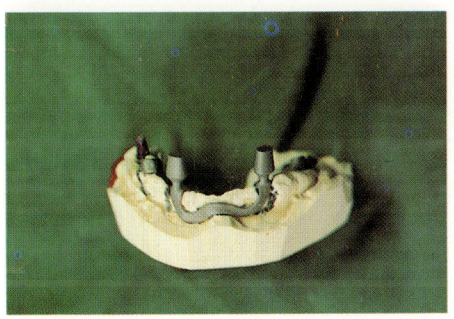

3.

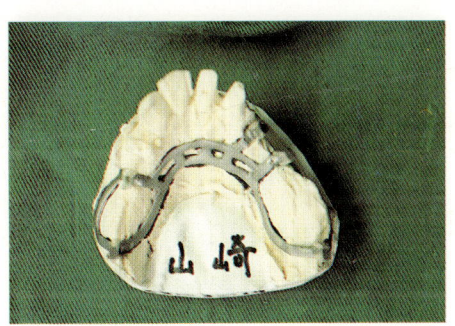

3.

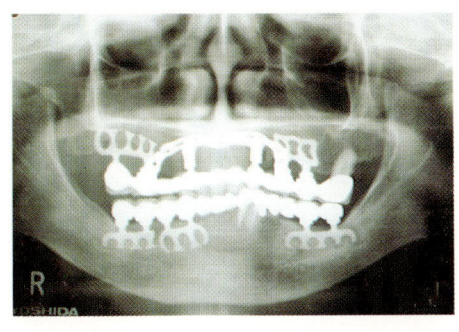

4.

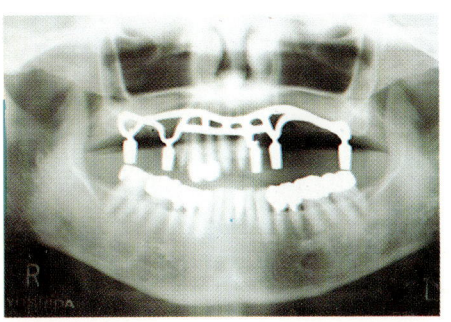

4.

Ramus frame implant
Case 9

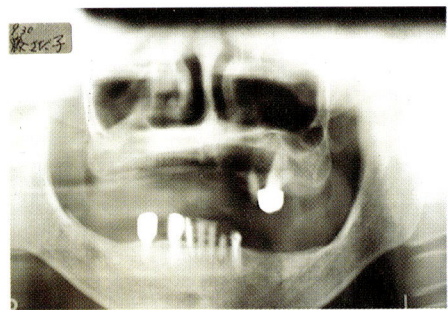

1.

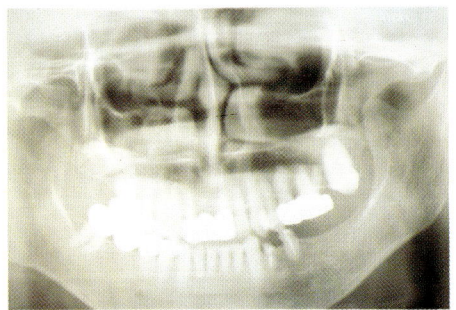

1.

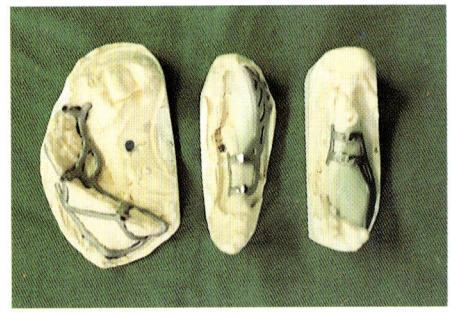

2.

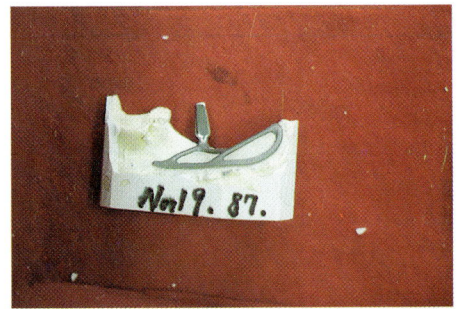

2.

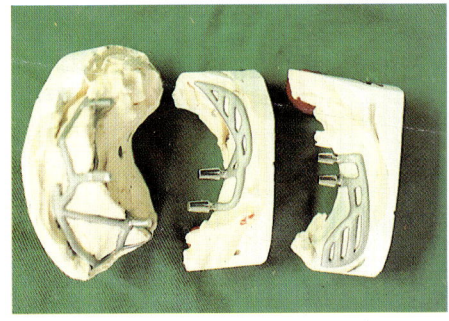

3.

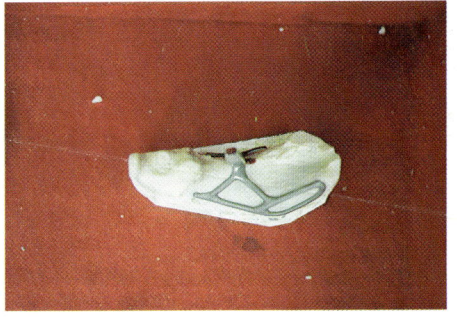

3.

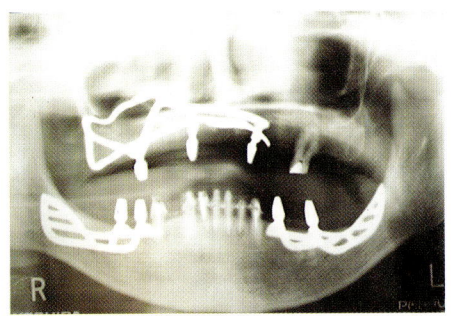

4.

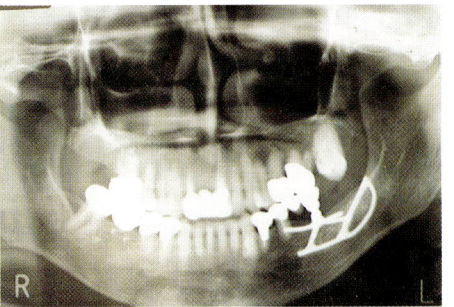

4.

Both side rami
Case 11

Rami
Case 12

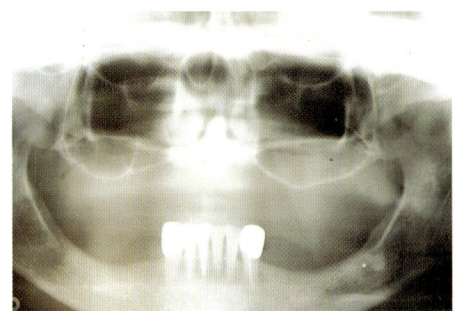

1.

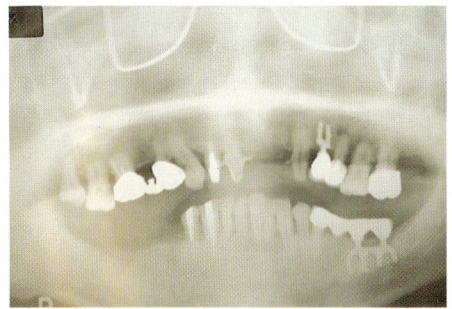

1.

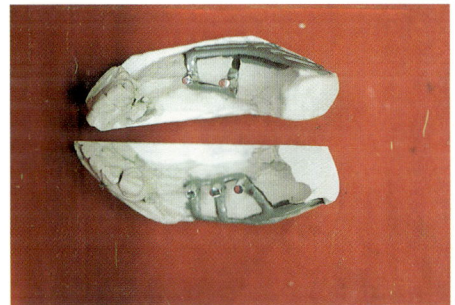

2.

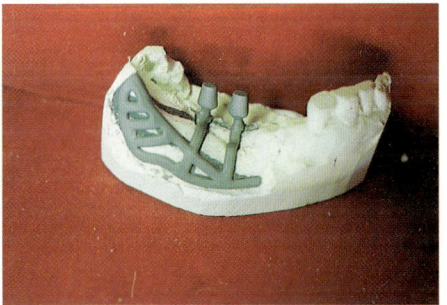

2.

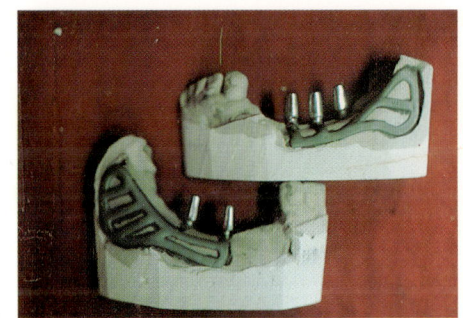

3.

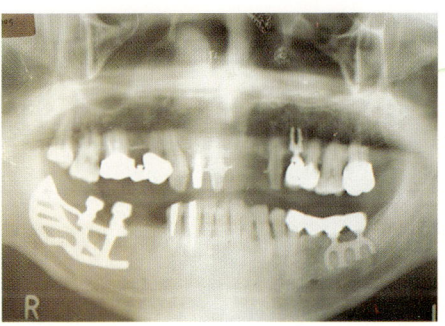

3.

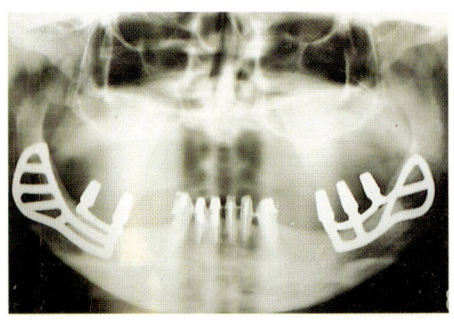

4.

**Full lower edentulous
Case 13**

**Full lower edentulous
Case 14**

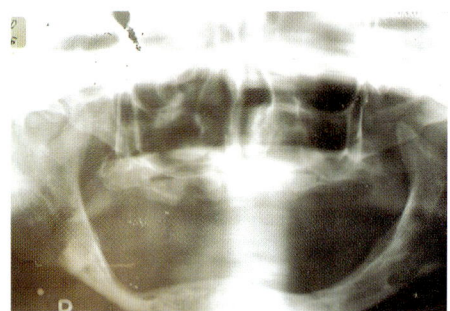

1.

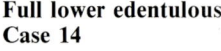
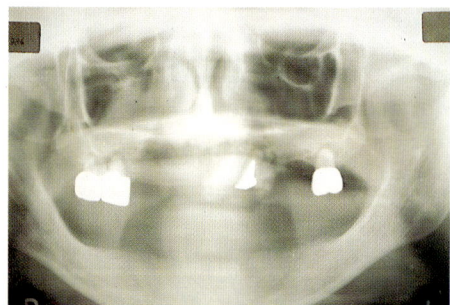

1.

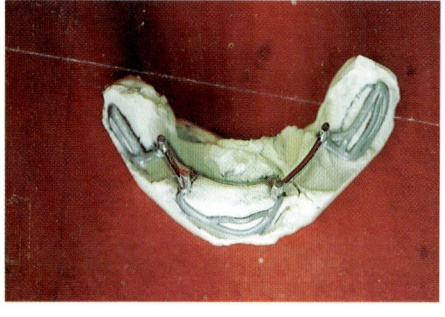

2.

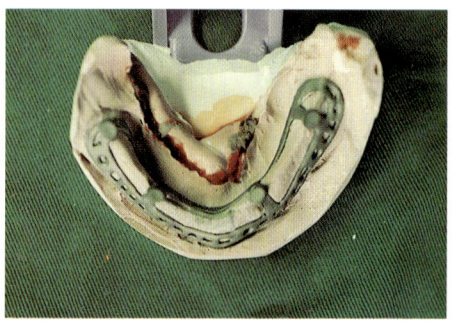

2.

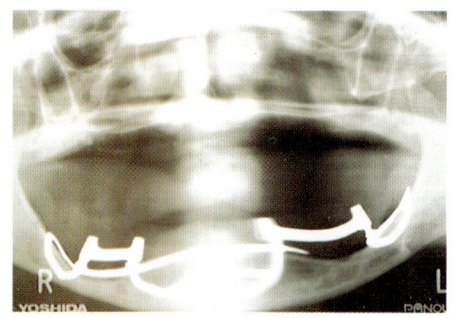

3.

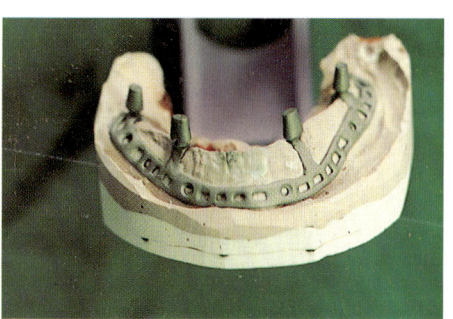

3.

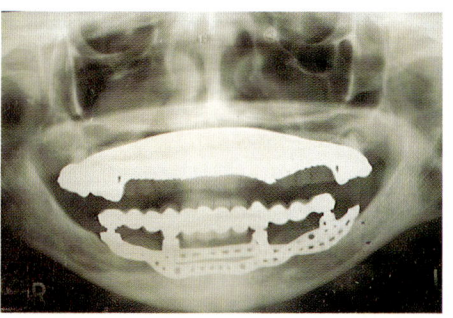

4.

4.

**Full lower edentulous
Case 15**

**Full lower edentulous
Case 16**

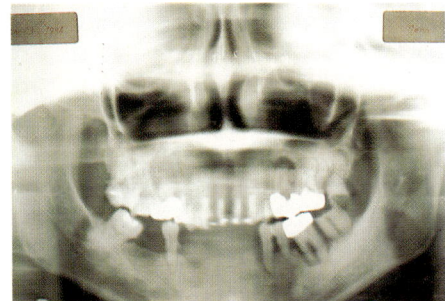

1.

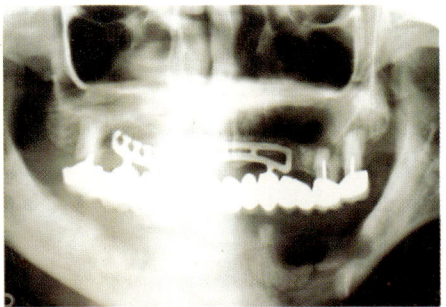

1.

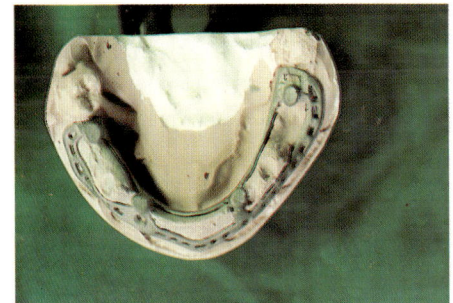

2.

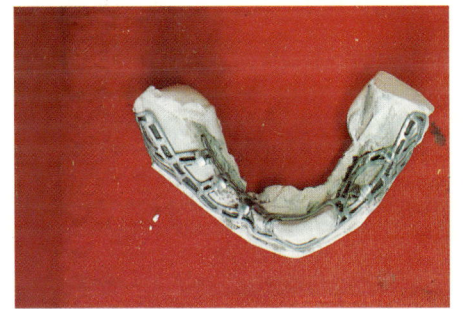

2.

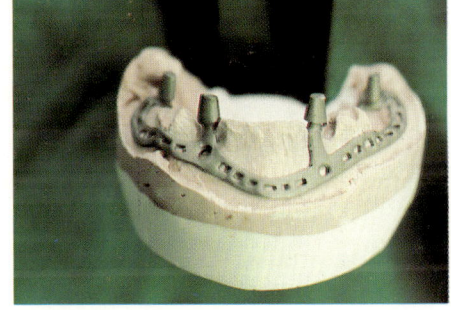

3.

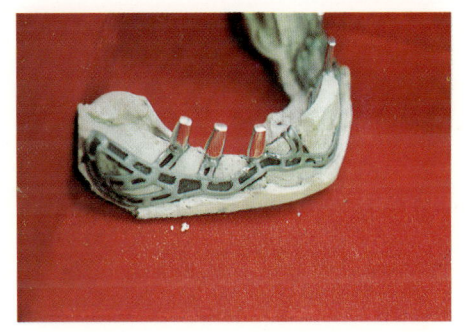

3.

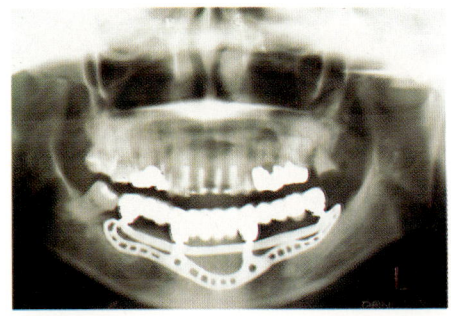

4.

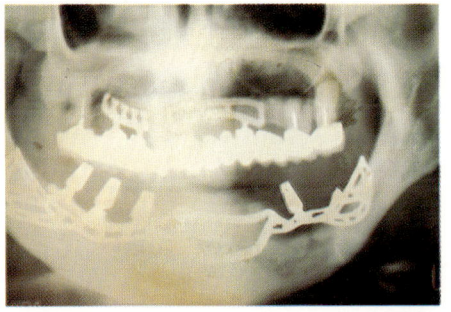

4.

Case 17   **Case 18**

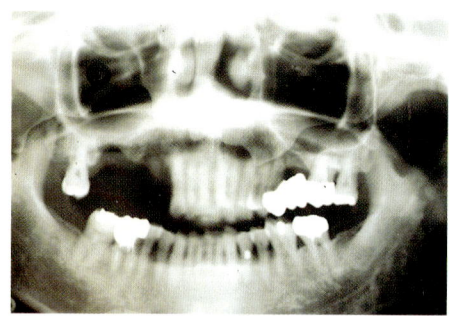

1.

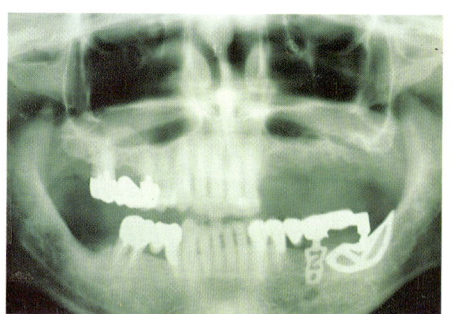

1.

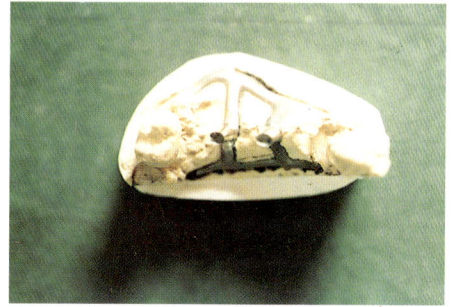

2.

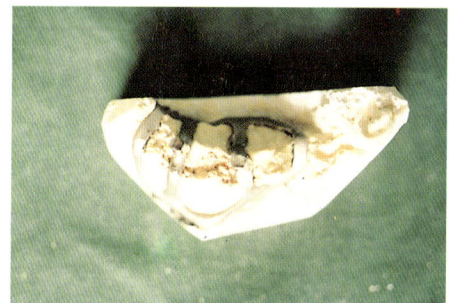

2.

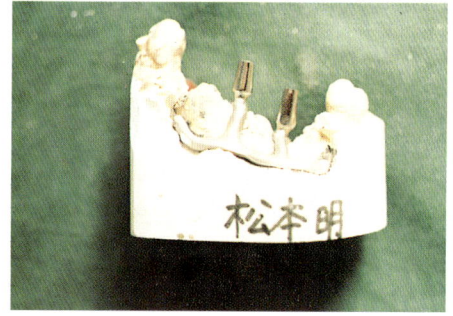

3.

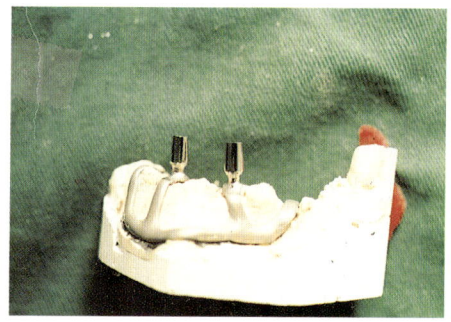

3.

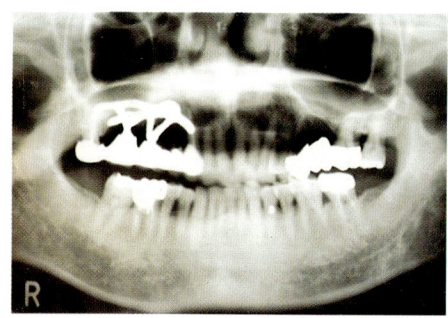

4.

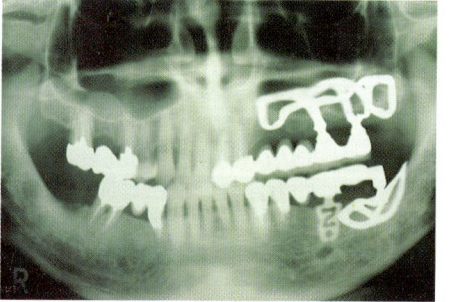

4.

Case 19

Case 20

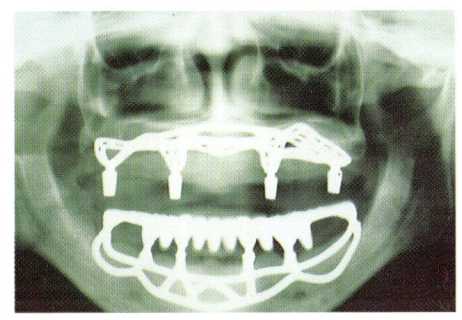

1.

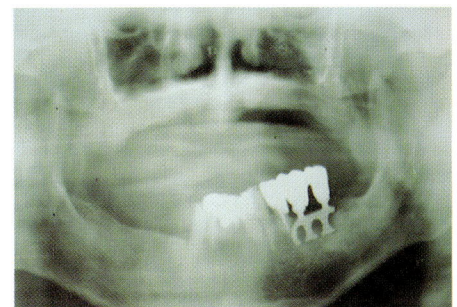

1.

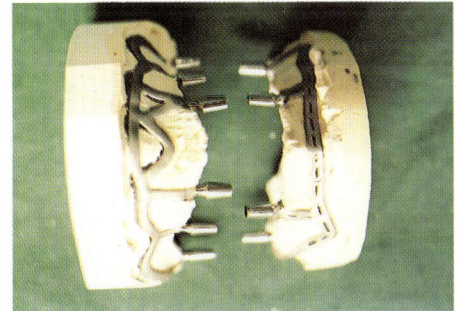

2.

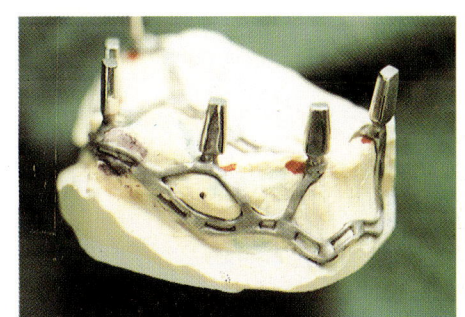

2.

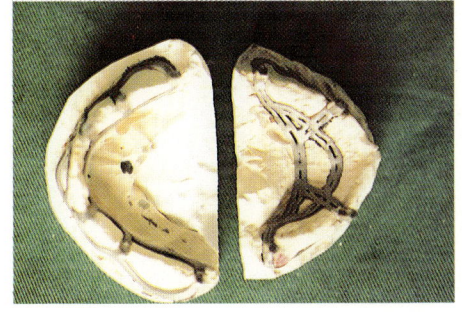

3.

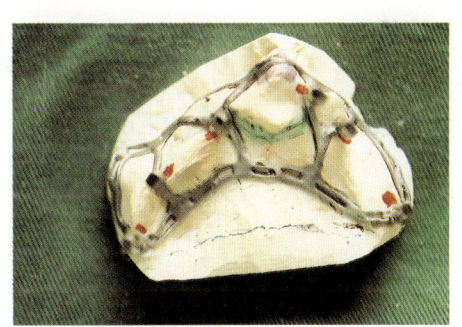

3.

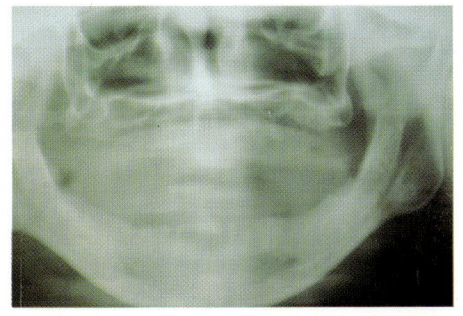

4.

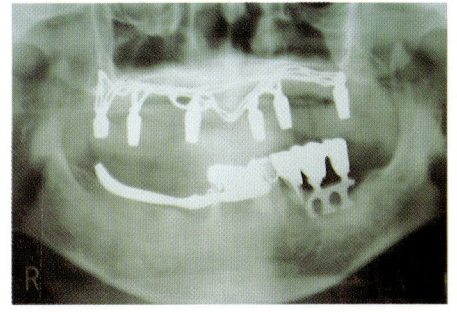

4.

Case 21

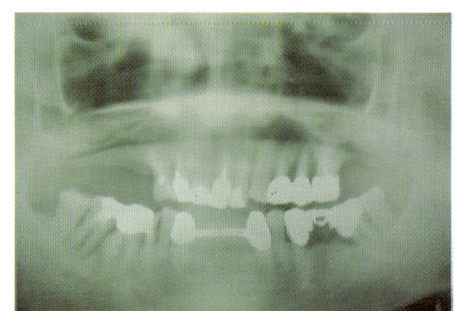

1.

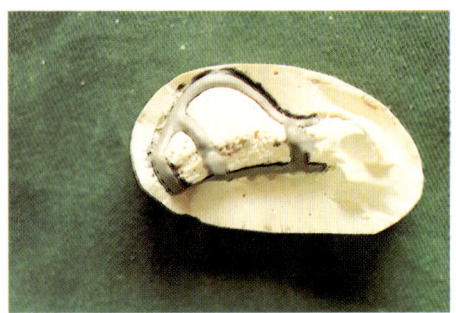

3.

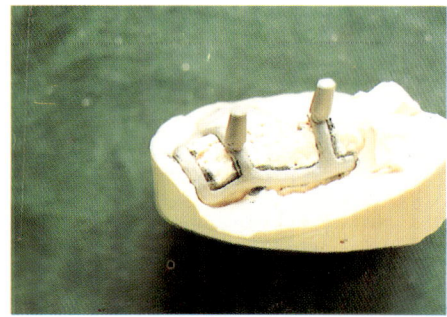

2.

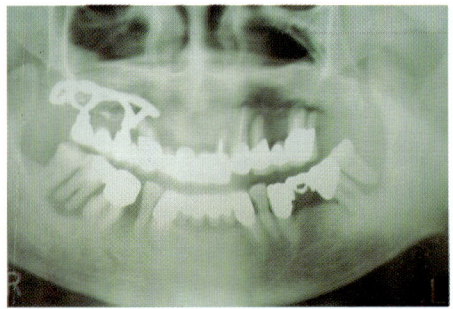

4.

Part 5

Other Implants

9. Ramus Frame Implant

9.1 INTRODUCTION

9.1.0 General

In the field of implant dentistry, several different methods, or systems, have been applied, such as intramucosal implants, endosteal blade implants, subperiosteal implants, and ramus frame implants.

Ramus frame implants are implants applied to the ramus, and were originally introduced by Roberts and Roberts about ten years ago. McSorley later reported his method of implanting wedge-shaped metal into the ramus, and since that time has remained one of the few specialists in ramus implantology. McEachen then reported on his ramus frame method, which combined ramus and metal.

In 1974, Linkow developed his system of five-piece ramus implants, or the so-called R2s5 system, with which ramus implant dentistry made a large step forward. Linkow's new method eliminated most of the defects, and nearly 80% of the unfavorable results of former methods. For the first time Linkow's system ensured a much easier and safer application of ramus implants.

Garefis discussed the historical development of ramus implantology in his work «From Roberts to Linkow» at the American Academy of Implant Dentistry (AAID) in Miami in 1977. According to Garefis, any implantologist using ramus implants tries hard to find the most suitable frame design in each individual case, for the benefits of ramus implants are thought to depend mainly on the shape and design of the frame. The author has used exclusively metallic materials for ramus implants and none of the new materials, such as ceramics or plastics.

Few implantologists have so far mastered the technique of clinically applying ramus implants. In Japan, the author is the only implantologist with a successful clinical experience in ramus implant operations, now numbering 16 cases. These cases were presented in a report at the AAID in 1977 and 1978, and, in the same years, at the Clinical Implant Society of Japan.

9.1.1 Endosteal blade implants

Most implantologists consider endosteal implants the most appropriate in cases of edentulous mandibles in which the osseous tissues of the mandible are sufficiently wide and deep. In cases where considerable resorption of the mandible is observed, they prefer subperiosteal implants. In fact, the cases in which endosteal implants are applicable are comparatively rare and, therefore, in most cases, the implantologist is obliged to apply a subperiosteal implant.

9.1.2 Subperiosteal implants

The probability of a successful subperiosteal implant is estimated about 70%. This figure would be quite satisfactory in laboratory experiments with dogs and apes, but for the clinical treatment of patients, the probability of success must be increased to 100%.

The main causes of the 30% failure rate in subperiosteal implant operations are the following:

1. incomplete stripping of the mucosa,
2. inaccurate impression-taking of the mandible surface,
3. incorrect design of the substructure, and
4. warping or deformation of the substructure metal.

There are various problems in the practical application of subperiosteal implants; a 100% success rate can only be achieved in this operation if these problems are solved. This is, of course, far easier in theory than practice.

9.1.3 Ramus frame implants

After the ramus frame implant operation, the patient can be expected to improve and recover rapidly. The probability of a successful operation should be nearly 100%, even though the operation itself is not really simple because of the deep operative field in the oral cavity. Once the wound has been closed and healed, recuperation is usually excellent. There should be no unfavorable prognosis or complications that occasionally occur with the subperiosteal implant operation. In fact, one of the reasons for turning to ramus implants is the difficulties involved in resolving the undesirable aftereffects of subperiosteal implants.

In addition, the probability of success with ramus implants has proved to be much higher than with other types of implant. This is because the ramus implant technique is actually based on the traditional and time-proven technique used for endosteal or blade implants: one end of the blade is implanted into the mandibular ramus by malleting, and the other end into the mental tubercle. Ramus implants can, therefore, be considered a modification or special application of endosteal implants. The success rate with endosteal or blade implants is known to be as high as 95%. We can therefore logically expect the same high rate of success with ramus implants, on the condition that the operator has sufficient experience and skill in the procedure and knowledge of oral anatomy.

One of the greatest advantages or merits of ramus implants is the elimination of the troublesome after-effects and complications that occasionally occur with subperiosteal implants. Please note, however, that these un-favorable prognoses will not occur in the 70% of successful cases of sub-periosteal implants.

9.2 INDICATIONS

The typical indications for ramus frame implants are:

1) a fully edentulous mandible, and
2) a defective mandible at the free end, particularly when notable re-sorption is observed in the mandibular bone.

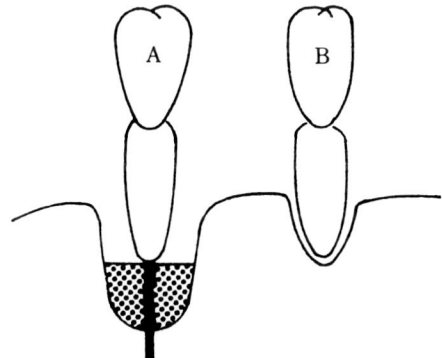

Fig. 204

With ramus implants, no occlusal pressure is exerted on the mandibu-lar body because there is no substructure or blade implanted in it (Fig. 204). The occlusal pressure is present at points A and B, whereas the region around point C, where bone resorption is probably most advanced, is prac-tically free of external pressure.

Please note that for the resorbed and involuted and, therefore, weak-ened mandible, other implant methods, such as endosteal blade implants, cannot be contemplated because of a possible fracture in this weak region when it is subjected to occlusal or any other external pressure.

9.3 CHANNEL FORMATION

Two important factors, from a clinical point of view, in successful ra-mus frame implant operations are the location and direction of the channel.

9.3.1 Location
The frame must be vertical, in whichever region of the ramus it is to be inserted (Fig. 205).

If the frame is inserted too high above the mandibular foramen, the possible complications include the following:

1. The patient can hardly close the mouth because the end of the in-serted frame would touch the maxillae.

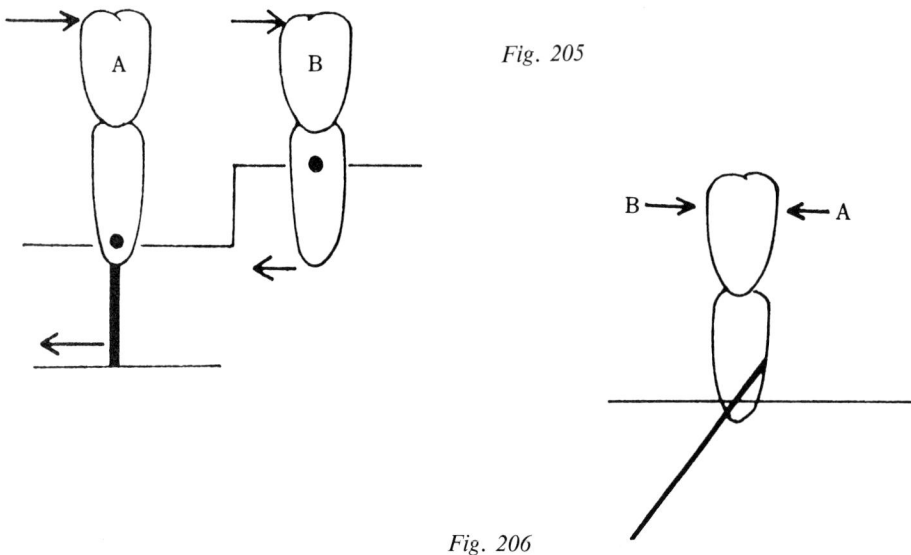

Fig. 205

Fig. 206

2. If the patient manages to close the mouth, problems may occur when opening and closing the mouth for the above reason. This is usually accompanied by considerable pain.
3. The inserted frame might become loose or descend after a certain period of time because the mandibular ramus, or the upper body connected to the mandibular foramen, is too thin, the amount of osseous tissues being too small to hold the frame securely (Fig. 206).
5. During the insert operation, the bone may crack due to an insufficient amount of osseous tissue. The weak region (the shaded area in Figure 206) is apt to crack, so that the inserted frame becomes loose and pain results. Eventually reoperation will be necessary.

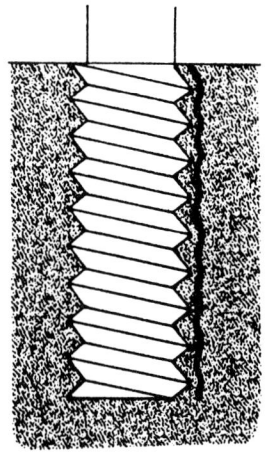

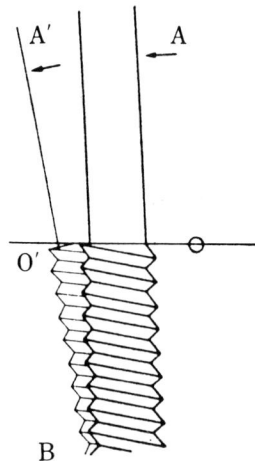

Fig. 207

Fig. 208

If, on the other hand, the frame is inserted too low, below the mandibular foramen, the possible complications are the following:

1. There is a constant fear that the frame should touch the mandibular canal, which is, of course, very dangerous.
2. The frame might press against the oral mucosa, also causing pain when the space between the mandibular body and the frame is too small.

To be sufficient the space should be at least twice as thick as the membrane; this is hardly possible when the frame is set too low, that is, below the mandibular foramen. Most inexpert dentists tend to set the frame too low when stripping the mucosa for channel setting. The best position for the frame is at the level of the mandibular foramen (Fig. 208).

During channel formation in the ramus, the operator should consider two important factors: the correct direction and depth of the channel. Otherwise, serious problems may arise. For instance, the inserted frame might touch the mandibular foramen, or, even worse, cut the nervous tissues of the lower alveolus. Judging the correct space is most important to prevent serious damage to the nervous tissues.

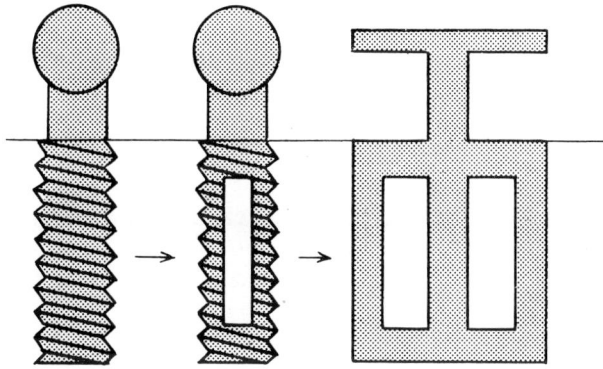

Fig. 209

9.3.2 Direction

After the optimal height for the frame has been determined, the next step is to calculate the correct direction for the channel. An incorrect direction of the channel for insertion in the ramus can sometimes cause the entire operation to fail, not only because the implant would not function effectively, but also because the ramus might become cracked or damaged.

In Figure 210, line R indicates channel formation parallel to the outer contours of the ramus, and line W channel formation in the thickest region of the ramus. The outer layer of the ramus consists of cortical bone, 2 mm thick and parallel to the outer contour of the ramus. It is most important that the depth of the channel lie between 8 and 10 mm inside the cortical bone of the ramus as shown in Figure 209.

After the operation the channel is ossified with cortical bone, making it sufficiently hard for the frame to be held firmly. This is one of the advantages of R-line channel setting, as is the reduced risk of perforating the ramus during channel formation. Care must also be taken, of course, dur-

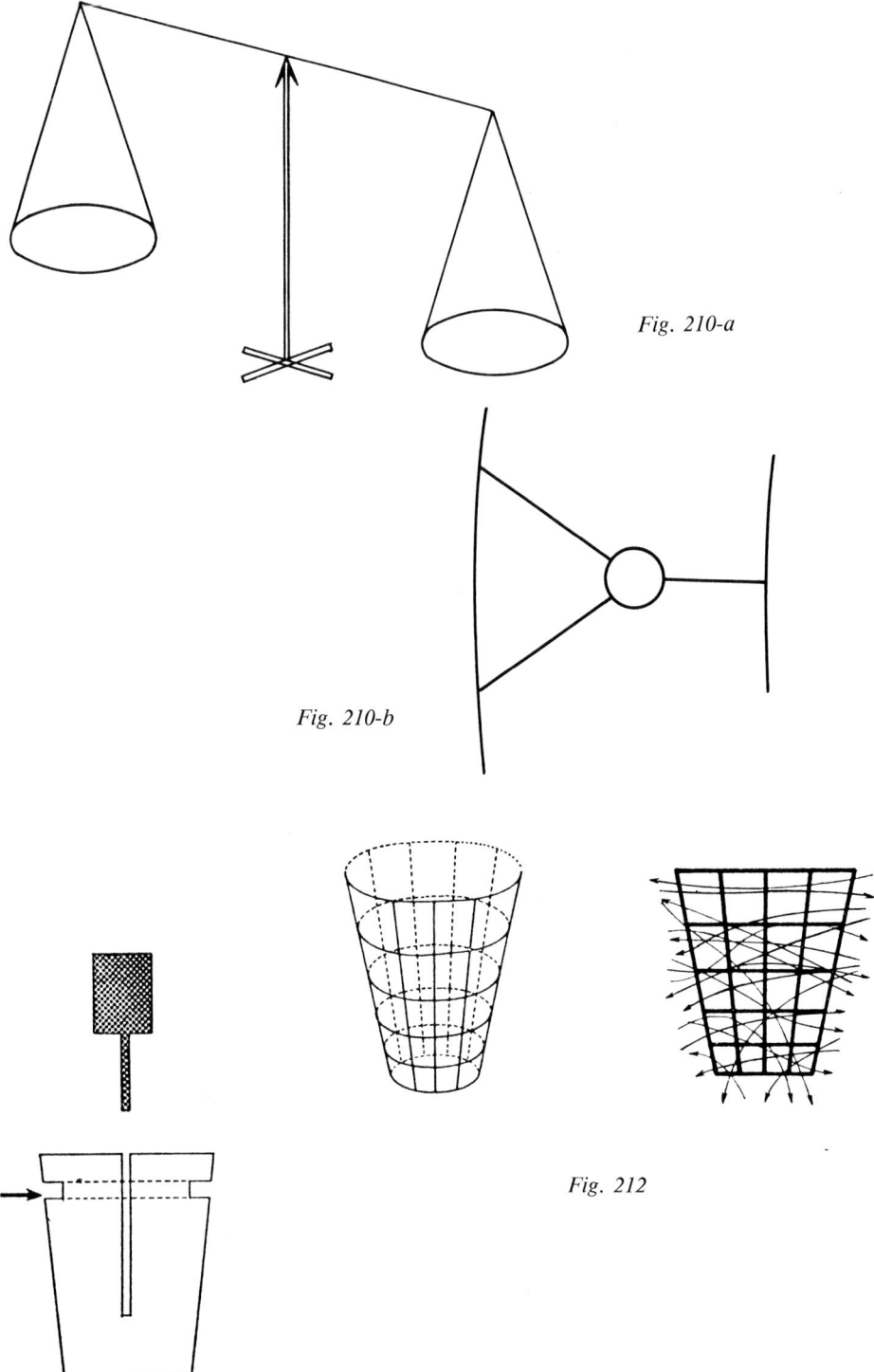

Fig. 210-a

Fig. 210-b

Fig. 212

Fig. 211

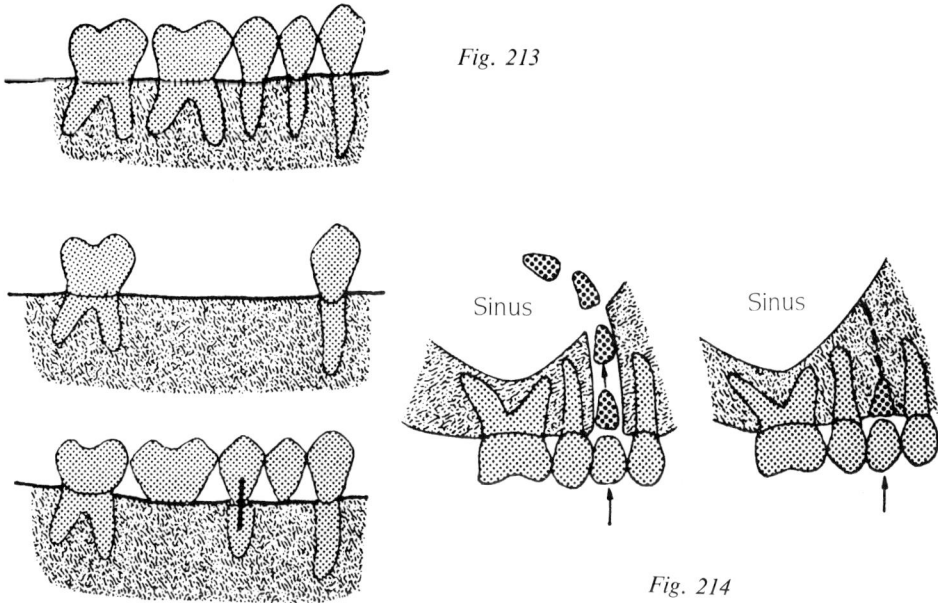

Fig. 213

Fig. 214

ing channel formation, not to make a hole into the outside of the ramus. If the R line is set too far from the outer contour, e.g. 5 mm or more instead of the standard 2 mm, the inner bone of the channel formed could be damaged. Furthermore, a channel formed too close to the inner ramus might cause undesirable contact of the frame against the mandibular canal. If the channel is too deep, the mandibular foramen might be struck.

The W line is set in the thickest part of the ramus so that, once inserted the frame can function most effectively. McSorley has already described this method.

Since the end of the ramus exposed in the oral cavity (point P in Fig. 213) is on the extension of the alveolar crest, the W-line method looks more favorable than the R-line method from the point of view of oral hygiene. However, the dangerous possibility of the frame end appearing outside the ramus still exists with the W-line method.

There is no mathematical means for determining the correct direction of the channel, so the suitability of the channel preparation depends largely on the skill, experience, and the intuition, or so-called sixth sense, of the operator. The author recommends the R-line rather than the W-line method in determining channel direction, although he should clarify that R does not indicate «right» and W «wrong».

POSTFACE

Implants are difficult. If insertion of a blade in the bone fails, the bone of the surrounding area of the inserted blade will be extensively damaged and the opportunity for a denture will be lost. Thus, utmost care is required in inserting a blade.

Subperiosteal implant is an especially difficult operation. To make the substructure fit precisely is also very difficult. In case the substructure does not fit tightly to the bone, it is recommended that the operator carry out another bone inspection.

At the beginning of one's experience, I recommend that the operator apply this implant technique to the small and easy case. Do not practice full edentulous operations. Only ample experience will make the operator able to perform difficult operations.

I decided to have this book published by an Italian publishing company because of my fondness for Italy.

On this occasion I express my sincere thanks to one of my old friends, Professor Muratori; to Professor Sebastiano LoBello, who extended his warm invitation to one of my daughters to study at one of the Italian universities; to Dr. Francesco Crescentini and his wife, who invited me and organized the Dr. Shumon Otobe Symposium in Pescara; to Dr. Domenico della Ventura and his wife, Dr. Paola Ebranati, who translated my book «Oral Implantology»; and also to Dr. Leonald I. Linkow, who has been my teacher. Finally my gratitude must be paid to Dr. Richard Guaccio for providing a careful editing of this text, and to Dr. Piccin, publisher of this book. I hope it will provide guidance to all its readers.

SHUMON OTOBE

BIBLIOGRAPHY

1. Linkow. L. I; Theories and techniques of oral Implantology; Mosby; 1970
2. Linkow. L. I.; Theories and techniques of oral Implantology; Mosby; 1970
3. Linkow. L. I.; Maxillary Implants; Glanus; 1977.
4. Linkow. L. I.; Mandibular Implants; Glanus; 1977.
5. Gershkoff A.; Implant Dentures; Lippincott; 1957.
6. Muratori. G.; The endosseous implant with removable and fixed superstructure; Parma; 1969.
7. Muratori G., Multi-type Oral Implantology; Parma; 1973.
8. Roberts H. D.; The Ramus, Single tooth, and Ramus Frame Implants; University supply; 1971.
9. Perel. M. L.; Dental implantology and prostheses; Lippincott; 1977.
10. Taylor. A. R.; Endosseous Dental Implants; Butterworths; 1970.
11. Pruin. E. H., Implantationskurs in der Odonto-Stomatologie; Quintessence; 1974.
12. Cranin. A. N., Oral Implantology; Thomas; 1970.
13. Scortecci. G.; Incidences parodontales et occlusales des implants à lames Linkow leur contention; Academie D'Aix; Marseille
14. Hansson. B. O.; Success and failure of Osseointegrated Implants in the Edentulous Jaw; Swedish Dental Journal; 1977.
15. Schwindliny. R.; Alloplastiche Implantate in der Zahnersatzkunde; Corl Hansen 1960.
16. 山根稔夫；歯科外科的矯正の臨床；医歯薬出版；1966.
17. 乙部朱門；臨床歯科インプラント埋入手術；一世出版；1973.
18. 根本 亘；ボタンインプラント歯肉内植歯術；東京インプラントリサーチ；1975.
19. 山根稔夫；形成歯科；医歯薬出版；1975.
20. 東海林芳郎；最新水平位診療アトラス；医歯薬出版；1973.
21. 宇賀春雄，園山昇；最新口腔外科小手術図説；医歯薬出版；1973.
22. 森崎益夫；歯科アシスタント教室；一世出版；1969.
23. 藤田恒太郎；人体解剖学；南江堂；1947.
24. Linkow. L. I.; Abutment for full mouth splinting: Journal of Prosthetic Dentistry Vol 11. No 5. 1961.
25. Linkow. L. I.; Full arch splint: Journal of Prosthetic Dentistry Vol 11. No 6. 1961.
26. Linkow. L. I.; Contact area in natural dentitions and fixed prosthodontics: Journal of Prosthetic Dentistry Vol 12. No 1. 1962.
27. Linkow L. I.; Mesially tipped mandibular molars: Journal of Prosthetic Dentistry, Vol 12 No 3. 1962.
28. Linkow. L. I.; Reconstruction of anterior teeth with extreme vertical and horizontal overlap: Journal of Prosthetic Dentistry Vol 12. No 5.
29. Linkow. L. I.; Importance of axial inclination of teeth in attainment of parallelism: Journal of Prosthetic Dentistry Vol 15. No 3. 1965.
30. Linkow. L. I.; Re-evaluation of mandibular unilateral subperiosteal implants. A 12 years report: Journal of Prosthetic Dentistry Vol 17. 1967.
31. Linkow. L. I.; Prefabricated mandibular prosthesis for intraosseous implants: Journal of Prosthetic Dentistry Vol 20. No. 4. 1968.
32. Linkow. L. I.; Prefabricated maxillary endosteal implant prosthesis: Journal of Prosthetic Dentistry Vol 23. No. 3. 1970.
33. Linkow. L. I.; Endosseous blade-implant - Two year report: Journal of Prosthetic Dentistry Vol 23. No. 4. 1970.

34. Linkow. L. I.; Some Variant Designs of the Subperiosteal Implant: Oral Implantology: Vol 2. No 3. 1972.
35. Linkow. L. I.; My Thoughts, Philosophies and Contributions Regarding Implantological Restorations for Several Atrophied Maxillae that are Partially or Totally Edentulous: Oral Implantology: Vol 4. No 1. 1973.
36. Linkow. L. I.; Further Evidence of the Compatibility of the Titanium Blade Implant with the Skeletal Structures: Oral Implantology Vol 4. No 2, 1974.
37. Linkow. L. I.; Factor Predisposing Implant Success - A Continuing Analysis of 173 Patients: Oral Implantology: Vol 5. No 3. 1975.
38. Linkow. L. I.; The Refinement of the Pterygoid Extension Implant Design for the Partially and Totally Edentulous Maxillae: Oral Implantology: Vol 6. No 3. 1976.
39. Linkow. L. I.; The endosseous blade implant and its use in orthodontics: International Journal of Orthodontics: Vol 8. No 4. 1969.
40. Linkow. L. I.; Implant Orthodontics: Jounal of Clinical Orthodontics: Vol 4. No 1. 1970.
41. Linkow. L. I.; An honest evaluation of blade type implants: Bulletin of the Hudson County Dental Society: Vol 41. No 6. 1972.
42. Linkow. L. I.; Endosseous Oral Implantology: A 7-year Progress Report: Dental Clinics of North America. Vol 14. No 1. 1970.
43. Linkow. L. I.; The Toroplant and Blade-Vents for the restoration of an edentulous maxilla with dehiscent nasal vestibule: Quintessence International Journal of Practical Dentistry Vol 2. May. 1971.
44. Linkow. L. I.; The Blade vent, a new dimension in endosseous implantology: Dental Concepts Spring 1968.
45. Linkow. L. I.; The two stage palato-labial juxta-endosteal implant intervention for severely atrophied edentulous maxillae. Dental Concepts: Vol 12. No 2. 1972.
46. Linkow. L. I.; Latest Development in Blade Implantology: Greater St. Louis Dental Society: Vol 42. No 11. 1971.
47. Linkow. L. I.; Principles and Pitfalls: Dental Survey (Pierre Fauchard Academy) September 1971.
48. Linkow. L. I.; The Status of Oral Implants 1969.
49. Cranin. N. A.; The anterior Vertical Transosteal Implant: Oral Implantology: Vol 1. No 1. 1670.
50. Robert & Robert; The Ramus Endosseous Implant: Oral Implantology; Vol 1. No 2. 1970.
51. Ashman. A.; Acrylic Resin Tooth Implant: Oral Implantology: Vol 1. No 2. 1970.
52. Baumhammers. A.; Scanning Electron Microscopy of Bladevent Implants: Oral Implantology: Vol 2. No 1. 1971.
53. Baumhammers. A.; Custom Modifications and Specifications for Bladevent Implants Designs to Increase their Biologic Compatibility: Oral Implantology: Vol 2. No 4. 1972.
54. Gershkoff. A.; The Implant Lower Denture: Oral Implantology: Vol 2. No 2. 1971.
55. Weinbeng. B. D.; Subperiosteal Implantation of a Vitallium Oral Implantology: Vol 3. No 2. 1972.
56. Beager. S.; Useful Adjunct to Two-Step Implant Surgery: Oral Implantology: Vol 3. No 3. 1973.
57. Babbush. C. A.; Endosseous Blade-Vent Implants: Oral Implantology: Vol 3. No 3. 1073.
58. James. R. A.; A Simplified Technique for Immediate Stabilization of Implants in Experimental; Oral Implantology: Vol 4. No 2. 1973.
59. Weber. S. P.; Implant Registration Program: Oral Implantology: Vol 4. No. 3. 1974.
60. Fagan. M. I.; Preventive Dentistry Concepts for Endosseous Implantology. Oral Implantology: Vol 4. No 3. 1974.
61. Weiss. C. M.; Severe Mandibular Atrophy - Biological Consideration of Routine Treatment with the Complete Subperiosteal: Oral Implantology: Vol 4. No 4. 1974.
62. Guaccio. R.; Endosteal Blade Implant: Abutments for Routine as well as Complicated Restorations: Oral Implantology: Vol 5. No 1. 1974.
63. Ricciardi. A.; Restoration of Function with a Implant Failure: Oral Implantology: Vol 5. No. 1. 1974.
64. McCoy. G.; Vitreous Carbon Implant: Oral Implantology: Vol 5. No 3. 1975.
65. Lemor. J. E.; Biomaterial Consideration for Dental Implants: Oral Implantology: Vol 5. No 4. 1975.
66. Muratori. G., Prevention of Osseous Atrophy and Fibrous Retention: Two New Concepts in Implantology: Oral Implantology: Vol 6. No 1. 1975.
67. Judy K. W. M.; A Typical Maxillary Prosthodontic Problems Solved Intra-Mucosal Inserts: Oral Implantology: Vol 6. No 2. 1926.
68. Franko. J. M.; Blood Scanning in Oral Implantology Patients: Oral Implantology: Vol 6. No 4. 1977.
69. Fagan. M. J.; The Fagan Endosseous Stabilizer (FES) Implant: A Preliminary Report: Oral Implantology: Vol 7. No 1.

70. Garefis. P. N.; The Full Upper Subperiosteal Implant, Pterygoid Extension Design for the Partial Edentulous Maxilla: Oral Implantology: Vol 7. No 4. 1977.

71. Muratori. G.; A 3-year Report on Human Bone Regeneration around or inside an Implant - The Lock Hinge Prosthesis: Oral Implantology: Vol 7. No 3. 1977.

72. Cullen. R.; The Subosseous Dental Implant Anglo-Continental; Dental Society, 1971.

72. 懸田利孝；嵌植義歯の一例　補綴誌　1巻1号 1957

73. 懸田利孝；嵌植下顎義歯について　補綴誌　2巻1号 1958

74. 小林俊三；Implant Button technique を応用した全部床義歯，補綴誌2．1958

75. 小林俊三；ボタン義歯について：補綴誌　9巻1号 1965

76. 山根稔夫；私の臨床（特にインプラントについて）日本歯科評論 362号，1972

77. 関谷昭雄・都筑億；歯内骨内インプラントの症例　補綴臨床　7巻2号 1974

78. 小嶋栄一；インプラント臨床症例　国際歯科ジャーナル　3巻4号 1976

79. 乙部朱門；下顎骨に発生した血管線維粘液腫の一例，日本口腔科学会雑誌　5巻2　　号 1956

80. 乙部朱門；上顎側切歯の形態異常（矯小型）について，歯科月報 36巻2号 1962

81. 乙部朱門；Kurer anchor system について　歯界展望 42巻1号 1973

82. 乙部朱門；Oral Implantology の診断の重要性　日本歯科評論 389号 1975

83. 乙部朱門；ピンインプラントとインプラントメタル　国際歯科ジャーナル　3巻3　　号 1976

84. 乙部朱門；ボタン・スクリュー・カーボンインプラントについて 国際歯科3巻4　　号 1976

85. 乙部朱門；歯科医師の要素・歯槽骨の性質　　　　　　ジャーナル3巻5号 1976

86. 乙部朱門；インプラントブレードについて　　　　　ジャーナル4巻1号 1976

87. 乙部朱門；ブレードインプラントで注意すべきこと　ジャーナル4巻2号 1976

88. 乙部朱門；骨膜下インプラント（診断）　　　　　　ジャーナル4巻3号 1976

89. 乙部朱門；上顎無歯顎の骨膜下インプラント　　　Quintessence　　　6／1977

90. 乙部朱門；下顎無歯顎の骨膜下インプラント　　　Quintessence　　　8／1977

INDEX

Finito di stampare
nel mese di luglio 1990
da « La Tipografica Varese » - Varese